**OUR OWN WAY
IN THIS PART
OF THE WORLD**

OUR OWN WAY IN THIS PART OF THE WORLD

Biography of an African Community, Culture, and Nation

KWASI KONADU

Duke University Press   Durham and London   2019

© 2019 KWASI KONADU. *All rights reserved*

Designed by Courtney Leigh Baker
Typeset in Avenir and Arno Pro by Westester Publishing Services

Library of Congress Cataloging-in-Publication Data

Names: Konadu, Kwasi, author.
Title: Our own way in this part of the world : biography of an African culture, community, and nation / Kwasi Konadu.
Description: Durham : Duke University Press, 2019. | Includes bibliographical references and index.
Identifiers: LCCN 2018047205 (print) | LCCN 2019010346 (ebook)
ISBN 9781478005636 (ebook)
ISBN 9781478004165 (hardcover)
ISBN 9781478004783 (pbk.)
Subjects: LCSH: Donkor, Kofi, Nana, 1913–1995. | Healers—Ghana—Biography. | Traditional medicine—Ghana. | Ghana—History—To 1957. | Decolonization—Ghana. | Ghana—Social life and customs.
Classification: LCC DT511.3.D66 (ebook) | LCC DT511.3.D66 K66 2019 (print) | DDC 966.7 [B]—dc23
LC record available at https://lccn.loc.gov/2018047205

Cover art: Kofi Dɔnkɔ carry ing the Asubɔnten Kwabena shrine at the Takyiman Fofie Festival, 6 October 1970. From the Dennis Michael Warren Slide Collection, Special Collections Department, University of Iowa Libraries.

To the lives and legacies of Kofi Dɔnkɔ, Adowa Asabea (Akumsa), Akua Asantewaa, Kofi Kyereme, Yaw Mensa, and Kofi Ɔboɔ

[For those] in search of past events and matters connected with our culture as well as matters about you, the [*abosom*, "spiritual forces," I . . .] will also let them know clearly how we go about things in our own way in this part of the world.
—Nana Kofi Dɔnkɔ

CONTENTS

Acknowledgments ix

Introduction 1

CHAPTER 1. Libation
"Matters Connected with Our Culture" 17

CHAPTER 2. Homelands
"In Search of Past Events" 44

CHAPTER 3. Tools of the Trade
"I was a Blacksmith ... Before I Became [a Healer]" 73

CHAPTER 4. Medicine, Marriage, and Politics
"Assist this State to have Progress" 107

CHAPTER 5. Independences
"Never Mingled Himself in Local Politics" 137

CHAPTER 6. Anthropologies of Medicine and Africa
"When the Whiteman First Came" 166

CHAPTER 7. Uncertain Moments and Memory
"Our Ancestral Spirits, Come and Have Drink" 195

Epilogue 228

Notes 239
Bibliography 287
Index 307

ACKNOWLEDGMENTS

Mpaeɛ. Onyankopɔn, Asase Yaa, abosompɛm, nananom nsamanfoɔ, m'abusuafoɔ, meda mo ase bebree. Na monim sɛ meresua, momma menhu da biara. To Ronnie (Amma), Abena, Sunkwa, and Afia, *monim sɛ ɔdɔ nyera fie kwan.* Beyond my family on several sides of the Atlantic Ocean, I owe a debt of gratitude to Nana Kwaku Sakyi, Kwame Ayiso, Kofi Sakyi Sapɔn, Nana Kwasi Amponsah Nkron Amoah, Nana Ama Akomaa, Nana Kwasi Appiah, Nana Akosua Antwiwaa, Nana Adwoa Asamoaa Nana Kwasi Owusu, Nana Yaa Kɔmfo, Owusu Brempong, Raymond Silverman, Peter Ventevogel, Therese Tindirugamu and Elaine Kohls of the Medical Mission Sisters, Edward Miner, and the staff of the Warren Collection at the University of Iowa. The staff at the Sunyani regional and the Holy Family Hospital archives were especially helpful. A postdoctoral fellowship from the West African Research Association supported research travel during the early stages of this project, and several grants from CUNY supported some of its research and writing.

For helpful and encouraging conversations over the years, let me register my thanks once more to Kweku Agyeman (Mwalimu Shujaa), Yaw Akyeaw, Scot Brown, Clifford Campbell, Reginald Campbell, Danny Dawson, Amari Johnson, Ọbádélé Kambon, Fallou Ngom, Dane Peters, Don Robotham, and Dr. James Turner. I am equally grateful to the anonymous reviewers for their critical and careful reading of the manuscript. For skillfully guiding this project, I thank Miriam Angress and her staff at Duke University Press. Finally, I thank you, the reader, for choosing this book. The usual disclaimers apply.

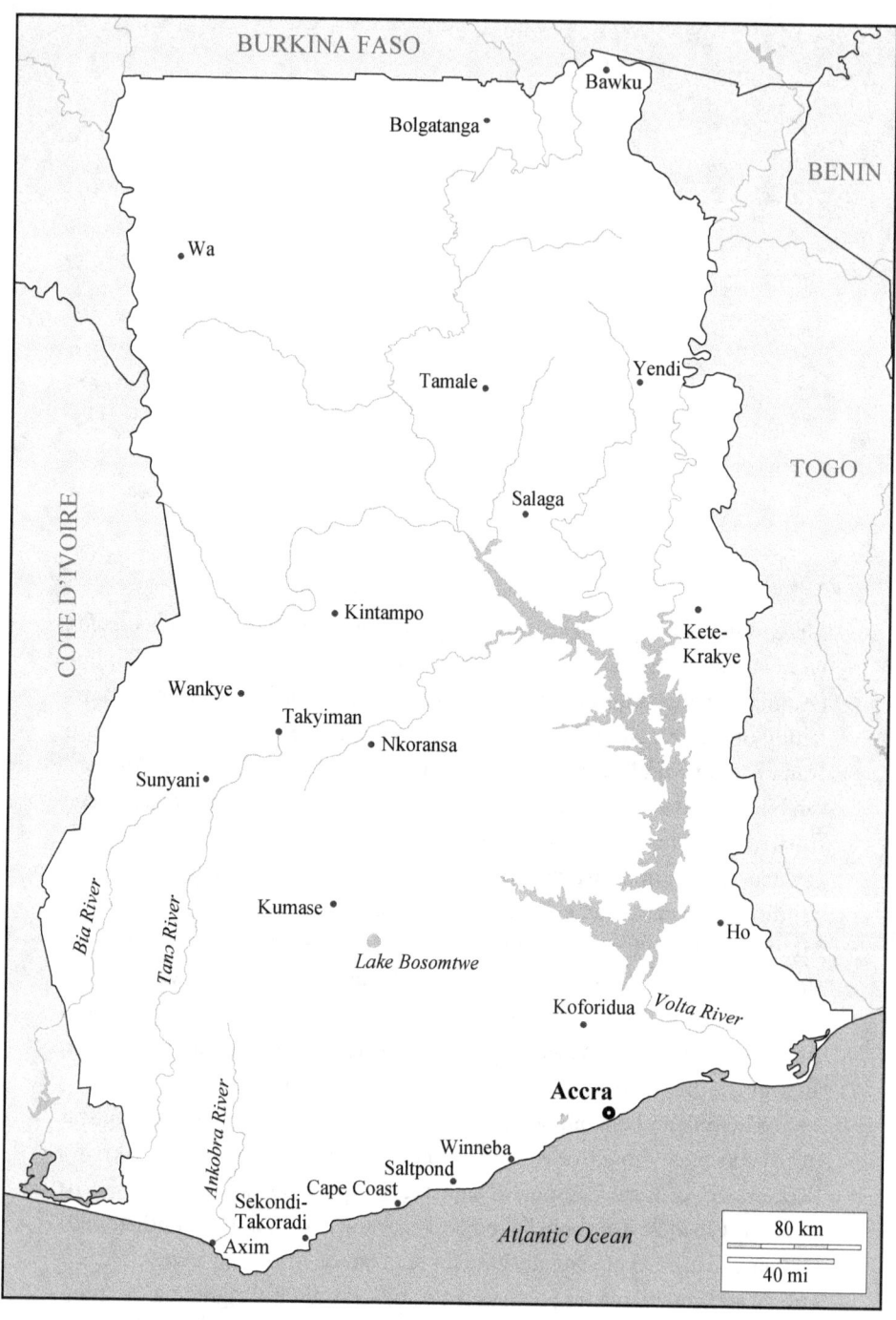

MAP I.1. Map of Ghana, featuring modern boundaries, major rivers, and towns.

INTRODUCTION

He who would be a healer must set great value on seeing truly, hearing truly, understanding truly, and acting truly. . . . You see why healing can't be a popular vocation?
—AYI KWEI ARMAH, *The Healers*

A cream-white casket was hoisted into the rear of a battered pickup truck, strapped onto its cargo bed, and secured by two young men who did their best to ensure the casket would remain in place. The truck then reversed onto the main road and positioned itself behind another vehicle that led the way through the main streets of the market town. Soon the truck joined a long procession of cars and minivans, each packed with kinfolk and townspeople, drivers blowing their horns. The night was upon them when they finally reached their destination—the home of the deceased. It was mobbed by hundreds, perhaps over a thousand, in bereavement. Mourners of all sizes and ages stood in and around the rectangular compound or sat on plastic chairs, exchanging greetings.

Inside a twelve-by-thirteen-foot room painted white, long lines of mourners proceeded slowly, single file. Making their way around the gold-painted headboard and foot posts, the women sobbed hysterically and sang funerary dirges, the men paid their respects in words and in silence to the body of the man resting in the double bed. That body commanded an enormous audience and even more respect—observers noticed tears rolling from the eyes of some men, for whom crying in public on such an occasion is culturally inappropriate.

But this was no ordinary funeral, nor was the occasion for an ordinary individual. On this mattress, the dark brown–skinned body—less than five feet ten inches tall and perhaps one hundred sixty pounds—was dressed in all white, the same color as the two pillows on which the head rested. White sheets covered the bed and the body up to its waist, and the finest handwoven *kente* cloth covered the body from the waist to the sternum. Goldpainted, black-handled ceremonial swords (*akofena*) were positioned on the thighs, two on the left and two on the right, pointing away from the body. He wore a white linen top, the forearms and elbows were adorned with gold ornaments, a black necklace with a large triangular disk hung around the neck, and a velvet headband along with gold ornamentation and rings on the fingers indicated his status as a healer. Individually—and certainly when taken together—these decorations told those in attendance something about the spirit or soul that had animated the body on view and the being who had occupied a central role in their lives.

Thunderous drumming and spiritually induced dancing and singing occurred outside the room, but the inside was more solemn, with several fans tilted toward the body and the viewers—and for good reason. The temperature that August day was 84 degrees Fahrenheit. The relatively high humidity was mitigated only by the cool evening breeze from the north. But the weather mattered little for the living. They had come to honor the life of the deceased. As the open casket laid adjacent to the double bed and as the unending flow of mourners encircled the bed, looking on the body, several spiritualist-healers (*akɔmfoɔ*), including relatives and trainees of the deceased, vigorously danced barefooted in a counterclockwise circle outside the room. The elder women akɔmfoɔ among these healers wore headbands made of green medicinal leaves.

Several male and female akɔmfoɔ joined the celebration. The spokesperson or speech intermediary (*ɔkyeame*) for the family of the deceased, Nana Kofi Ɔboɔ, poured some gin on the floor next to the bed, invoking the spiritual presence of the deceased's ancestors, the earth, the spiritual forces located in nature, and the cosmic force by which temporal life and death exist. Periodically, a cow horn (*aben*) transformed into an instrument was blown and gunshots from an old shotgun were fired ceremonially in the air. Morning came and more mourners found their way to the deceased. Nana Ɔboɔ poured yet another libation. Mourners screamed "old man" (an affectionate term for the deceased during his later years), while highlife music from a small, black AM/FM radio played in the background. The deceased was eventually buried not in a plot of land, but rather in a room on his family compound, fittingly next to the abode of the particular spiritual force (ɔbosom) to which he owed his life and by which he forged a life worth remembering.

Nana Kofi Dɔnkɔ passed on nkyikwasi (Sunday, 6 August 1995), and with his temporal transition also passed a life story worth sharing with a world wider than his own, beyond those who paid their respects as the cream-white casket was covered and the door to his final resting room closed. This healer—and the figure of the healer in African and world history—was versatile, operating fluidly as custodian and interpreter of shared values, facilitator of spiritual renewal, promoter of social cohesion, settler of disputes, and assessor and planner of the community's growth. Kofi Dɔnkɔ's composite human history, however, survives what rests in the white casket. That history persists in the genes of his great-grandchildren, in the memories of kin and community, in the hundreds of healers he trained, in the tens of thousands of patients he treated, in the academics he enriched through his intellect and compassion, in the cultural quilt of a community he enlarged, and in a world where healers of his caliber and character are sorely needed. This book tells his and their composite story.

❈

FOR REASONS I CANNOT fully explain nor necessarily understand, these facets of Kofi Dɔnkɔ's life, these integral roles he played in so many lives, these social and intellectual histories filtered through one person, spoke to me, so much so that in spite of not meeting Kofi Dɔnkɔ, I refused to throw away the aforementioned vignette of his videotaped funeral rites. I was a sophomore in college when Kofi Dɔnkɔ transitioned toward that ancestral village. I was also born in Jamaica and had only my grandfather, a healer himself, to make sense of Kofi Dɔnkɔ and his cultural homeland. In 2001 I boarded a Ghana Airways flight at Baltimore's BWI airport. The wheels retracted and the cabin, spiced with Akan/Twi and English, shook as the plane made its way through the layers of clouds. The Airbus A320–200 aircraft and I soon reached a comfortable altitude, moving effortlessly over the Atlantic. After landing at Kotoka International Airport in a sticky Accra morning, I stayed in the capital overnight before spending a few days each in Koforidua and Kumase, and finally reaching Takyiman. Armed with only a beginner's command of the Akan/Twi language, I did not use it during my initial encounters with my hosts, with whom Nana Kwaku Sakyi had put me in contact and who turned out to be family of Kofi Dɔnkɔ.

Having only a vague sense of a research plan, I wanted to study indigenous medicine for my doctoral research but had little clue about how and where exactly. Kofi Dɔnkɔ's son, Kofi Sakyi Sapɔn, helped refine my ideas and provided access—made possible by his relation to Kofi Dɔnkɔ—to several healers. As I moved around town on my own, and during my conversations with healers and townspeople, I increasingly heard stories about Kofi Dɔnkɔ. Although deceased, he was omnipresent. Patients from afar still visited his compound, expecting to see him. My Akan/Twi improved because I respectfully refused to speak English, and as it did I began to ask questions in the language, and again Kofi Dɔnkɔ resurfaced. Eventually I completed my research and tried to pay little attention to Kofi Dɔnkɔ or stories about him, but without success—he turned up in almost every interview, although he was invisible in the regional and national archives. Finally, I wanted to know more about this haunting figure and the lore surrounding him.

Who was Kofi Dɔnkɔ? And how might this person made invisible through recordkeeping and archiving become legible with only a slight documentary trail? How might his life and that of his community and his nation become a useful window to understand culture, health, and healing, and well-known transformations of the twentieth-century world, such as colonial empire, religious and medical missionaries, and nationalist and military governments, from everyday human perspectives? Beginning with that first trip to Ghana in 2001, I have traveled there every year until 2014, spending a month or two each time and vacuuming up all details I can about Kofi Dɔnkɔ's life and times, seeking to answer these questions and more. I have written other books since. But as the years passed, that certain video footage of Kofi Dɔnkɔ's funerary rites and the unending lines of the bereaved still lurked around the corner of each completed project. It was not the memory of the recorded events that haunted me; I had no intimate memory of the funeral because I was not there. It was the memory people kept of Kofi Dɔnkɔ, and the persistent fear, ricocheting in my mind, that the best of my skill might not do justice to the story those memories represented. The outlining and writing of the first drafts of that story in August 2015, precisely twenty years after Kofi Dɔnkɔ's passing and a century after his birth, signaled an end to that fear. But little did I know the endgame of this story, and how it might all turn out.

Kofi Sakyi (Dɔnkɔ) was a healer, blacksmith, drummer, woodcarver, farmer, and head of the family born to Yaw Badu of Nkoransa and Akosua Toa of Takyiman, into a Bono (Akan) family, around 1913 (figure I.1). Kofi's

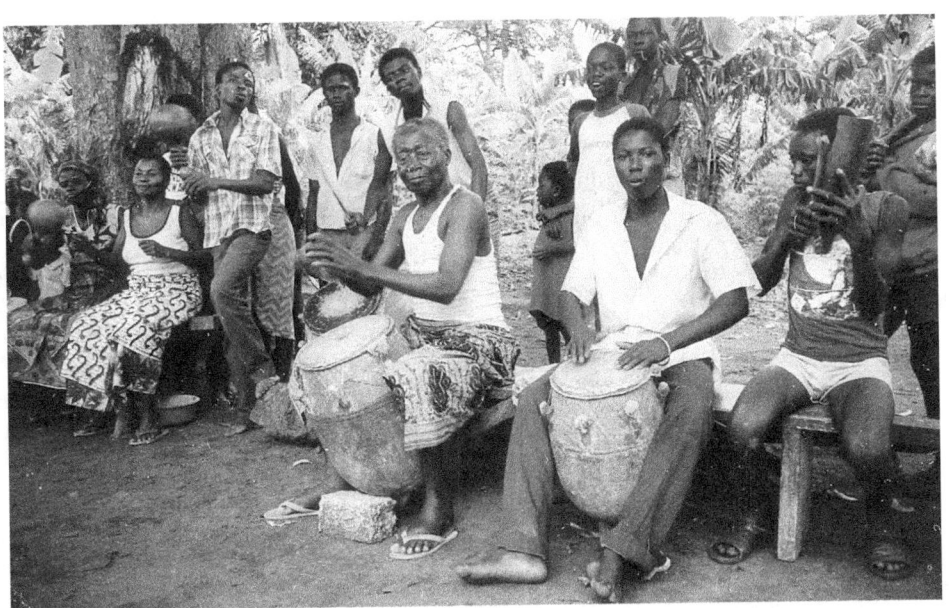

FIGURE I.1. Nana Kofi Dɔnkɔ (left) drumming at Asuotipa Festival, Takyiman, ca. 1989. From the privately owned Nana Kwaku Sakyi Collection, Miami, Florida. Used courtesy of Nana Kwaku Sakyi, photographer.

early years and socialization in a family of well-respected healers and blacksmiths foreshadowed his eventual vocation, for while he engaged matters of spiritual culture and healing through a family that nurtured those passions, other young men in the tripartite Gold Coast colony were being socialized by the forces of latent empire, capitalism, and Christian missionaries. It is not that Kofi Dɔnkɔ, as a fellow member of the colony, was immune to these forces, but he was less seduced by them and thus thought about them differently.

Kofi Dɔnkɔ's path as a prominent healer was baked into the circumstances of his birth. After his two elder sisters were born, the next five children died shortly after birth, disturbing Kofi's parents and prompting a consultation with the family's ɔbosom, Asubɔnten Kwabena. Yaw and Akosua made several ritual sacrifices and petitioned Asubɔnten for the long and healthy life of their newborn son, who in this circumstance received the name "Dɔnkɔ," an allegory for service to Asubɔnten Kwabena. Although reluctant to join a cast of healers during his early teenage years, Kofi Dɔnkɔ would become the most significant healer for the spiritual force that protected his early and long life.

The healer-to-be spent his early years with his father, a skilled herbalist and blacksmith, in the Nkoransa village of Akumsa Odumase. There, Kofi Dɔnkɔ began to learn rudiments of the healing arts and blacksmithing before departing in the late 1920s for his mother's town of Takyiman to begin his almost seven-year training to become a healer. In the early 1920s, before Kofi's training, British colonial anthropologist Robert S. Rattray visited Takyiman and devoted a significant part of his writing to Bono cultural life, with a view that Takyiman was "the ideal ground upon which to study Akan customs and beliefs."[1] No evidence indicates that Kofi Dɔnkɔ crossed paths with Rattray, but anthropologists from Margaret Field to Eva Meyerowitz to Dennis Warren would pursue Rattray's claim over the next fifty years. The intervening years were punctuated by a series of local and regional transformations graphed onto global empire and the periodic crises of "indirect" British rule in the colony. British colonial imposition translated into the dual subjugation of Takyiman under Asante and British hegemony, and heavy social tensions brought on by a colonial economy anchored in cocoa corresponded to the rival popularity of "enforcer" spiritual forces, accompanying migrant cocoa laborers from the northern savanna that clashed with Christian missions and colonial officials from the southern region. Takyiman was the gateway between the northern and southern halves of the colony, and the town's and Kofi Dɔnkɔ's positionality—cultural, ecological, and economic—offer fertile ground upon which to examine those transformations and their human experiences.

Although Kofi Dɔnkɔ stayed away from politics, he too was ensnared in the morass of land and legal disputes that pervaded the colony, and he participated as a farmer with hired migrant laborers in the cocoa boom between the 1930s and 1950s. Yet Kofi Dɔnkɔ suffered an all-too-common fate: the exploitation of his labor and product by cocoa brokers during the boom years, and that of this intellectual history and vast healing knowledge during the coming-of-age for Ghana and African studies in the 1960s and 1970s. More than any Africanist anthropologist, Dennis Warren can be credited with bringing Kofi Dɔnkɔ's ideas to the academic marketplace. But Warren's pioneering research in Takyiman on Bono disease classification and medicines relied crucially on some 1,500 disease lexemes articulated by "one venerated Bono priest-healer"—Kofi Dɔnkɔ. This multiyear research constituted a foundation for Warren's later writings and his admirable academic career—he received promotion, tenure, and World Bank expert status along the way—whereas Kofi Dɔnkɔ was memorialized as an "informant" and certainly not an intellectual in his own right. Kofi Dɔnkɔ could justifiably be written off as a victim of the politics of knowledge and of history, but this would be shortsighted. Two recently discovered record books for patients Kofi Dɔnkɔ treated during the 1980s certify Kofi Dɔnkɔ as an intellectual whose history contributes to our understanding of health and healing in Africa and the world.

Kofi Dɔnkɔ was a marginal peasant-farmer whose fortune and misfortune rode the tides of the cocoa boom, an everyday person who gives us a window into the social lives and networks of rural dwellers, and an exceptional and important person who articulated a profound understanding of disease and therapeutics to trainees who resided in West Africa and throughout the African diaspora as well as a notable group of scholars. Location and an integral cultural heritage stand out as two of several factors that shaped the life of Kofi Dɔnkɔ and Takyiman. Situated at a crossroad, his and his town's positionalities invite us to think of Takyiman as a gateway for cultural contact and exchanges, rather than solely the coastal region of the Gold Coast/Ghana; a gateway that does not presuppose a European presence and as a counterpoint to scholarly accounts that valorize the perspective of Christianized and "modernizing" individuals along the Atlantic seaboard. Rather than prop up Kofi Dɔnkɔ as some cultural nationalist whom Black Atlanticists would love to topple, it is precisely Kofi Dɔnkɔ's deep devotion to his craft, his culture, his community that framed his transcendence of academic boundaries—African/diasporic, indigenous/allopathic, colonial/postcolonial—and that makes him a figure from whom we might learn to heal the traumas caused by those binary, yet artificial, categories.

❁

KOFI DƆNKƆ'S FUNERARY rites, described at the opening of this introduction, were recorded on video, but for technological and cultural reasons—each with their own episteme and logic—a great deal of the rites, the preparations leading up to them, and the collective and individual meanings, feelings, and immaterial participants were not and could not be recorded. Most recordings of human action—the basis of human history—capture only episodic fractions of it, leaving aside an interlaced range of human emotions, ideas, exchanges, and connections. It is not that persons like Kofi Dɔnkɔ, who are often categorized as "marginal" or "the poor," are difficult historical subjects because they leave behind insufficient evidence of their lives. Instead, we tend to reduce historical evidence to documents and consequently consecrate documents as the beginning and the end of a story. Through this act, we make historically marginalized subjects ghost-like figures, haunting but never full revealed; said another way, history writing has been an act of making illegible certain categories and constituents of humanity.[2] That Kofi Dɔnkɔ, like most of humanity before the digital age, did not (and may not) leave a dense documentary trail means that such persons will remain hidden to those of us who are ill equipped to reconstruct or are unreceptive to alternative ways of thinking about their stories. The story of Kofi Dɔnkɔ and his community invites us to imagine history as a craft, an intellectual platform to help write/right the world.

The more I watched the video recording of Kofi Dɔnkɔ's funerary rites, the more I saw filmmaking as a methodological analog to standard history writing. Filmmaking is like history writing in that both establish an artificial order on a story (or a series of stories), on time and space, and much of this is done after shooting, during the postproduction process of editing the frames, angles, and shots to create a product that will draw a paying audience. If history is the long shot (the scene-setting, general impression), biography is the close-up (the most detailed view). Here and in the book's subtitle, I use the familiar term *biography* only to draw the reader's attention to a new approach, "communography." In this way, *biography* is simply a placeholder. I have chosen to tell the story of Kofi Dɔnkɔ and his community and homeland through an approach to writing meaningful history that I call communography, in that my concern is *not* with an individual life story but rather with the thousands of kin, community members, and strangers who knew, interacted with, and lived during historic moments Kofi Dɔnkɔ shared. I choose also to tell this story through the evocative and varied moments in which humans live, rather than through the predictable and artificial plots historians devise. Staying with our filming metaphor, professional actors who act in plots are poor actors, in sharp contrast with those who act in the moment. Great actors who consistently work on their craft all indicate losing themselves in the moment—most do not remember the details of their performance. Prominent healers like Kofi Dɔnkɔ, who enter into conversation with spiritual forces in a trance-like state and access another archive while performing the roles of medium and interpreter, also do not remember much of their "possession" once the extended moment is over. The spiritual forces in conversation with healers show us life and temporal death in each trance experience, as each force enters and hyperanimates the human body and then, after the force's "human" moment, leaves it exhausted. Humans, likewise, do not live their lives in plots. We live in moments, and in a series of moments strung together that we call our temporal lives.

By "moments strung together," I mean that human beings live *in* historical moments and those moments—the contexts in which the contents of our lives are generated—come to form our temporal lives. Certainly, this is not the only way to think about the ebb and flow of human lives, but it is one way to envision those lives, since human experiences do not often subscribe to plots or the sequential order of events in which a life story is (re)presented. Thinking about human history in terms of moments—in all their variation—means that each story about a person or community does not necessarily have two sides. A story may have five sides or one, depending on the moment and the kinds of human action involved. Kofi Dɔnkɔ became a remarkably skilled healer, blacksmith, and family and community leader—and these constitute multifarious sides of a story—but he also remained an "ordinary" person, embedded in the mundane ebb and flow of community life. (The quotation marks around *ordinary* indicate that this descriptor and category, on its own, inadequately characterizes the composite person that was Kofi Dɔnkɔ.) Through neither celebrity nor individual triumph, he took a selfless position that placed community above self-interest and that minimized social breakdown by fighting for wholeness. In effect, the ordinary, the marginalized, and the proverbial "people without history" are precisely the historical subjects who give us a wide-angle view of moments both mundane and cross-fertilized by local and global events. To interpret Kofi Dɔnkɔ's multitiered story is to do so in ways he, if alive, may not have chosen, especially through my approach and words. A communography is therefore a composite production, and the subjects of this approach are composite persons to the extent that their lives can be revealed through documentary fragments, repositories of ideas, memory, language, ritual, and material culture.

The story of Kofi Dɔnkɔ and his community began from a ground zero in published knowledge, where no earlier historical works existed on which to build, and so I had to develop a map for his life and his community's life, research nearly everything around them, take it all in, and then process all on three intersecting scales: individual, village/township, and homeland/world.[3] Although most of us strain against evidentiary limitations, trying to recover bits of human experience and to place content in context, I took the methodological position of a detective unrestricted by disciplinary practice and ideological boundaries. My quest for Kofi Dɔnkɔ's life and times brought me to institutional archives in England, Ghana, Switzerland, and the United States. I consulted collections of the International Committee of the Red Cross, Salvation Army, Wesleyan Methodist Missionary Society, Roman Catholic Mission, and Holy Family Medical Mission; the Basel Mission Archives; the Bodleian Library of Commonwealth and African Studies at Oxford University; the University of London's School of African and Oriental Studies archives; the British Museum library and archives; the British Library; the National Archives of the UK (Kew); the Indiana University Archives of Traditional Music; the Melville J. Herskovits Library of African Studies at Northwestern University; and other African studies collections in the United States.[4] In Ghana I raided the national archives (Public Records and Archives Administration Department), the Manhyia Archives in Kumase, and the regional archives at Sunyani and Kumase. From these archives I assembled maps, land surveys, photographs, legal and religious documents, typeset and published oral histories, letters, newspapers, regional and local court cases, published ethnographies, historical accounts, and annual reports for the Gold Coast region (ca. 1895–1939), which was then divided into the three colonial holdings of the Gold Coast Colony, Crown Colony of Ashanti, and the Northern Territories. In all these repositories, there was no evidentiary trace of Kofi Dɔnkɔ, although he was a prominent person in locations where several of the aforementioned organizations worked and where records about those communities were kept.

The most helpful repositories, however, were the local archives in Sunyani, the records of the Holy Family Hospital that operated in Kofi Dɔnkɔ's Takyiman, and more than anything else, the photos, documentary fragments, family and shrine histories, interviews, songs, and oral and video recordings that came from people who knew him in some capacity and at some moments of his life. The strength of these sources is that they help bring Kofi Dɔnkɔ and his sociopolitical world vividly to life, while archival and published sources, especially rarely used and locally produced Akan/Twi-language texts, make up for what the former lack in distilling Kofi Dɔnkɔ's life by filling out the broader social, cultural, and political contexts of well- and lesser-known historical events. I examine a bevy of Akan/Twi terms that appear in the archival and oral sources specific to Kofi Dɔnkɔ, fleshing out key concepts he put to work and that worked to translate his therapeutic knowledge into social practice.[5] This attention to language serves the purpose of explicating cultural practice, following orthography and conventions established by the Ghana Bureau of Languages (but I have left spellings as they appear in the sources), and grounding the subject in a world he would have easily recognized.[6] This is, after all, his and his community's story.

But for all this, there are instances in the book where Kofi Dɔnkɔ's specific role or place in historical events is less than certain, and he unfortunately disappears briefly because of limitations in the sources. Then again, the life of an individual or community will always have gaps in its recorded and remembered histories. Some of these expected gaps in this case are fortunately filled by a remarkable set of patient records kept by Kofi Dɔnkɔ's secretary or scribe, but almost nothing about Kofi Dɔnkɔ himself except for frail scraps of paper where a scribe jotted down spare lines Kofi Dɔnkɔ dictated about his children, his family, and his community work. In sum, my decade-long journey through national, missionary, university, family, and individual (re)collections revealed that had I made the usual research commitment to institutional archives fashioned by empire, I would not have found Kofi Dɔnkɔ and his place in the history of his community, homeland, and the world.

❋

THAT HUMANITY IS divided into "races," the geography of the world into continents and nation-states, and historical time into moments dubbed "precolonial" or "postcolonial" is commonplace. But if we filter these conceptual divisions through the ideas and lived experiences of historical subjects such as Kofi Dɔnkɔ, they might amount to semantic nonsense. Kofi Dɔnkɔ offered his therapeutic services and knowledge to all, regardless of "ethnicity/race," religion, and other markers of human-devised boundaries. On the one hand, Kofi Dɔnkɔ was one of the first to train as healers diasporic Africans from the Americas and to actively participate in early health projects that sought to integrate indigenous and biomedical practitioners in Africa. In doing so, he transcended cultural boundaries between "Africa" and "diasporic Africa," between Christians and Muslims, and between so-called traditional and allopathic medicine. On the other hand, healers like Kofi Dɔnkɔ were problematized in such health projects because they often supported a one-way transmission rather than a mutual exchange of knowledge. This part of Kofi Dɔnkɔ's story underscores how cultural and hegemonic boundaries are both porous and reinforced, and how individuals both transcend and resign themselves to the "fact" of those boundaries. For Kofi Dɔnkɔ's part, there is no evidence that he exploited the boundaries he transcended. His ideas were born in specific contexts, but they did break out of those contexts, thereby transforming the condition of his life and work, and that of his community's engagement with the broader world. In fact, Kofi Dɔnkɔ might be considered global in the sense that his ideas, healing practices, and reputation touched people in West Africa, Europe, and the Americas.

Kofi Dɔnkɔ lived in moments scholars have trademarked "colonial" and "postcolonial," but his life story demonstrates that the ruptures signaling these eras are overexaggerated, and more so because they take their cue from a European script of imperial rule—in his case, the British/English variety.[7] Kofi Dɔnkɔ and many Africans like him never folded their historical moments and lived experiences under the tent of precolonial or postcolonial. In fact, Kofi Dɔnkɔ and his Akan/Bono peoples have *their own* understandings of time (*berɛ*), history (*abakɔsɛm*, "matters that have come and gone"), calendar (*adaduanan*), and their place in a historicized culture and forest-savanna ecology.[8] Further, his peoples' coded wisdom proverbially provides a method for locating those understandings: *Onipa bɛhwɛ yie a, na ɛfiri nea wahunuiɛ* ("If a person looks well, it is from what s/he has seen"). Viewed from this theoretical position, Ghana is less a nation-state defined by homogeneity and a citizenry of "one nation" than it is a geography populated by kin, strangers, and antagonists, all of whom are connected to communities and locations and to internal and external diasporic formations. Rather than simply ask how Kofi Dɔnkɔ's life story maps onto major themes in twentieth-century Ghana/Africa/world, we might also ask what specifically is revealed through the lived experiences and ideas of Kofi Dɔnkɔ and his community about the standard themes of colonialism, religion, disease, independence, global war, and human culture. The story of Kofi Dɔnkɔ and his homeland encourages us to take the cues and constructs in our narrations from the lived experiences, ideas, and optics of the people we seek to interpret.

THIS BOOK PRESENTS the contents and formative conditions of Kofi Dɔnkɔ's life in a narrative that demonstrates, on a broader scale, three principal themes in the human experience: (1) individuals cannot be representatives of the culture and communities to which they belong, but those who occupy different roles in that culture can offer integral, wide-angle perspectives on the lives of cultural and community members and a protracted commentary on an evolving culture or society; (2) African and world history can be greatly enriched by focusing more on communal histories or communographies that take as their focus multifarious people rather than exceptional individuals; and (3) shared genetics and behaviors aside, humans are distinguished by their culture and the ideas and practices that flow from it. These themes take on greater shape in this communography, which is divided into seven chapters and an epilogue detailing the culture, community, and homeland that shaped the temporal life of Kofi Dɔnkɔ.

The first chapter is concerned with Kofi Dɔnkɔ's ontological world, that is, the world of spiritual forces, their variety and interrelationships, and how these conceptions formed senses of the world, organized societies, and histories, and how they fashioned the social world and work of a healer. Its aim is to understand key ideas that saturated this social world in the era in which Kofi Dɔnkɔ was born. With his own influential spiritual force called Asubɔnten Kwabena, Kofi Dɔnkɔ used a historically constituted partnership between spiritual forces and their human hosts for the "common good," constantly translating his ontological world into social practice and enabling his multifaceted culture to move through the history of his homelands.

The second chapter extends the ontological and social worlds outlined in chapter 1 to the entangled histories of Takyiman, Nkoransa, Asante, and the British from the late nineteenth century to the birth and adolescence of Kofi Dɔnkɔ in the early twentieth century. Although born in the Nkoransa village of Akumsa Odumase, Kofi Dɔnkɔ's mother was from Takyiman, where Kofi Dɔnkɔ would live most of his life but which was under a dual hegemony of Asante control and British colonial rule. Nkoransa, Takyiman, and a tripartite colony constituted the multiple (home)lands of Kofi Dɔnkɔ, and the clear majority of his and his family's lives oscillated among these locations. Although scholars tend to speak of one colony, in fact the three colonial territories (Gold Coast Colony, Crown Colony of Ashanti, and the Northern Territories), excluding the later addition of British Togoland, were administered, resourced, and viewed differently though the machinations of imperial Britain.[9]

In chapter 3, Kofi Dɔnkɔ's homelands of Nkoransa and Takyiman provide two poignant cases for examining the ways in which the emergent themes of religion/spirituality, education, health, and family took shape in them and in the broader tripartite colony during Kofi's late adolescence and early adulthood. As Kofi Dɔnkɔ and a new class of healers worked for the prosperity of his adopted town of Takyiman, the major themes of religion/spirituality, health, and family continued to take more intimate shape as

Kofi Dɔnkɔ grew into a life of medicine and marriage and navigated the politics of colonial life.

Chapter 4 focuses on the politics and competing claims to land, religious authority, and decolonization as cocoa and other natural resources buoyed the tripartite colony during Kofi Dɔnkɔ's adulthood. It pays specific attention to his layered role as blacksmith, healer, farmer, husband, and father. In chapter 5, the patterns of life for Kofi Dɔnkɔ, Takyiman, and the colony/nation ran on analogous tracks, revealing a series of relationships, freedoms sought, and twists of fortune around the evolving story of Kofi Dɔnkɔ, his community, and his nation to be.

Kofi Dɔnkɔ's and his sister's known expertise enabled their family to turn a community tragedy into an independent "healer's village," while a Takyiman-led Bonokyɛmpem Federation, a movement that consolidated Bono identity and independence from Asante, partnered with Kwame Nkrumah to forge a nation independent of British colonial rule. While competing national factions fought over independence, similar conflicts at the local level underscored the move by Kofi Dɔnkɔ and his colleagues to form their own autonomous healing association, although he helped shaped the cooperative relations with Takyiman's new hospital and the creation of new "customary laws" promulgated in the early republic. The new republic ironically inhibited "traditional" institutions but provided the conditions for "independent" African churches and an Islamic organization to take root under one-party rule. Because Kofi Dɔnkɔ did not take sides in religion or politics, he was sought out by Christian and Muslim patients and avoided much of the politics that fomented military coups and crises.

While the nation found itself in crisis, increasingly enthralled by Christianity and capitalism, Kofi Dɔnkɔ's healing knowledge gave life to the career of an anthropologist who would share Kofi Dɔnkɔ's intellect and remarkable skill with the world beyond Ghana. More than any other anthropologist, Dennis Warren would circulate and profit from Kofi Dɔnkɔ's accrued knowledge and reputation, placing in sharp contrast an independent Ghana claiming control over its human and material resources and a Ghana still exposed to the exploits of capitalists, neocolonialists, and the coming-of-age of African studies. Rather than cast Kofi Dɔnkɔ as a victim, chapter 6 considers the relations between Dɔnkɔ and Warren as an allegory to the intertwined comings-of-age of independent African nations such as Ghana and the academic study of Africa, set against global power relations and forces of exploitation. Within this setting, the chapter examines the politics of health and healing—more precisely, attempts to integrate biomedical and indigenous approaches amid a series of military coups and economic crises.

Although these conflicts and succession disputes plagued the nation, there was no sign that Ghana was immune from coups or the uncertainty and unrest that would require remedy during the years Jerry Rawlings ruled Ghana. Chapter 7 considers the recurrent theme of uncertainty in the lives of Ghana citizens. Flanked by national politics and unrest, this chapter argues, an aging Kofi Dɔnkɔ showed no sign of yielding to either volatility or mental decline. Takyiman and Kofi Dɔnkɔ were mutual gateways for migrants fleeing conflict and seeking therapy, and Kofi elevated and expanded his healing practice independent of Takyiman's foremost hospital. If Kofi Dɔnkɔ held in place community bonds and partnerships with local and foreign actors, so too did his passing in 1995 occasion a reverse in the partnership between that hospital and healers and a resurfacing of tensions within his family, community, and nation. The epilogue considers a few ways in which the major themes of this book resonate in the world in which we live, thinking through the watershed moments of 1948, the consequences of forced intimacy occasioned by colonial rule, the opportunities missed by independence leaders, and what the figure of the healer might mean for our present era.

CHAPTER 1. **LIBATION**

"Matters Connected with Our Culture"

The healer must first have a healer's nature.
—AYI KWEI ARMAH, *The Healers*

Kofi Dɔnkɔ cheated a death that devoured five potential siblings, entering the corporal world as a child of Yaw Badu and Akosua Toa around 1913. As an infant he stood between spiritual and mundane worlds, nestled in the arms of his afflicted parents, while his natal town of Nkoransa and his mother's (and later his own adopted) town of Takyiman lay situated between two empires—one local, one foreign—under Asante hegemony and British colonial rule. In 1913 Richard C. Temple, president of the Anthropological Section of the British Association for the Advancement of Science, made the case in his presidential address for "the administrative value of anthropology," a sort of applied anthropology training for colonial administrators and servicemen.[1] The Royal Commission on University Education in London issued around the same time a report echoing Temple's view. Theirs was a message that insisted "An accurate acquaintance with the nature, habits, and customs of alien populations is necessary to all who have to live and work amongst them in any official capacity, whether administrators, executive officers, missionaries, or merchants."[2] A former customs officer and assistant district commissioner in the northern Asante town of Ejura, the Scotsman Robert S. Rattray was brought into this world of applied (colonial) anthropology between stints

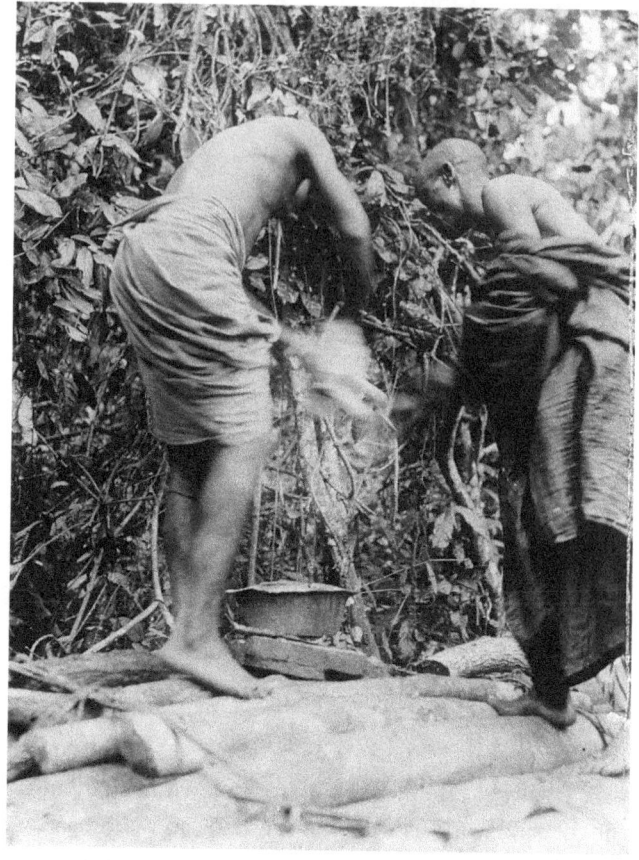

FIGURE 1.1. Sacrificing a white fowl to Asubonten. Photographed by Robert Sutherland Rattray, ca. 1923 (MS 445), © Royal Anthropological Institute, London, 300.445–03–093. Used with permission.

of colonial service and studies at Oxford University, and he became head of the first "Anthropological Department" of Asante in 1921.[3] Convinced by Temple's position and by his fluency in African languages (including Akan/Twi), Rattray started to pay more attention to culture while in the Asante region, beginning with his stay at Ejura, where down a dirt road to the west laid Takyiman and Nkoransa.[4] As early as 1913 Rattray's anthropology fixed on "social and religious beliefs, rites, and customs," as evidenced by his "many years' residence in Ashanti" that culminated in *Ashanti* (published in 1923), but he saw the Takyiman region as a source of Asante "religion" and saw religion as inseparable from "almost any aspect of social life."[5] It was in the Takyiman region where Rattray received the nickname *Oboruni Okomfo*, a "foreign/European ɔkɔmfoɔ."[6] Although the European ɔkɔmfoɔ did not meet the soon-to-be-healer Kofi Dɔnkɔ, Rattray certainly encountered an Asubɔnten Kwabena (figure 1.1), the same spiritual force (ɔbosom; pl. *abosom*) Kofi Dɔnkɔ would inherit, on his way to the Tanɔ River—the incubator for such river-bound spiritual forces.

Driven as he was by the idea of progress and his access to culture through language, Rattray warned indigenous peoples that his European culture, "ideas, arts, customs, dress, should not be embraced by them blindly," lest they "become pseudo-European, but [rather they should] ... aim at progress for their race based upon what is best in their own institutions, religion, their manners and customs."[7] These best practices ultimately were to be grafted onto European (British) ones, enabling the Asante/African peoples "to take their place in the commonwealth of civilized nations ... who will become the greater force and power in the Empire because they have not bartered the wealth of their past."[8] The fog of empire aside, Rattray in his time and as a serviceman in the empire was struck by something beyond his job description, in fact beyond the mandate of the Anthropological Department—the arena of belief, or what I call spiritual culture, and how it, like power, ran thoroughly through social and political life. Rattray's quest for belief through observation and for fluency in the Akan/Twi language echoed some of the nineteenth- and early twentieth-century Basel missionaries who followed his research, styling him "our reporter Mr. Rattray."[9] But rather than evangelical aims, his objectives were less published results or their political uses and included a more respectful adventure to understand the Asante/Akan peoples beyond the cranial measurements and classificatory schemes in vogue in the early twentieth century. But as Rattray soon discovered, the locus of Asante belief, specifically a range of spiritual forces, was not in the Asante capital of Kumase. Instead "the great *obosom* (god) of all Ashanti" lay in the Takyiman region, that is, "the Tano river, from which are derived countless of 'his children' as lesser *abosom*, and ... is considered as the 'son of the Supreme God.'"[10] This chapter is concerned with this world of spiritual forces, in their variety and interrelationships, and how these "religious conceptions of the Twi-speaking peoples" formed senses of the world that manifested in societies and their histories, fashioning the social world and work of healer Kofi Dɔnkɔ.[11] The aim is to understand key ideas that saturated this social world in the context of when Kofi Dɔnkɔ entered his human community in the early twentieth century, leaving behind a spiritual one.

After visiting Nkoransa and Takyiman in 1921, Rattray compared his research against historic representations of "non-human spiritual powers" and concluded the Africans' "beliefs have for centuries been described as 'fetishism' or 'fetish worship,' but the[se] religious conceptions ... [had]

been grievously misrepresented."[12] For Rattray misrepresentation flowed from "semi-educated Africans" uninterested in their culture informing Europeans and other foreigners, problematic interpreters, and "inappropriate European words . . . employed to describe objects and actions," which, adopted and adapted by Africans who learned European languages, "were used again by [Africans] when interpreting."[13] Starting from this perspective, Rattray eliminated the use of interpreters through his own fluency and bypassed "educated Africans" through direct contact with elderly women and men. But for all his skill and embeddedness Rattray, despite his diagnosis, could not escape the trappings inherent in translating culture from one idiom to another. Although, for instance, he rejected the caricature "fetish" and "rigidly confined [it] to designate" charms and talismans—rather than what the Akan/Twi speaker "calls *suman*"—Rattray rendered as "god" the category of "non-human spirits" that these speakers called "*abosom*."[14] Although called a European ɔkɔmfoɔ, Rattray was not one of the Akan/Twi-speaking healers he engaged, and although his understanding of belief and indigenous language was far more advanced for his time and, when compared with that of previous interlopers, his knowledge could not stand in for experience, socialization within a healing family, and the abilities that made a Kofi Dɔnkɔ possible. Rattray's explication of the ideas and spiritual forces Kofi Dɔnkɔ would translate into social practice, which Rattray investigated during his visits to the Takyiman region, therefore function as both a source to be mined and a guide to the evidence that set out the ontological world of Kofi Dɔnkɔ.[15]

The ontological world of Kofi Dɔnkɔ was coded in ideas and practices expressed in various ways. Perhaps the most evocative was ritual libation (*mpaeɛ*), for in its "text" appear the names, praise names, and specific utilization of spiritual forces invoked. Libation, as prelude to an event, involved the ritual pouring of palm wine or a local or imported alcoholic drink on the ground, accompanied by invocative words within well-rehearsed structures that permit improvisation. Libation therefore symbolizes a connective tissue between material and immaterial worlds. In these instances and others the text of libations goes some way toward explaining those spiritual forces— of nature or ancestry—because their form adheres to standard categories of beings while nimbly accommodating different social circumstances. The iterations of these libation texts tell us something about their authors and, from a purely cultural perspective, offer an untapped source for the ideas of healers who understandably operated in some secrecy. Although we do not have textual evidence from Kofi Dɔnkɔ's earliest libations, we can surmise that his text, recorded later in life (and set off in the next section), resembled very much ones he heard in his healing family and around his trainers as a teenager, and those that Rattray and others recorded at the start of each festive, formal, or ritual occasion.

Whereas Rattray engaged his informants without an interpreter, all the researchers who interviewed Kofi Dɔnkɔ required one, filtering our impression of Kofi Dɔnkɔ's ideas and work in ways that might misrepresent. As tempting as it might be to dismiss such interviews, a closer look at these third-party sources almost certainly reflects the pitfalls of translating culture and the conceptual frames of both interpreter and interviewee. It is possible to determine the approximate meanings of Kofi Dɔnkɔ's ideas through such sources, but the prospect of making those ideas comprehensible lies precisely in the structural form of libations and suggests how they were made all the more salient in social and cultural life. Rattray's corpus of Akan/Twi libation texts collected in Takyiman and in Greater Asante should not surprise us, nor should their very close adherence to one such rare text articulated by Kofi Dɔnkɔ.

❋

ONE SUNDAY IN April, around the time of the annual Apoɔ festival in Takyiman, Kofi Dɔnkɔ received two visitors to his compound, presumably having made an appointment for a day when healing work was proscribed. The white graduate student from the United States and his Ghanaian interpreter brought with them an alcoholic drink that Kofi Dɔnkɔ used to pour libation. The libation formally introduced the foreign student to the cast of ancestors and spiritual forces with which the healer worked in collaboration and served to petition those forces to ensure the young researcher's safety and success. The interview was prefaced by a requisite opening libation, divided here into five sequential parts for closer analysis.[16] On that Sunday Kofi Dɔnkɔ presented the student and his customary gift of alcoholic drink, offering these words:

> Nana Saman Kwadwo, come and take drink.
> Silverman is a whiteman....
> Silverman is in search of past events and matters connected with our
>   culture as well as matters about you, the [abosom].
> Through that, he will obtain a high position so that in [the] future
>   his descendants may narrate his deeds as I am talking to you now.

Here is his drink.
We pray for health and strength, long life and glory, long life and good luck.
Protect him against a bad companion, an evil spirit, a witch, a wizard, a vicious fetish priest/priestess, a tyrant and a wicked Muslim.
I pray you to guide and guard him so that while he is here he may be able to assist this state to have progress.

By invoking "Nana Saman Kwadwo," Kofi Dɔnkɔ suffused the occasion with an initial category of spiritual forces, namely ancestors, and specifically the spirit of his grandfather Kwadwo Owusu. A title for elders, office-holders, and ancestors, "Nana" signified the status of the departed being called "Saman." *Saman* is the linguistic root for the terms *nsamanfoɔ* (ancestors; sg. *ɔsaman*) and their indeterminate abode, *asamandɔ*, "which means," according to a group of early twentieth-century healers, "there is no more town. No town exists there anymore."[17] But the term *saman* also alerts us to a cluster of ancestral spirits who each correspond to the ethical contents of their human lives and to the way they transitioned. Within four identifiable categories of ancestry, *asamanpa* are "good-natured" ancestors who experienced a natural death en route to asamandoɔ, *asaman twɛn-twɛn* linger near the earth as ineligible candidates for asamandoɔ because of their unethical existence, and the acutely negative *asamanbɔne* or *ɔtɔfo* ("lingering spirit") experienced a violent death or improper burial and consequently they boldly and aggressively wander about.[18] Death by suicide is viewed as culturally unacceptable and debars a deceased person from asamandoɔ; such spirits return to the human world as *ɔtɔfo sasa*—individuals incarnate with a cruel or homicidal character, leading to the same end.[19] The *nananom nsamanfoɔ* (sg. *nana saman*) are "evolved ancestors" in the sense they have achieved their life's mission (*hyɛbea*) and transitioned across waters or up a hill to asamandoɔ; thus they are the ones invoked through libation for the provision of blessings, children, prosperity, health, healing, and long life.[20] If "ancestorhood" is an epochal stage in human development, then the nananom nsamanfoɔ embody the idea of becoming fully human in terms of life cycle—or at least a crucial node in that cycle.[21]

That Nana Kwadwo was called upon as "Nana Saman" specifies two likely, yet closely related occurrences: he lived an ethical life, fulfilling his earthly mission according to standards set by his ancestors and human community, and therefore he found a place in asamandɔ among the nananom nsamanfoɔ targeted for invocation. At an *adae* (ancestral) ceremony witnessed in 1922, Rattray recorded a libation initiated with the words "Me nananom nsamanfo, nne ye Awukuade," which he translated as "My spirit grandfathers [i.e., ancestors], to-day is the Wednesday *Adae*."[22] For Bono societies, the Wednesday adae ceremony fell on *monowukuo*, a "new or fresh" Wednesday.[23] Moreover, in the early twentieth century Basel missionaries, who studied and published literature in Akan/Twi while erecting mission schools across broad regions like Asante, recorded another libation, this time by ɔkɔmfoɔ Kwame Dapa of Nsuta, who announced, "Today is Adae. . . . spirits of the grandfathers, come and receive the palm wine and drink."[24] A Basel missionary named Owusu asked several healers why they venerate the deceased. They responded: "The reason why we have to serve the deceased is the following: When the dead person was living, he was my father or she my mother, during his or her life I honored him or her very much and appreciated him or her. Now he or she has died and I have to present the same veneration to his or her spirit. If I have [palm] wine and food I have to also give some of it to him or her."[25] Nana Kwadwo's invitation to "come and take drink" and the invocation of his spiritual presence served to bear witness to the meeting, introduce him to the "whiteman," and petition him and his kind to protect the student "against a bad companion, an evil spirit, a witch, a wizard, a vicious fetish priest/priestess, a tyrant and a wicked Muslim."

The plea for protection in exchange for "libations of palm wine and liquor," among other offerings, in part explains the enlarged net ancestry cast over family and community life.[26] But the petition also adheres to an early twentieth-century observation made by foreign evangelists of the Basel mission (BM), or their local coverts and informants, at a time when BM mission schools were the predominant Christian institutions in the interior, doubling and in some cases tripling the numbers of Wesleyan, Roman Catholic, Bremen, and other mission schools.[27] The Basel missionaries' remark, supposedly anchored in "the Asante point of view," reckoned, "The [local] person senses himself from the cradle to the grave under the influence of good and bad spirit powers whose hostile attitude he will try to mitigate through sacrificial offerings and prayers and whose protection and assistance he is seeking to win."[28] Christian filtrations aside, the mitigation of unseen but experientially real forces, some of which were viewed with hostility, accord very much with the reasons for protection, made transparent by the (translated) keywords *bad, evil, vicious,* and *wicked*.

If the world of asamandoɔ was a solar system, then there existed a galaxy of spiritual forces. We will return later to some of these forces indicated by

Kofi Dɔnkɔ—the "bad companion," "vicious fetish priest/priestess," and "tyrant and a wicked Muslim." For other, nonhuman forces, English language glosses such as "evil spirit" and "witch" or "wizard" shroud the deep resonance of these beings who pervade the forest environs, no less the healer's world. The first of such beings is the well-known *mmoatia* ("short creatures"), citizens of the tropical forest and occupants of the sacred *odum* tree (*Chlorophora excelsa*) that possess backward feet with the heels toward the front, a high-pitched voice, an appetite for bananas, a jovial attitude toward children, and, for the healer, an unrivaled knowledge of plant medicines. As medicinal procurers par excellence, the mmoatia have their own healers who communicate with them, but like any tool they can be an asset or troublesome, invoking passions of fear rather than facilitation.

The second and perhaps most recognizable of the lot is *sasabonsam* or *kasampere*, a fearsome creature of the dense forest; the term is often translated as "the devil" by Christians, who view its accomplices as "witches." We know *Sasabonsam Kwaku* (Sasabonsam born on Wednesday) through its missionary-induced profile: a forest monster with long hair, dangling legs, feet pointing in both directions, and bloodshot eyes. Invoking fear and awe, sasabonsam purportedly sits on the high branches of an *odum* or *onyina* tree (*Ceiba pentandra*), in cahoots with mmoatia and wielders of "witchcraft," the alleged *abayifoɔ*. This graphic portrayal of sasabonsam is not completely inaccurate, but it is a grave mischaracterization, for sasabonsam is solicited to detect and defeat the very "evil" with which it is thought to be associated.[29] Rattray defined *sasa* as the "spirit surviving after death" and *bonsam* as a "male witch."[30] However, sasa is not just any spirit but rather the negative or ill-reconciled spirit of a deceased creature that is able to cause harm, whereas bonsam is an acute malevolent force that can be used to harm or heal—by attacking the very antisocial forces it represents. In sum, sasabonsam is a spirit-dweller of the deep forest that assumes the form of a creature that may capture or endanger humans, but it also infiltrates and arrests destructive forces. For these reasons, the forest-dwelling Akan peoples have great respect for sasabonsam and mmoatia.[31]

What of the "witches" and "wizards"? One of the most central ideas and objects of missionary furor was the notion of *bayi(e)*. Often caricaturized as "witchcraft," bayi is best described as an undetermined power shaped by a user's intent, producing a constructive or adverse outcome that users and recipients view differently. Cases involving bayi (called *abayisɛm*) are infamous and long-standing. Although chronicled since the sixteenth century and habitually through Christian optics, bayi may have little to do with our

Cartesian grasp of "witchcraft" and all that this term—no pun intended—conjures. The concept of bayi takes its ideational root from the utterance *ɛbɛyɛ yie* ("it will be all right"), spoken while one optimistically seeks out the *ɔbayifoɔ* ("one who deploys bayi"), but it might also originate from the "unnatural" removal (death) of a child of the matriclan, where bayi notoriously inflicts the most havoc. Bayi, like the mmoatia or even sasabonsam, is a neutral power, recourse, or means through which individuals serve their communities or fracture them. There are lawyers who represent unequivocal murderers, rapists, and corporate criminals and unleash into society rather than help imprison these socially destructive individuals. Conversely, there exist lawyers who work for the public good and with dense caseloads to free the wrongfully convicted and political prisoners, or to fight against the malignant forces of injustice. Both types of attorney matriculate through the same educational requirements, pass the bar exam, and practice in court systems governed by the same laws. Spiritualist-healers like Kofi Dɔnkɔ are lawyers of a sort in the sense that in each instance a healer works with the tools of their vocation and they balance the weight of their competencies and what clients want against the public good.

Although ɔbayifoɔ (pl. abayifoɔ) is a gender-neutral category, it is usually reserved for female practitioners, whereas their male counterparts are called *abayi-bonsam*. In Takyiman, female abayifoɔ typically outnumber the male abayi-bonsam; the matriclan (*abusua*) is her habitat, goes the popular view, where she does the most harm among her "blood" relatives.[32] For matrilineally structured societies where inheritance, succession, and identity flow through the mother's lineage, the potentially antisocial force of bayi is most potent in the hands of female clan members because only they can be mothers who confer (clan) identity, decide inheritance, and authenticate family and community leadership. Conversely, the abayifoɔ are powerless outside of their own clan, although their desire to feed on blood—the metaphysical and relational connective tissue of the matriclan—makes bayi an ambivalent force because it could potentially destroy the very family structure that sustains it.[33] One may never know the identity of an ɔbayifoɔ—even the abayifoɔ themselves. Healers have long argued that *bayie* is imbued with a capacity for constructive ends, but intentionality shapes bayi into a destructive force.[34] Freedom from the consuming powers of bayi, however, may come by way of confession: if abayifoɔ confesses their deeds, they typically do so when caught by one of several "ɔbayifoɔ-catching" spiritual forces called *ɔbosombrafoɔ* (pl. *abosommerafoɔ*).[35] After warnings fail to elicit a confession or if the ɔbayifoɔ refuses to confess, they may be ostracized as an outcast and banished to the outskirts of town or to another town of similar individuals, or spiritually "killed" by the ɔbosombrafoɔ. Ultimately, the origins or uses of bayi (d)evolve into complex claims centered around social inclusion or exclusion.

※

THE SECOND STANZA of Kofi Dɔnkɔ's libation picks up where the first ended, requesting protection and "careful guidance" for the graduate student against the covetous and slanderous. In his aged and shifting voice, tenor to soprano, Kofi Dɔnkɔ uttered:[36]

> That will in [the] future enable his descendants to realize the sort of historical events which he came to study from the Techiman state.
> That will also let them know clearly how we go about things in our own way in this part of the world.
> I pray you to guide and protect him against a tempter, a covetous person and a slanderer.
> Anybody who wishes his downfall and does not want him to return to America in success must be given a most bitter punishment by you.
> Give him careful guidance so that he may come back again to meet Kofi Donkor and his sister as well as his followers in good health—that is all that we are asking for.
> Do not permit any misfortune to occur.
> Take this drink and destroy any person who wishes our downfall.

Through his grandfather and a cast of spiritual forces, Kofi Dɔnkɔ's concern about posterity, for his community and the reputations of himself and his elder sister, went beyond the foreign student. The healer contemplated a future in which generations of foreigners—coded as the student's descendants—would know, if not grasp, a society where history, culture, and spirituality were tightly braided; this goes some way toward explaining why Kofi Dɔnkɔ emphasized "how we go about things in our own way in this part of the world." And to ensure this, in the same way he petitioned for protection, he made a case for the student's success and his extended family's good health while deflecting misfortune and seeking ruin for the forces of destruction. To destroy destruction is bold, but perhaps the healer was emboldened by his ability to temper, even work in his favor, human and immaterial forces ranging from negligible powers to cosmic forces. The next stanza takes up these wide-angled, spiritual forces located in nature.

The first two stanzas were prefatory but important material. In some ways, after these stanzas the petition seems elevated to a larger, more powerful court of appeal, where most healers and townspeople view these spiritual forces as "parcels" of a cosmic life force. Christians, Muslims, and the graduate student's interpreter call this force "God," but there might be significant differences between the "God" idea and conceptions Kofi Dɔnkɔ had in mind, especially in view of the third stanza. Kofi Dɔnkɔ continued:

> Oh Almighty God, take this drink.
> Earth [Asase Yaa], take this drink.
> Kranka Afua, here is drink.
> Mirikisi, come and take drink.
> Boɔmuhene, take drink.
> It is just a while ago that I came and rendered thanks to you and returned to this place.
> When I returned here, I met good news at home; I must therefore give you something to eat.
> I am very thankful to you for guiding me safely to this place; please permit no evil to befall us.
> Any enemy of mine who wishes my downfall must be handed over to Kune by you for punishment.

What are we to make of this "Almighty God," Earth, and the spiritual forces that headline stanza 3? There is an order to this list, a sort of hierarchy of powers organized by the principle of seniority.

Rattray was "convinced that the conception, in the Ashanti mind, of a Supreme Being has nothing whatever to do with missionary influence, nor is it to be ascribed to contact with Christians or even, I believe, with Mohammedans [i.e., Muslims]."[37] In this "Supreme Being" Rattray saw "one great God" akin to "Jehovah of the Israelites," a masculine and remote figure who "delegated His powers to His lieutenants, the *abosom*."[38] Through Rattray's "one God" hypothesis the "Sky God" interpolation of *Onyame* was born, a caricature enjoying an absurd afterlife in recent scholarship.[39] Like Rattray, the BM began collecting large tracts of ethnographic material soon after they established themselves in Akuapem. Among them stories of God, of creation, and about the origin of the abosom took priority. In one story missionaries were informed by their Akuapem hosts, "When God created the world he first created a woman ... [and then] a man. ... he started with it on Saturday and created until Friday all things. But on Saturday he did not create anything. First he created the human beings and brought them into the world ... then he created trees and stones and all other things." Having completed "the act of creating he appointed the fetish [i.e., abosom] as his interpreter and representative on earth. Thus the creation was complete."[40] In the same way Kofi Dɔnkɔ began his third stanza, so too did another early twentieth-century healer utter, "Unique great Onyame, who does not waver! Earth, born on Thursday, receive the palm wine! Tanno, receive the palm wine!"[41] Certainly the synergy between the creation story and the healers' libations would suggest a hierarchy of spiritual forces, at least after the earth and Onyame.

But who or what was this "Almighty" force called Onyame? The answer may lie in confusion. In one instance, as Basel missionaries understood it, "God sent Ɔdomankama and Bɔrebɔre with the mission to create the entire world," but in another instance in the same report "God" is "Nyankopon" and "Odomankama."[42] How could "God" have created, yet simultaneously dispatched other beings to engineer the same creation? How could the "one great God" of Rattray and the BM's "creating god Onyame" be also Nyankopon, Odomankama, and Bɔrebɔre?[43] Fortunately, that group of healers interviewed by the BM teacher Owusu have something to say about this confusion. Bear in mind, the "utterances of [the] priest," or the healers' ideas, have been filtered through a gender-neutral Akan/Twi language to the gender-specific German language and on to English, making the translations of nouns, pronouns, and some verbs understandably suspect.[44]

When Owusu asked, "What do you know about God, the creator?" They responded, "We know that Onyankopong exists. We know him, that it is him who made heaven and earth and everything." Owusu followed up, "How do you pray to him?" The healers responded, "We have no particular time in which we would only worship him. But when we go to our fetishes we call him first because we know 'he is the elder'—ruler." As is the case in society, hierarchies of settlements, custodianship of land, power, and authority rested on seniority. When asked, "How do you serve him?" the healers replied as before, but added, "But when we go to our fetishes then we worship him first and give him food, before we bring it to the fetishes." The questions about "God" then hit a climax. Owusu asked, "What names of honor do you give to God?" The healers replied, "We call him Onyankopong Kwame—The great gleaming one, who is born on Saturday." If creation commenced on a Saturday, it bears to reason that this day would be associated with a creative force. The healers continued naming the characteristics of this indeterminate force: "Borebore, Oboadee! The creator who has made everything," "Totrobosu ama su ama wia! The creator of rain and sunshine," "Odomankoma Anase Kokroko—The one who overshadows everything," and "Tweduapong! Lean against the tree, it does not waver."[45] These honorifics point to a more compelling explanation for who or what was this Onyame. Bɔrebɔre Bɔadeɛ translates to "the creator of all things"; *Tobrobonsu*, "the one who causes plentiful rains"; *Amosu*, "the giver of rain"; *Amowia*, "the giver of sunlight"; *Odomankoma*, "the benefactor of multitudes"; *Ananse Kokroko*, "the great spider"; and *Tweduapɔn*, "the tree which when leaned against does not break."[46] What, therefore, stands as significant is not the dominance of an "animist worldview" concluded by the BM nor Rattray's "one great God," but something more developed and that could not be so easily dismissed as "primitive."[47]

In a BM report entitled "Names for God of the Twi Blacks of the Gold Coast," written around the 1920s, the Akan/Twi-speaking peoples in dialogue with the missionaries listed the following honorifics or praise names (*mmraneɛ*): "The dazzling one, the splendorous one; the manifold one, the super-rich one; counselor; creator; great friend; satisfier; giver of water; bringer of light, giver of sun; giver of rain; the Almighty; if one leans against a tree (then it does not break) . . . ; when one looks at him, one becomes alive!; the one who extends himself over the town; protector of nations; immortal one; and the one who remains eternally."[48] These descriptions adhere very closely to those given by the healers interviewed, strongly suggesting that those ideas had wide circulation and broad resonance. Although it might be tempting to dismiss this cultural salience, a closer look at British colonial rule at the turn of the twentieth century reveals, according to colonial reports, the "very slight advance of Christianity in the Colony during the past ten years, the mass of people still retaining fetish worship. . . . In Ashanti, Christianity has made no headway."[49] Writing during the same period the BM, as the missionary society with the greatest reach and having recently established a mission station in Asante, had to concede, "The missionary never needs to particularly prove the uniqueness of God the creator, it is considered a known factor."[50]

From a purely cultural perspective, two working conclusions can be drawn about a multidimensional creative force and its atomization into multitudes of spiritual "representatives." In the first place, the futility of the "one God" hypothesis seems obvious and trite in light of a multifarious and unfixed creative force. Rather than names that define in unilateral ways, honorific and adjectival phrases spell out how indigenes perceived that force. In turn cultural-cum-ritual practices built around spiritual forces accessible through nature—and thus what was created—made the experience of positively and negatively charged forces possible. Second, if we are to believe that once "God was finished with the creation of the world, he brought the fetishes to earth so that they would be his representatives and judges," then the abosom, "a name for that which one otherwise calls a fetish," is no less a representation of real and historicized forces than the world and everything else created in it.[51] Organic materials of the earth—soil, plants, animal parts, gold, clay from rivers, and so on—formed the canvas from which shrines were wrought as technologies for engaging the abosom, such as a clay or brass vessel (*ayawa*), a clay pot or earthenware vessel (*kukuo*), or a cluster of medicines formed around a wooden club (*akonti*). In this world of coexistence, healers lived and worked in partnership, using all available tools, including most conspicuously abosom, a reference to that which is precious, is valuable, or serves an unlimited purpose. To be sure, the term *abosom* takes its ideational starting point from "the Twi word *sombo*, 'something of value.' The [abosom] were heavy and people valued them highly."[52]

Cognizant of this world order, Kofi Dɔnkɔ poured a libation charged with words delivered to an "Almighty," the earth, and then to abosom named Kranka Afua, Mirikisi, and Boɔmuhene.[53] As the creative force is infinite in its manifestations, so too are the abosom in their reproduction, classified by their source or point of origin and the day they revealed themselves.[54] It would seem, then, that the creative force revealed itself on Saturday (Onyankopɔn Kwame), the earth on Thursday (Asase Yaa), and the two thus considered in conjugal terms, in that "the Earth is invoked always after God and also before the fetish because she is ... God's wife, who produces everything that God desires."[55] Revealed on Friday at the town of Kranka, some four miles east of Tanɔboase, where Taa Kora resides (figure 1.2), Kranka Afua is also referenced as "wife" to Taa Kora, the "father" of all Tanɔ River or water-derived abosom. In both cases "wife" and "father" stand for specific relationships and for seniority among masculine and feminine understandings of spiritual forces. Indeed the interwoven world of spirits and humans, life and afterlife, parallel each other: "The condition after death," the group of healers declared, "will be the same in which you were when you died.... As you were here, you will be there."[56]

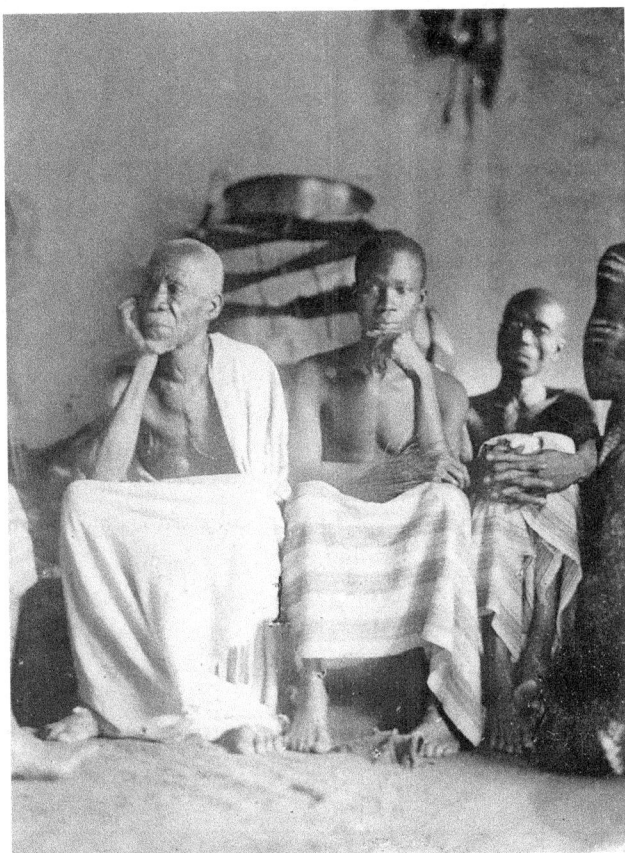

FIGURE 1.2. The shrine and altar of Taa Kora. Photographed by Robert Sutherland Rattray, ca. 1923 (MS 445), © Royal Anthropological Institute, London, 300.445–03–080. Used with permission.

THE FOURTH STANZA flows naturally from the preceding one, focusing almost exclusively on Taa Kora and its "children" diffused across Takyiman and a region wider than the present boundaries of Ghana. Kofi Dɔnkɔ spoke once more:

> Oh Abanemhene, take some drink.
> Twumpuduo, take drink.
> Taa Koraa, take drink.
> Abanem Tano, come and get drink.
> Agyentoa the hunter, come and get drink.
> I pray for your benevolence.
> It is stated that no one should seek for an equal partner before he
>   plays with him.
> What we most tenderly desire is to become one people with the
>   whitemen.

Libation 31

Both the blackmen and whitemen have same type of blood and we
should therefore unite and become one people.
They should also show us all their good habits and we should also
show them ours.
Anybody who wants our friendship and unity to be strained should
be destroyed by you.

During Rattray's research in northern Asante, perhaps the Takyiman region, he came upon a "popular myth" that he believed formed "the very basis of Ashanti theological beliefs."[57] The story recounts how multifarious Onyame or Onyankopɔn had various "children" who were sent "to the earth in order that they might receive benefits from, and confer them upon, mankind. All these [children] bore the names of water are now rivers or lakes: Tano (the great river of that name), Bosomtwe (the great lake near Coomassie), Bea (a river), Opo (the sea) ... and every other river or water of any importance."[58] Whether still or running, "waters in Ashanti ... are all looked upon as containing the power or spirit of the divine Creator, and thus as being a great life-giving force."[59] It was no hyperbolic view that Rattray considered the embodiment of the Tanɔ River, "Ta Kora, the greatest of the Ashanti [abosom] upon earth."[60]

As one of the first abosom created by Onyame, Taa Kora stands as a significant force for several reasons. First, there is an order to the aforementioned list of offspring. Taa Kora is the firstborn and eldest "child" of Onyame, electing to reveal itself at a cave in Tanɔboase, "Tanɔ [River] under the rock."[61] (Boɔtwerewa Kwaku guards the mouth of the Tanɔ River at the village of Traa; it the only indigenous ɔbosombrafoɔ and, like Taa Kora, "the senior of all *abosommerafoɔ*" in Takyiman) (figure 1.3).[62] The Tanɔ River emerges in Takyiman and makes its southerly way past Bosomtwe rock and lake, paralleling river Bea or Bia in present-day Ivory Coast before entering the Atlantic Ocean.[63] Second, from Tanɔ the river to Opo (*ɔbosompo*) the sea there exist thousands of Taa Kora's "children," discernable by the prefix *Ta* or *Taa* (a contraction of *Tanɔ*), such as multitudes of Taa Kofi or Taa Kwasi, but no reduplications for Taa Kora or its thirdborn offspring Taa Mensa Kwabena of Takyiman.[64] Third and most important, Kofi Dɔnkɔ's principal *ɔbosom*, Asubɔnten Kwabena, can be traced to Taa Kora. Among the Tanɔ abosom found in Taa Mensa Kwabena's shrine house (*bosomfie*) in 1922, Rattray also found Atiokosaa, "the mouthpiece [i.e., ɔkyeame] of the great Ta Kora," and "Asubonten."[65] Revealed to the founder of Tanɔso village, Nana Amea Ampromfi, Asubɔnten Kwabena was the first ɔbosom

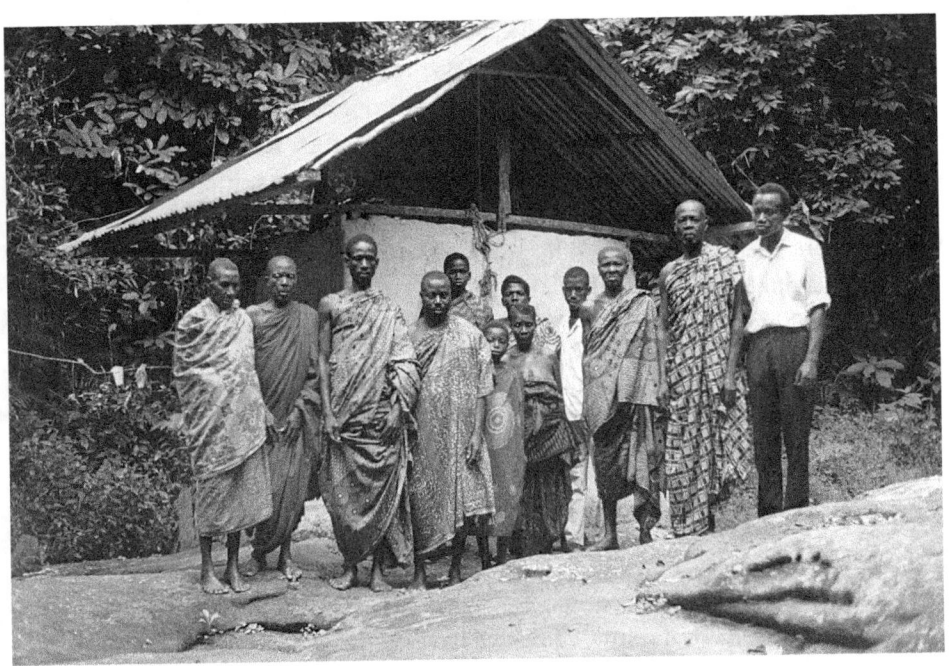

FIGURE 1.3. Bɔɔtwerewa's house by the mouth of the Tanɔ River, 9 September 1970. From the Dennis Michael Warren Slide Collection, Special Collections Department, University of Iowa Libraries. Used courtesy of Greg Prickman, Head of Special Collections.

harvested by Nana Ampromfi from the Tanɔ River, at a shallow crossing place where its permanent abode—a shrine platform—remains on the bank of the river. According to Rattray, Asubɔnten Kwabena was both "the father of the [ɔbosom] Ati Akosua" and a "son of Ta Kora."[66]

Of Taa Kora's progenies, (Bonse) Taa Kofi was the first, followed by Twumpuduo Kwadwo at the town of Tuobodom and then Taa Mensa Kwabena of Takyiman. Kofi Dɔnkɔ's fourth stanza begins with Abanemhene ("ruler inside the forbidden place"), a praise name for Taa Mensa Kwabena, state ɔbosom for Takyiman. Taa Mensa's authority counterintuitively superseded the ruler of the polity, the Takyimanhene, and reverence for it in Takyiman surpassed that for Taa Kora. This partly explains why Taa Mensa Kwabena is also called Taa Kɛseɛ ("Tanɔ [Mensa Kwabena] the great") and Abanem Tanɔ; *abanem* (der. *ban*, "fenced area or forbidden place") refers to an interior section of Takyiman where its physical shrine is kept. Invoking such powerful abosom therefore symbolizes a social contract between humans (spiritualist-healers among them) and the nonhuman forces or powers at work. Kofi Dɔnkɔ the healer made a case for benevolence, friendship, and unity but based on the "good habits" of all parties, including the spiritual forces called upon as witnesses and as consecrators of the occasion. In these instances one might ask, as BM teacher Owusu did, why propitiate—or better yet, engage—the abosom as (spiritual) partners in a social contract disposed toward community and life's challenges? The healers interviewed replied this way, and we might suspect their colleague Kofi Dɔnkɔ would have also: "We consider them as our masters, who protect our life and equip us with all we need."[67]

> Oh Tunsuo Kofi, take some drink.
> Bura Kofi, take some drink.
> Oh Buruku, take some drink.
> Adɔpe, here is drink.
> Oh Atia Digya, here is yours.
> Boo, here is drink.
> Nantee come and get drink.
> Oh our ancestral spirits, come and have drink.
> All of you, the three thousand three hundred and thirty traditional healers (herbalists), come and have drink.
> I pray for your benevolence.
> Finally, I pray [to] you!
> It is said that if a person comes to a place and meets disgrace, anybody who follows him is also equally disgraced; he even becomes disgraced forever as he is left behind.
> I further pray [to] you, this is to the health of this gentleman (the interpreter) who is accompanying him.
> Kindly guide and protect him.
> Wherever the whiteman will take him for any transaction, let his performance be attended with success and glory.
> Do not permit any misfortune to befall him. . . .

In this fifth and final stanza of his libation text, Kofi Dɔnkɔ summarizes his petition. In it he invokes benevolence, guidance, and protection—not to mention "success and glory" for the graduate student's interpreter—against the potentiality of disgrace and misfortune. He brings together all the previously named categories of spiritual forces but also includes some new cast members that show both geographical and chronological depth. While Nanteɛ resided at Tanɔso in Atiokosaa's shrine room and Boɔ was found in Bamiri, Offuman, Asueyi, and Taakofiano, Buruku Biakuru ("builder of towns") was an "old" ɔbosom and the first brought from the Amowi caves where the Bono people trace their ancestral origin. Out of the Amowi ancestral rock shelter, the Bono people settled centuries ago at Yɛfiri after leaving Pinehi, a settlement in present-day Nkoransa near the old grounds of Amowi and where Biakuru resides.[68] Although some stayed at Pinehi and even Yɛfiri, others proceeded on a southwesterly path to Manso, the capital of the Bono kingdom founded sometime during the thirteenth century, and within the Manso area to what became the village of Tanɔboase—site of Taa Kora. It is impossible to determine the "age" of Biakuru and Taa Kora or decide whether the "old" Biakuru revealed itself before or after the first "child" of Onyame. On the one hand, on its face the logic of Onyame's "children" and their birthing order excludes Biakuru; on the other hand, that logic might clarify early history in that Biakuru was known to the Bono people first, but as migrants they encountered Taa Kora at Tanɔboase, who revealed itself to be the "first" offspring of Onyame and by extension the eldest of all abosom, including Biakuru.

Both the closing of Kofi Dɔnkɔ's libation text and BM informants suggest a key distinction in antiquity, power, and authority drawn among these spiritual forces. In Kofi Dɔnkɔ's fifth stanza, the ancient Biakuru stands out against less prominent spiritual forces such as Tunsuo Kofi, Bura Kofi, and Adɔpe. Likewise, BM informants divided the abosom into two broad categories: *abosompɔn*, "great *abosom*," and *abosomma*, "children [of those great] *abosom*" (considered "lesser" spiritual forces).[69] While reminding us the abosom in general were "falsely so-called fetishes," those informants went on to say the abosompɔn were "primordial" spiritual forces "created with the universe and actually before other creatures. They therefore are the highest-ranking children of God, and therefore most similar to God in every way. They can live among the human beings where God sends them." That these abosompɔn were created with the universe underscores a crucial understanding about the sequence of creation and the interwoven texture of the world Bono peoples inhabited. Although we do not know exactly when or how Onyame was created, we can surmise that this multifarious creative force created the universe with the abosom, then the earth (world), women, men, plant life, rock formations, "all other things," and finally brought the abosom to earth and appointed them Onyame's "interpreter[s] and representative[s] on earth."[70]

In this schema of creation the abosompɔn are thought be "most similar to God in every way," and thus "they reside in the air, they are invisible, not tied to a place or a space, almost omniscient, constantly present and they are immortal. Without God's will they do neither good nor bad to the human beings, but they wait for His orders at all times. They favor most to take up their residence deep in the forest under large trees, in romantic regions, on rocky inclines and in caves." We have already seen how caves functioned as loci for Biakuru and Taa Kora, and how trees, the dense forest, and moving or still bodies of water do the same for other spiritual forces. Once these forces reveal themselves at a point or source of origin, that

> Location can no longer to be entered without that of a sacrifice offered.... Reasons for sacrifices are illnesses of individual persons, as well as general illnesses such as small pox and measles, persisting droughts, misfortunes befalling individual families as well as the entire land and infertility of women. In such and similar adversities the [abosompɔn]... are asked for recovery, rain, fertility and wealth, as well as victory over the enemies. When these petitions are answered the promised sacrifices are obligatorily offered, which however cannot be done by everybody, but only by the high priest [i.e., ɔbosomfoɔ] appointed for it.[71]

As the abosom were referenced as "interpreters" for Onyame, at another, more proximate level healers were also understood to be interpreters of the abosom. It is precisely in this sense that ɔbosomfoɔ Kofi Dɔnkɔ invoked "the three thousand three hundred and thirty traditional healers" and offered that they too "have [a] drink."

Of the many spirits—ancestral and otherwise—invoked in the closing stanza, none was more crucial than the reference to 3,330 past healers. This number is not meant to have literal meaning; instead it refers to an enormous multitude, in the sense that the number three has deep ritual significance and the number thirty means that which is sufficient. By casting attention on these ancestral healers, Kofi Dɔnkɔ was necessarily calling attention to himself and his vocation while drawing upon their cumulative wisdom and vantage point. In the same way he called on a range of spiritual forces, it seems logical to do so for past healers, who during their lifetimes occupied three distinct yet overlapping healing categories. Indeed, whether in a sparsely populated village or a sprawling town, an individual could readily find one of the three principal categories of healers. Although most families included competent adults and some older children conversant in a range of common ailments and their medicinal remedies, they often turned to healing specialists when those ailments persisted or reoccurred or perplexed local clinic and hospital staff in the early or mid-twentieth century.

From the early twentieth century onward, a handful of missionary societies in the tripartite colony dominated provisions for schooling, religious indoctrination, and health care through mission schools, a few seminaries, clinics, and later hospitals. Their monopoly on education, health, and religion was made possible by a hands-off colonial government policy, which provided grants that supported such mission schools. With this relative free rein, Basel and other missionaries targeted a categorical nemesis standing in the way of their proselytization and progress—the healers who were at once health care providers, bearers of cultural knowledge and traditions, spiritualists, marriage and naming ceremony officiants, therapists, advisors, and more. The missionary strategy was ideological, and the tool was disinformation to undermine such healers as dishonest and fraudulent, and to offer themselves as purveyors of the "true" God and the "right" ethics. What concerns us here is not so much the outcome of disinformation campaigns, though evangelization clearly had consequences, but rather what we can learn about these healers who stood in the bull's-eye of missionary crossfire from, ironically, missionary accounts that paid added attention to them.

Basel missionaries believed that "Each disease is according to the point of view of the Blacks caused by a superhuman power. The sick person therefore goes first to the Summani—magician, or Oduruyefo—medicine-man, as he is also called. That one heals with herbs and roots. He has in individual cases really good remedies."[72] This first member of a healing ensemble was the herbalist or *ɔdunsinni* (pl. *nnunsinfoɔ*; "one who works with parts of a tree"). The ɔdunsinni specialized in herbal medicines for diseases, leaving psychosomatic and other serious illnesses for the *akɔmfoɔ* and *abosomfoɔ*. Rather than divination or communication with an ɔbosom, these herbalists created instead *asuman* ("talismans"), earning the name "Summani" (*suman* person) and the reputation of *aduroyɛfoɔ* ("one who makes medicine").[73] Although some used asuman for malicious purposes—on their own or at the behest of a client—most herbalists operated out of their homes and served their community with "really good remedies." In cases where their "remedy does not work," Basel missionaries reasoned, "a witch is at play, who caused the disease and one calls now the Bosam-komfo [i.e., ɔkɔmfoɔ]. That one looks for the witch who caused the disease and kills her and thus the sick person becomes healthy again."[74]

Unlike the herbalist who might harm through his patented asuman, the ɔkɔmfoɔ was morally forbidden by their ɔbosom from such acts, except for "witches" to be handled by an abosommerafoɔ.[75] The BM had conflicting accounts of the ɔkɔmfoɔ ("one who does akɔm"). On the one hand, the "ɔkomfo (prophet) is wise and stands in exact contact with the fetish-world," but on the other hand, the akɔmfoɔ were "private persons," "either owners of a fetish or rather those talented with the gift of soothsaying, man or woman," and usually traveling, "morally imperfect, true deceivers." They were further described as "magic healers . . . often summoned from far away and taken into service by a village or a family for some specific purpose," being "their own bosses" and leading "a wild and boisterous life!"[76] Certainly mobile, enterprising, and skilled in the arts of divination and medicine, most akɔmfoɔ served their communities rather than their self-interests.[77] The root of ɔkɔmfoɔ is -kɔm, a concept denoting "hunger" (ɔkɔm) and connoting "making revelations" or "prophesizing" (nkɔm) in the sense that hunger created through fasting and mediation prepared the ɔkɔmfoɔ to be satiated by a spiritual force. Through that spiritual force, "revelations" and healing for the public good were dispensed.[78]

The BM considered the akɔmfoɔ and asɔfoɔ the "immediate servants" of the abosom, the asɔfoɔ in Akuapem being equivalent to the ɔbosomfoɔ in Takyiman. Though appropriated by Christian sects to mean "pastor," the term ɔsɔfo (pl. asɔfoɔ) undoubtedly predates Christian missions on the Gold Coast/Ghana, and likewise its meanings have a local provenance. Basel missionaries wrote, "ɔsɔfo means worshipper, caretaker . . . derived from sɔre [meaning] to treat with care . . . [and] to venerate through words and actions." The ɔsɔfoɔ/ɔbosomfoɔ was further an advocate for those seeking protection, supervisor of all activities concerning the abosom, and the highest-ranking healer with "the same prestige as the ruler of the land."[79] In fact, sharp contrasts were drawn between them and the akɔmfoɔ. Unlike the akɔmfoɔ, ɔsɔfoɔ/ɔbosomfoɔ did not prophesize and thus were considered to be "more venerable and not of such a deceitful type."[80] Moreover, as the "official person assigned to the sacrificial service and the necessary [spiritual] actions," and "chosen by the town, the village, or the family," the ɔsɔfoɔ/ɔbosomfoɔ were "respected people, as high in rank as the kings or the chieftains . . . [but they] act on behalf of their town and family for the common good."[81] The abosom under their custodianship belonged to their matriclan, not to the individual, as they worked for the "common good." In Akuapem and Takyiman, the abosomfoɔ were of high stature, so much so the authority of the ɔbosomfoɔ for Taa Mensa Kwabena surpassed that of the ruler of Takyiman. How authority took shape in this way is the story of the Bono kingdom, its capital of Bono-Manso, and its subsequent capital and independent polity of Takyiman. It is also a story of how communities arose around the sources of Tanɔ-based spiritual forces brought from nature into human culture, how specific matriclans assumed custodianship over those primordial forces for the public good, and how the ontological world outlined thus far became the social world of Takyiman. But Takyiman became home to Taa Kora and ɔbosomfoɔ Kofi Dɔnkɔ in different epochs and through its trailblazing founders, a hunter named Takyi Firi and his sister Afia Ankomaa.

❉

TAKYIMAN'S CHARTER FLOWS from orally preserved accounts about Takyi Firi and Afia Ankomaa, the centrality of Taa Kora, and the establishment of Tanɔboase. Bono histories concerned with temporal origins point unanimously to the Amowi caves inhabited in late antiquity. Ubiquitous references to ancient "holes in the ground" signaled caves and adjacent watering holes. Far from mythological, the mnemonic "holes in the ground" pointed to shelter and accessible water supply—the rudiments of human life. Amowi is thus memorialized as a temporary shelter: After emerging from a hole in the ground, Afia Ankomaa migrated with her siblings—Kokotipa, Amoa Sanka, Takyi Firi, and Amma Ako Ntoa—settling first at Nkwakuro ("town of life") near Yɛfiri. Kokotipa and Amoa Sanka died at Nkwakuro, leaving Afia Ankomaa, Amma Ako Ntoa, and Takyi Firi. Their migration was part of the larger movement of Bono peoples, seemingly orchestrated by their leader, Nana Asaman, after the collapse of the Amowi caves.[82] The migrants settled at Manso, some eleven miles north of the town that would bear Takyi Firi's name—Takyiman.

Manso became the capital of the Bono kingdom, where rivers and streams marked its eastern boundary in Kete Krakye, its southern limits in Mampɔn and Offinso, its western limits in Bonduku and Banda, and its northern limits near the Black Volta River and possibly Yendi. Nana Asaman ensured his people were strategically stationed at each of these cardinal points to secure the kingdom's frontiers. Following the paths and hunting grounds around Manso, Takyi Firi and his sisters found provisional shelter around the cave of Taa Kora, surrounded by dense forest.[83] Walking through the forest near Taa Kora's cave (figure 1.4), Afia Ankomaa went into spiritual communion or trance with the "spirit" of Taa Kora. As she reached their budding village, the spirit revealed itself and that it was designed for

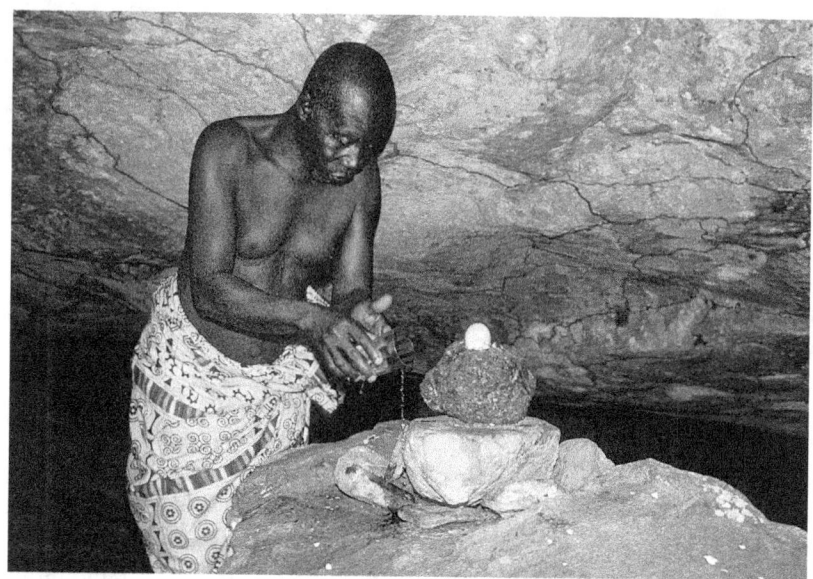

FIGURE 1.4. Tanɔboase Krontihene pouring libation for Taa Kora, 3 September 1970. From the Dennis Michael Warren Slide Collection, Special Collections Department, University of Iowa Libraries. Used courtesy of Greg Prickman, Head of Special Collections.

protection and peacekeeping—hence *Tanɔ a ɔkora adeɛ* ("Tanɔ that preserves a thing"). Over time, *Tanɔ a ɔkora adeɛ* simply became Taa Kora. Initially Takyi Firi became the settlement's male leader (*ɔhene*) and the ɔbosomfoɔ for Taa Kora, while Afia Ankomaa became the first ɔkɔmfoɔ for Taa Kora and the settlement's female leader (*ɔhemmaa*). Takyi Firi decided, at some unknowable point, to leave the settlement he constructed for his sisters in order to build a community around the presence and utility of Taa Kora. A sacred grove was also constructed in what became Tanɔboase. Takyi Firi then moved farther southwest to hunt for elephants in an area named Akyease, then on to a site that became Takyiman. The scenario of finding primordial spiritual forces and founding settlements around them reoccurred as often as the paths in the forest were crossed. It is thus not surprising that the abosom assumed pivotal roles in the development of villages and towns.

As Tanɔboase grew, Afia Ankomaa's son Fosu Aduanwoma became its leader. Upon their transition to *asamandoɔ*, Afia Ankomaa and Amma Ako Ntoa had their wooden stools—symbols of leadership—ritually "blackened" and stored in the bosomfie of Taa Kora, while the "blackened" stools for the immediate male heirs to Ankomaa were kept in the stool room of the founding family's residence (*ahemfie*).[84] The life of Afia Ankomaa's daughter Nsoaa Agyekuo or those of Amma Ako Ntoa's children remain unclear and poorly memorialized. While compelling oral sources tell us much about Takyi Firi the trailblazing hunter, unfortunately little about his own family exists either in memory or in the documentary sources. We know he belonged to the *ɛkoɔna* clan and that the village that blossomed into Takyiman ("Takyi's nation") developed out of the nucleus of his family.[85] After his death Takyi Firi moved from founder to foundational archetype: he became the masculine model of trailblazing leadership, embodying the overlapping identities of hunter, ɔbosomfoɔ, and sociopolitical leader. To be sure, the place of the hunter in community development became so central that the itchy body from hunters skillfully traversing the forest (*ne ho yɛ hene*, "his body is itchy") became the foremost expression of male political leadership (ɔhene) and the term for hunter (ɔbɔfoɔ) developed into a title—Takyi Firi is commemorated as Bofoɔ Takyi.[86]

One of the early rulers of Tuobodom, a town between Tanɔboase and Takyiman and home to Taa Kora's second offspring Twumpuduo Kwadwo (*twe mpini me*, "draw near me" [Tuesday-born]), was a skilled hunter who is credited with "discovering" Twumpuduo on a hunting expedition.[87] Other accounts credit Takyi Firi for finding Twumpuduo. Although the edge may go to Takyi Firi as custodian for Taa Kora, the important point is that the tripartite qualities defining male leadership in Bono societies was established during Takyi Firi's life—and afterlife—and often one person embodies them.[88] Likewise, the birth of the abosom into human society became coterminous with the establishment of villages and towns. This was true for villages such as Tanɔso, where settlements were literally built around spiritual forces and by extension the leader of the settlement was usually the ɔbosomfoɔ for its principal Tanɔ ɔbosom.[89]

Villages expanded into towns and towns became polities under more refined, but no less challenging, bureaucracies that remained attentive to the presence of Taa Kora's numerous offspring. These spiritual offspring flowed through the Takyiman polity and demarcated some of its most important villages and towns. Although Takyi Firi founded Takyiman, the oral histories for the town—and later the polity—indicate the ɔbosom Taa Mensa Kwabena revealed itself to ɔbosomfoɔ and ɔhene Ameyaw, one of the earliest rulers of Takyiman. Ameyaw belonged to the Adonten royal family, the custodian for Taa Mensa Kwabena. The symbol of Adonten leadership, its stool, is said to have originated from the Amowi caves, along with other stools represented by specific officeholder, such as the *atomfohene* ("head of blacksmiths"). This head of blacksmiths, most of whom resided in the Tunsuase quarter of town, was subordinated under ɔhene Ameyaw's ruling Adonten family and remains so today. How Taa Mensa Kwabena became the "national" ɔbosom of Takyiman remains a vexing question, but the abosom themselves plainly reveal Taa Mensa's place in the birthing order of the Tanɔ abosom, in the history of Takyiman and its residents, and in the very spatial organization of the polity. We have already seen how the Bono peoples migrated from Amowi in a southwesterly direction, building (transitory) settlements at Pinehi and Yɛfiri, Manso, and finally Tanɔboase. They brought with them from Amowi to Pinehi and Yɛfiri one of their oldest ɔbosom named Buruku Biakuru, the "builder of towns."[90] This builder of towns makes clear the immediate task in front of the cave-dwelling Bono. Biakuru remained at Pinehi near Amowi and perhaps at Yɛfiri under the Krontire family.[91]

Moving southwest, under the leadership of Takyi Firi and Afia Ankomaa, Taa Kora elected to reveal itself, and the village of Tanɔboase was born. The main road from Manso to Takyiman was marked with the offspring of Taa Kora in a sequence indicating when and where they chose to reveal themselves: Twumpuduo Kwadwo at Tuobodom, Taa Kofi at Taakofiano, and Taa Mensa Kwabena at Takyiman. Although Taa Kofi is referenced as the firstborn offspring, the area of Taakofiano is farther south than Tuobodom, casting doubt on the "firstborn" claim yet supporting the aforementioned order of self-revelation. Nevertheless, once the Bono kingdom collapsed in 1722–23, Takyiman became its successor polity, situated, as it were, between the southern edge of arid savanna terrains and the northern edge of dense forests, punctuated by hills and rivers. Takyiman replaced Manso as the new capital, with five cardinal roads crisscrossing the polity. Each of these roads were placed under the spiritual custodianship of specific Tanɔ abosom: Taa Kwasi for the Wenchi road (west); Taa Atoa, the Oforikrom and Nkoransa roads (east); Taa Kuntunu and Atiokosaa, the Kumase road (south); and Taa Kofi and Twimia, the Sunyani road (southwest) (map 1.1).

The fifth road, the Tamale road, stood under the custodianship of principal Tanɔ abosom located along it—Taa Kofi, Twumpuduo Kwadwo, and Taa Kora. These Tanɔ abosom oversaw these roads and all the abosom situated along them.[92] Over time and throughout the forest, the offspring of Taa Kora migrated and settled with their human hosts and custodians.

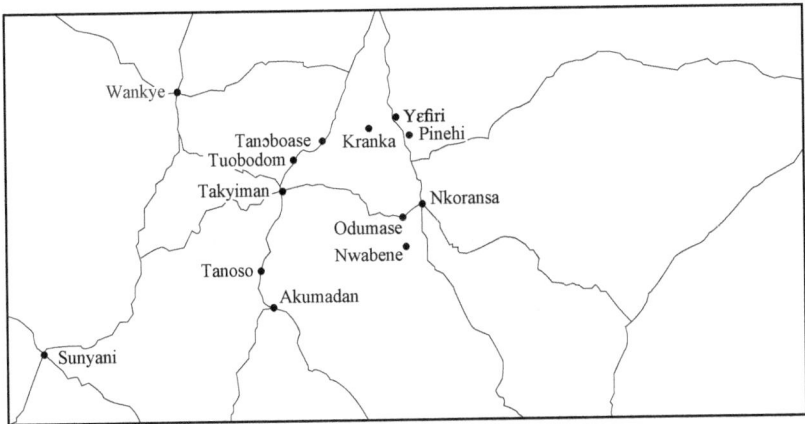

MAP 1.1. Map of the Takyiman region.

Because the Tanɔ abosom could reproduce without limit, forest and coastal settlements venerated, for instance, a multitude of Taa Kofi. As Thomas Kyei recalled of his childhood in Agogo, the welfare and health of the community was the concern of all, and the abosom were central to this. The oldest ɔbosom in Agogo was Taa Kofi.[93] Through Taa Kofi, most diseases and social discord were healed and the progress of the town, like so many populated by Tanɔ abosom, was calibrated by the partnership between these spiritual forces and their human hosts. With his own influential Tanɔ ɔbosom, Asubɔnten Kwabena, ɔbosomfoɔ Kofi Dɔnkɔ used that partnership for the "common good," constantly translating his ontological world into social practice and enabling his multifaceted culture to move through the history of his homelands.

CHAPTER 2. **HOMELANDS**

"In Search of Past Events"

The healer would rather see and hear and understand than have power over men. Most people would rather have power over men than see and hear.
—AYI KWEI ARMAH, *The Healers*

Toward the end of the nineteenth century, assistant colonial surgeon Richard A. Freeman described Takyiman as a region filled with "several considerable streams . . . beautiful little forest rivers meandering quietly among the trees, between high banks of crumbling sandstone thickly covered with soft velvety moss and delicate fern." Of those rivers, he noticed one "that rises near to Tekiman is the . . . [Tanɔ] river in a place called Boasi ('under the rock')."[1] Freeman's description of the Tanɔ River as "the most important of the streams of the Gold Coast" adhered very close to local understandings.[2] Freeman further described the area as one with "patches of forest that occurred alternating with orchard-like country," marked by red and yellow soil and with populous and numerous villages as he and his party marched south. South of Tanɔso, Freeman stopped at Akomadan on the Takyiman-Kumase road and observed "small parties of slaves bearing the wicker sacks and the bundles covered with green leaves in which the kola-nuts are packed for transport" through the commercial crossroads of Takyiman and on to the north.[3] Although defeated and in partial ruin, life continued to the extent its people could rebuild their lives under a twin hegemony—Asante and British rule. The Takyiman polity was literally caught in a historic and geographical middle. But how was Takyiman defeated (again) and what became of the polity? How did this twin hegemony shape its peoples, including a Bono identity crafted in opposition to Asante and a new cocoa regime run by colonists? If Nkoransa's treachery facilitated the first defeat of the Bono kingdom and thus Takyiman, how would a son of Nkoransa and Takyiman manage being born into two distinct ecologies, hegemonies, and citizenships, and among a defeated and ruined people? This chapter takes aim at these questions, extending the ontological and social world outlined in the previous one into the entangled histories of Takyiman, Nkoransa, Asante, and the British from the late nineteenth century to the birth and adolescence of Kofi Dɔnkɔ in the early twentieth century.

❈

THE CENTRAL GOLD Coast/Ghana region has been a crucial locus of Bono histories, besides their long-standing partnership with Taa Kora and its Tanɔ River offspring. At the crossroads of two predominant ecologies and cultural tapestries, the tropical forest in the south and savanna grasslands in the north, inhabitants of the Bono kingdom viewed their in-between position not as a restriction but as a recourse to the finest of both worlds. And as the colonial moniker for the broader region—"the Gold Coast"—implied, gold extraction, manufacture, and trade through these worlds made the kingdom prosperous. The kingdom and its capitals at Manso and then Takyiman had access to gold from the savanna Banda region and the northern reaches of the deciduous forest. Oral histories collected in the 1940s offer some perspectives on the place of gold in early societies and the limits placed on gold production and commerce owing to the sacred rivers and mountains that lined the Takyiman landscape. They suggest that gold in Takyiman was not exploited owing to the premium place on the Tanɔ and associated rivers as well as the sacred highlands in and around the town. Although some gold was procured from what would become Kofi Dɔnkɔ's natal town of Nkoransa, the main sources of gold were the Tain River and Banda region.[4] Free and captive individuals apparently extracted and washed gold throughout the year, although a prescribed division of labor meant only men excavated and only women washed. Discovered quantities of gold dust or nugget were then presented to the head treasurer on the sovereign's behalf; the gold was weighed and one-third went to the town's treasury and the remaining two-thirds to the prospectors. That two-thirds, however, was then divided: one-third went to the prospector's family head and two-thirds remained in the prospector's possession, which was now less than half of the original. This one-third system applied to natural resources (e.g., gold, cocoa, timber, or spiritual forces) found on land under the custodianship of a ruling family; unoccupied lands in Bono territories were also brought under this system through claims made by "founding" clans.

Restrictions, however, were placed on gold discovery and its uses. In cases where captive individuals discovered gold, they would give the gold to their holder, who in turn would provide them a small amount and keep the rest in trust until the captive needed it. Male captives with wives were given two-thirds "as the married slave was liable for taxes (a married man was responsible for his family and therefore had to be in full control of his money)." Prospecting for gold was prohibited on Fridays, "the day of Asase Afua ['earth which revealed itself on Friday']" and who was held to be "the 'mistress' of gold."[5] Once gold was brought to market, it was traded without restriction, and producers or merchants traveled to and exchanged their gold for goods in Kaniamase (now Buipe), Bona, Bonduku, Djenne, Timbuktu, and Gao. Caravans from some of these savanna trading centers visited Takyiman only in the dry season. In their transactions, elders recalled, "gold was weighed against Bodom beads. Later, people were given definite weights [*mmrammuo*, 'brass weights used in measuring gold dust currency'] which were officially tested. Common people would devise their own weights which could depict all kinds of things but had to be officially acknowledged."[6] Although Manso was situated closest to the cave and river of Tanɔ—the solid and liquid embodiments of Taa Kora—gold prospecting was deeply prohibited in and around this river. Indeed, defiling or killing fish described as decorated in gold in the Tanɔ River was forbidden, and transgressors received severe penalties.[7] Although Taa Kora's sanctions, counsel, and spiritual intervention might have been vital to the kingdom and its prosperity, oral sources indicate Bono elite abandoned such counsel and pursued their self-interest with impunity, foreshadowing the kingdom's collapse.

At the start of the eighteenth century, the Bono kingdom began to fracture through a series of succession disputes, the arrogance of the governing family, excessive taxation, and the immoral practices of Bono ruler

Ameyaw Kwakye (r. 1712–23).⁸ Of the many errors the kingdom's leadership committed, none was more fatal than these. An emboldened Asante confederation led by its ruler Opoku Ware (r. 1720–50) had empire on its mind, and an invasion of the Bono kingdom, made possible by the treachery of Baafo Pim, soon followed. Baafo Pim was a nephew of Opoku Ware and leader of a group of Asante refugees domiciled in the Bono town of Nkoransa; he apparently deceived Ameyaw Kwakye into declaring war against Asante.⁹ In the end Ameyaw Kwakye committed suicide in the forest after an Asante victory over his kingdom and its citizens—rituals at his gravesite are performed at midnight before the start of Takyiman's *Apoɔ* festival. Nonetheless, nine Bono villages were seized by Asante and placed under the jurisdiction of specific Kumase leaders to collect taxes, including spoils of war, on behalf of the Asante ruler.¹⁰ The villages in question included Tuobodom, Tanɔboase, Buoyem, Offuman, Nkyeraa, Braman, Nwoase, Subinso, and Tanɔso.¹¹ We have already seen how these villages were sacred sites of revered and powerful Tanɔ *abosom*. While a subjugated status compelled Takyiman to provide soldiers to fight on Asante's behalf against Gonja, Banda, Gyaman, and others in succeeding wars, Taa Kora at Tanɔboase and Taa Mensa Kwabena of Takyiman were also conscripted to facilitate Asante victories.

In the aftermath of defeat, followed by the destruction of Manso and its abandonment in the second half of the eighteenth century, Takyiman succeeded Manso as the new capital and commercial hub, and Nkoransa became an independent town. Baafo Pim was rewarded with the leadership of Nkoransa, which remained autonomous and Asante's most strident ally until it "revolted against Asante in 1892 . . . [and] its towns and villages [were] destroyed." Nkoransa was then "included within the [British] protectorate by treaty," as British imperialists fought with Asante as well as with French and German rivals to consolidate its colonial holdings while seeking to revive the north-south commerce diverted by the revolts against Asante.¹² Two Bono revolts stand out. In 1875 a group of provinces under the aegis of a Bono confederation seceded from Asante and remained an independent polity under the leadership *ɔbosomfoɔ* Kwasi Gyantrubi (r. 1875–94) until British and German acquisition in the mid-1890s. The confederation was a mutual defense pact against Asante attack—and one that Nkoransa, fearing Asante retribution, almost joined—but it also stood in the path of British and German colonization. By colonial necessity, Gyantrubi was executed in 1894 because his political power was irreconcilable with

European imperialism.[13] The other revolt originated from Takyiman. Takyiman, however, like Nkoransa, failed in its rebellion against Asante. Asante defeated Takyiman a second time in 1877.

Takyiman's defeat triggered a self-imposed exile for some 25 years, through which most of its townspeople and their male and female rulers Kwabena Fofie (r. 1864–86) and Kuruwaa (r. 1874–95) migrated to Gyaman in Ivory Coast.[14] Ironically, Gyaman's ruler Nana Agyeman welcomed these migrants after Takyiman had helped Asante defeat Gyaman on two previous occasions. Perhaps shared affinities as Bono people trumped their conscripted roles in fighting each other. Some families decided to stay in the demoralized Takyiman region, and this was true for about half of Kofi Dɔnkɔ's family.[15] How they fared is not quite clear, but colonial reports provide some perspective. In 1883 British officials described the "large town of Tekima or Tekiman ... [as] only represented by three ruined houses, and one in [the] course of construction. This town was partly destroyed, and partly fell into ruins after the flight of King Kwabina Fufia [Kwabena Fofie] and his people to Gaman [Gyaman], which occurred about eight years ago."[16] Rupert LaTrobe Lonsdale, special commissioner to Asante, Gyaman, and other locales, further reported, "In connexion with the claim by the Gaman King in this dispute, Kwabina Fufia, King of the Tekiman people, asks to be permitted to return to his country, and to remain there uninterferred [sic] by the Ashantis."[17] A return to Takyiman would have to wait until 1896.

While Takyiman laid in ruins and its exiles waited for an opportunity to return to their homeland, their Asante overlords were facing dissolution brought about by a British incursion in 1873–74, a protracted and bloody civil war (1884–88), a loss of key trade routes and markets, and power struggles—all while under increased British colonial pressure. British colonialism began on the Atlantic littoral by consolidating its own and acquired slaving forts; using commerce, Christianity, military aid, and treaties to ally with—and then subjugate—anti-Asante coastal and hinterland polities; incorporating those polities into the Gold Coast Colony in 1874; and then, under the pretense of commerce, offering treaties of "protection" to bring the savanna region within the colonial orbit. This colonial process would end with a fourth and final invasion of Asante in 1896. The seeds of Asante's demise, however, were sown in the 1874 Anglo-Asante war and the subsequent Treaty of Fomena. The treaty made provision for an independent Asante heartland but ceded conquered territories south of Asante to the British, who converted these "protected" territories into the Gold Coast

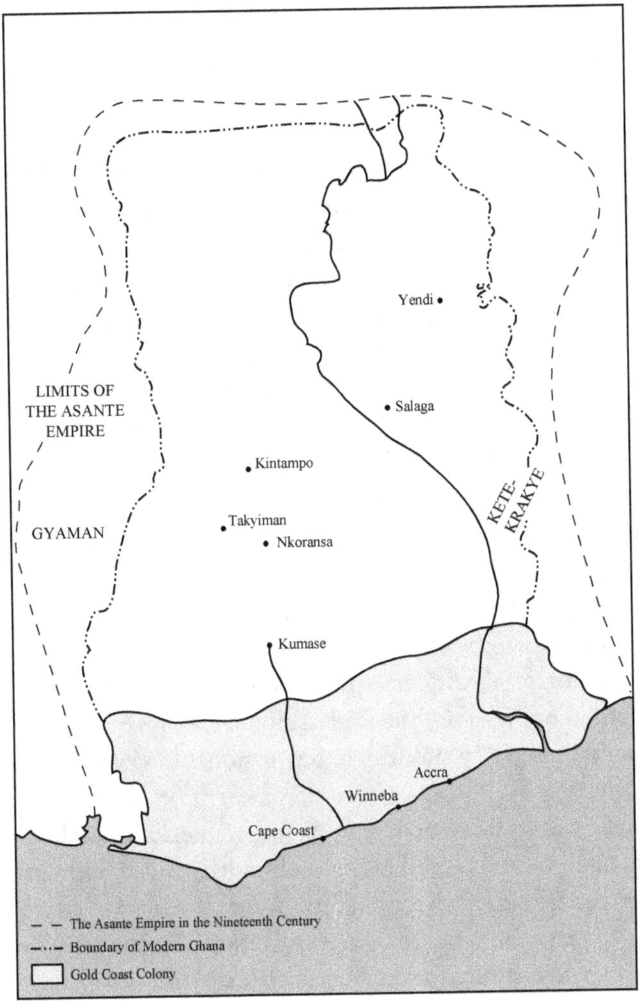

MAP 2.1. Map of Asante empire (Greater Asante).

Colony.[18] Soon the British signed treaties of protection with territories north of Asante to further destabilize it and to keep German and French rivals at bay. By severing the northern and southern portions of "Greater Asante," an empire larger in size than present-day Ghana, British imperialists simply reconfigured a region politically united under one empire (Asante) into the colonial territory under another (Britain) (map 2.1). The British strategically isolated the Asante heartland and helped to populate its capital with pro-British radicals who had exiled themselves to the Gold Coast Colony but returned to an Asante court headed by Agyeman Perempe. The

Homelands 49

radicals and conservatives clashed over the future of Asante. But during this turmoil and Asante's attempt to regain political stability under Perempe, the British entered Kumase unopposed and extended protection over it in 1896, exiling Perempe and many members of the Asante court.

Against these tidal transformations, Takyiman remained committed, almost counterintuitively, to its Tanɔ abosom. This commitment was made even more salient by the evolution of sociopolitical authority: the state *ɔbosom* Taa Mensa Kwabena wielded more authority than the Takyimanhene, which reflected a marriage between spiritual and temporal power on one hand, and how that power was diffused on the other, through foundational Tanɔ abosom. These Tanɔ abosom played no minor role in the earliest accounts of social organization and cultural innovation, and Taa Mensa Kwabena and Asubɔnten Kwabena were crucial in guiding the Bono peoples' departure from Takyiman in 1877 and their return in 1896. That year Takyimanhene Kwaku Gyako II (r. 1886–99) brought his people back from exile and opened a Methodist school in Takyiman—one of the few mission schools to open inland. The school failed and the first Methodist church in the Takyiman township collapsed. The timing of this missionary incursion and the return from exile corresponded to Asante capitulation to British rule in 1896, an opportunity the leadership of Takyiman exploited to return and rebuild their polity and which the missionaries saw as an opportunity to proselytize.

Whatever benefit was to be gained from Asante implosion was short-term and shortsighted, for in the end all the polities that sided with and against Asante surrendered their sovereignty to another (foreign) overlord. Be that as it may, to mark the return and reconstitution of its peoples, an annual Apoɔ festival was instituted at the behest of Taa Mensa Kwabena to publicly narrate and settle grievances, criticize leadership, and reaffirm Taa Mensa Kwabena and the Takyimanhene (figure 2.1). These ritualized exercises of holding leadership accountable hark back to the role elites played in the collapse of the Bono kingdom. Throughout the festival, therefore, normative laws were relaxed, farming and funerals were suspended, and insults were tolerated. Not surprisingly, the largest corpus of insult songs target Nkoransa and Asante, and Bono identity in Takyiman has been (re) defined in anti-Asante terms.[19]

Beyond the performance of retribution, neither the Apoɔ festival nor Taa Mensa Kwabena could relieve the memory and lived experiences of Asante hegemony—both of which weighed heavily on Takyiman's leadership. On 7 October 1896, Takyimanhene Kwaku Gyako II was summoned

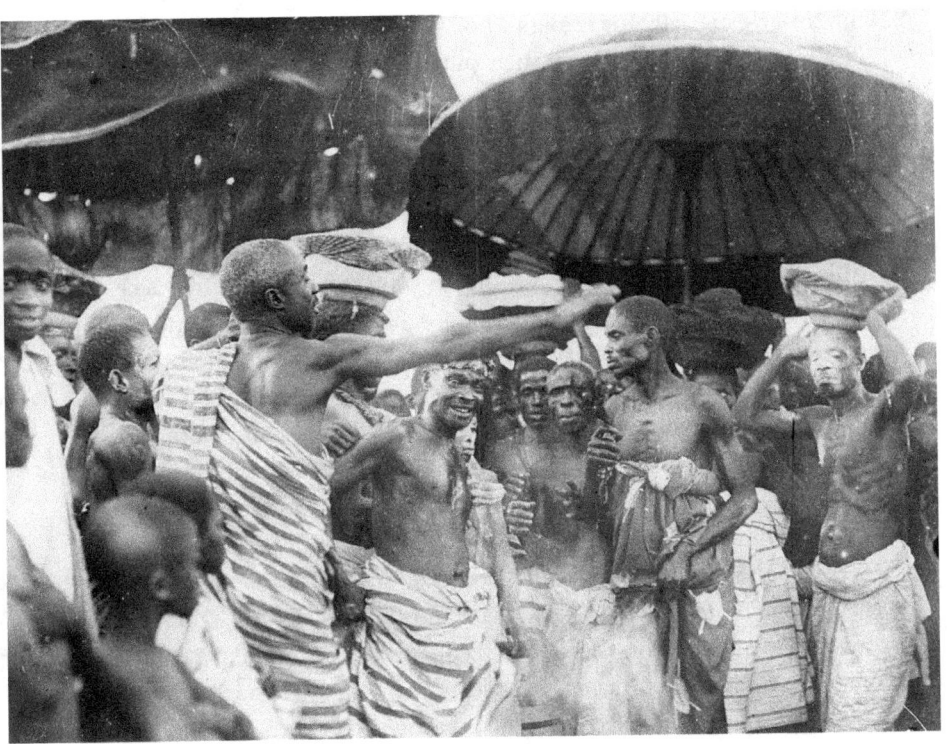

FIGURE 2.1. The Apoɔ festival at Tekiman. Photographed by Robert Sutherland Rattray, ca. 1923 (MS 445), © Royal Anthropological Institute, London, 300.445-03-056. Used with permission.

to Nkoransa to sign a treaty of protection with the British; Gyako II said he would do so in Kumase.[20] He was detained in Kumase until the British officer in charge, Captain Stewart, arrived. Meanwhile, Kwadwo Konkroma, the heir to Gyako II, "was appointed to look after the country in his absence." When Stewart arrived in Kumase, Gyako II expressed remorse for not heeding the directive. After a stern warning, Gyako II returned to Takyiman.[21] Less than a year later Stewart "entered into a treaty of protection with the King of Tekiman," Kwaku Gyako II, in Nkoransa. Stewart reported, "The King of Tekiman is an old man and is dying fast, so he was represented by his heir," Kwadwo Konkroma.[22] The "treaty of friendship and protection," executed 5 June 1897 on behalf of the British monarch and Kwaku Gyako II, "King of the country of Tekiman, and the Chiefs and principal headmen of that country," was a standard document used to align anti-Asante polities with British imperialist interests.[23] The articles of

Homelands 51

the treaty, especially for readers who are unfamiliar with these quasi-legal instruments, make clear that their purpose had little to do with "friendship" or "protection." The treaty precluded entering "any treaty with any other foreign power," precluded engaging in war with bordering groups "by which trade of the country shall be interrupted" or "the safety and property of the subjects" shall be endangered, and stipulated conflicts were to be arbitrated by the "Governor of the Gold Coast Colony" or "the nearest British authority." Furthermore, "British subjects shall have free access to all parts of Tekiman, and shall have the right to build houses and possess property according to the law in force in the Gold Coast Colony," and the Takyimanhene and officials shall "keep their main roads in good order, that they will encourage trade, and give facilities to traders."[24] In return for these crucial concessions the colonial government would "respect the habits and customs of the country, but will not permit human sacrifices; and slave dealing when brought to the notice of the Government will be punished according to the laws of the Gold Coast Colony."[25]

As the colony was "attracting the attention of capitalists," colonists immediately pounced on the valued recourses in Takyiman, particularly its rubber endowments during the rise of the British rubber industry.[26] In 1899 a proposed rubber concession agreement between Claude Beddington and colonial governor Frederic M. Hodgson to "forest lands producing rubber and as belong... to the Chief of Tekiman" failed to materialize.[27] This initial setback was an issue of protocol rather than hostility between the colonial apparatus and commercial interests. As a consequence Beddington was instructed by the Colonial Office in London, through Hodgson, to get "a grant of the land from the native owners in the *usual way*."[28] As the foundation for business the "usual way" and the rail lines transporting raw materials were being laid, the associated mining boom and the influx of migrant workers continued to disturb the ecologies tapped for capitalist exploitation. Futile attempts were made to enlist local people, through their village leaders, to seek out and destroy mosquito larvae in and around cities connected by rail and by new roads between Sekondi, Accra, and Kumase.[29] Indeed, railways between the coast and Kumase signaled the inroads made by the colonial administration, but also a necessary political stability required to establish mining and other capital-intensive industries. The rails transported mining equipment, gold, and other valuables to the coastal gold-producing areas in the west at Sekondi, and the cocoa-producing areas in the east at Accra.[30] The ports at Accra and Sekondi were the two most vital in the Gold Coast Colony, with the Gold Coast

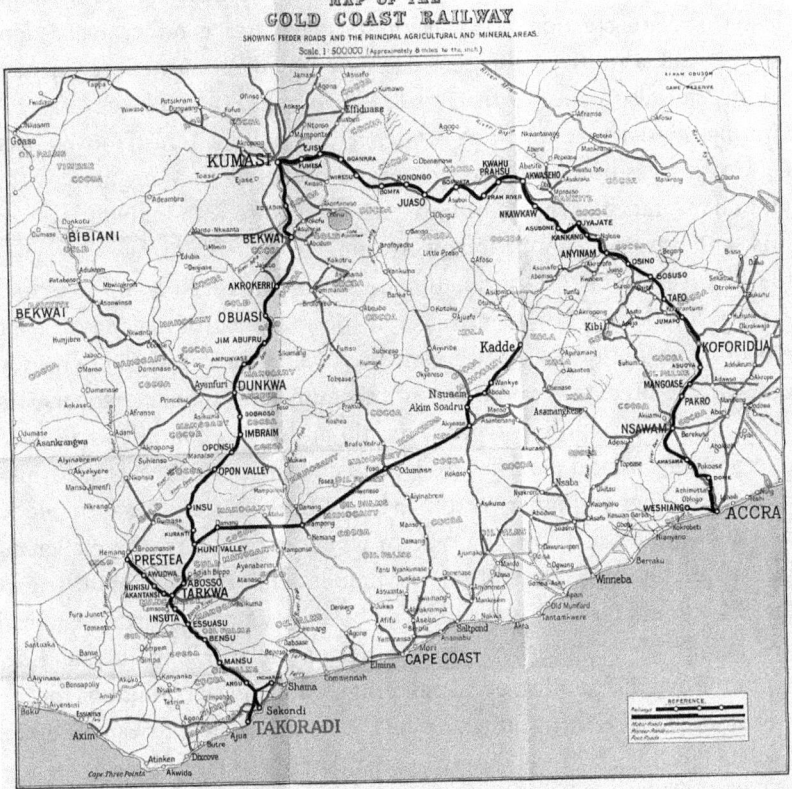

FIGURE 2.2. The Gold Coast Railway, showing feeder roads and the principal agriculture and mineral areas, March 1922. National Archives of the UK, Colonial Office 1069/42/89. Creative Commons.

railways headquartered at Sekondi and the colonial government at Accra (figure 2.2). Accompanying the entrenchment of the colonial government into existing political communities and ecologies were economic and environmental transformations tied to the very premise of colonization.

❧

AS THE NINETEENTH CENTURY ended, a broader look at the landgrabs and concessions made in Takyiman and throughout the tripartite colony reveals that natural resources were targeted and cocoa was becoming king. To be sure, mining for gold and other minerals, harvesting timber and rubber, and sequestering prime real estate were crucial, but in some ways they paled in comparison to the burgeoning cocoa industry. This partly explains the colonial government asserting control over this industry. The cocoa industry owed its creation or expansion to cocoa farmers rather than sedentary peasant farmers, yet this expansion generated not only unprecedented profits, but also parasites that caused serious health challenges. Cocoa-farming migrants, despite long residence in the dense forest, moved back and forth so as not to lose attachment to hometowns. Many merged the mutual insurance of the matrilineal Akan structure with individual enterprise and private accumulation by investing proceeds from one cocoa farm to purchase another.[31] Deforestation caused by the cocoa boom and commercial lumbering, however, triggered the spawning of malaria-carrying mosquitoes. The removal the forest canopy and the subsequent creation of favorable breeding conditions for mosquitoes made matters worse. In the central and southern regions humid and warm conditions allowed microorganisms and parasites to live outside their normal hosts, permitting mosquitoes and other vectors to breed freely. Malaria, a severe blood disease—the most dangerous type of which is caused by the malignant parasite *Plasmodium falciparum*—was holoendemic throughout the tripartite colony, and clearing forested lands for cocoa farming further enabled the major vector to thrive. High temperatures, relative humidity, and decent monthly distribution of rainfall provided the ideal conditions for the mosquitoes that transmit the parasite.[32] Europeans and Africans suffered and died from malaria, yellow fever, and other diseases endemic to the forest. The virulent outbreaks of yellow fever in 1895–96 are a case in point, making quite clear the intimate and shifting balance between transformations in society, its ecologies, and the public's body.[33]

The rise in industrial cocoa production led to sharp declines in palm oil and coffee production, but more importantly it occasioned one of the most crucial vicissitudes of late nineteenth- and twentieth-century societies. Thousands of farmers prospered, creating tremendous income gaps between them and the urban professionals on the one hand, and subsistence farmers and underemployed migrant laborers on the other.[34] The outward expansion of the cocoa industry from the Akuapem area initiated an unprecedented movement of farmers who sought new lands for cocoa trees. These lands-turned-cocoa regions hinged on tens of thousands of migrant laborers who came from the northern Gold Coast, Upper Volta (Burkina Faso), and elsewhere.[35] The sheer increase and popular use of the *abosommerafoɔ*, so-called witch-catching shrines, matched the upsurge in the cocoa cash crop, which itself brought heavy social tensions and the profits of which challenged the very social structure that provided security for its members.³⁶ Major socioeconomic changes often alter disease patterns within a society, and the expansion of the cocoa industry in the southern Gold Coast provided a stimulus for opening roads and clearing forestlands, which further widened the distribution of malaria.³⁷

Cocoa-generated industrialism, economic growth, and living standards ironically did not produce better health or living conditions. With urban growth came a decline in human health and quality of life; armed with higher incomes, African consumers did not choose more nutritious foods but rather (imported) white bread, sugar, tea, tinned milk, and other foodstuff of dubious value. Consumers now incorporated into the cash (crop) economy also chose to consult not the ancient Tanɔ abosom but the newly imported abosommerafoɔ. What stands as significant is the psychic shift from the peace and prosperity, and from the matrilineally anchored Tanɔ abosom, to the individually owned abosommerafoɔ "witch-catching" abosom and *asuman* originating from what Akan peoples and colonial officials viewed as "wild tribes" of the savanna in order to combat the chaos in their "ordered" societies.³⁸ More than a difference in ecology or cultural arrogance, this shift provided a mirror to the decisive and divergent development of the resource-impoverished northern region and the comparatively prosperous, urbanized southern portion of the Gold Coast/Ghana from the late nineteenth century onward.

By 1900, colonial economic activities created wage laborers and a "rural capitalism" through rubber, mining, timber, and foremost, cocoa production. Organized on a capitalist basis, peasant cocoa farmers cultivated the crop for themselves, for their families, and for sale and export. In so doing they hired laborers and became part of a circuit of producers, nonworking landholders, distribution agents, buyers, intermediaries, transport owners and employees, and porters.³⁹ With the success of cocoa on the world market, local cocoa farmers enjoyed higher prices and could pay a rapidly expanding migrant labor force, drawing labor away from the mines and transforming average farmers into employers imbued with an individualistic sense of success and self. All this commercial success, however, came at a price, and at a time of numerous shifts in early colonial society. First, the influx of migrant workers (viewed as cultural "strangers" or "temporary visitors") paralleled the cultural shift from leaving property to a sister's son—in line with matrilineal inheritance—to leaving it to the son of a characteristically male owner. Second, in the process communal ownership shifted to individual ownership and sale of land. Finally, the shift from Asante to British overlordship was signaled by the abortive Yaa Asantewaa war of 1900, which marked, symbolically and for all practical purposes, the last major resistance effort against British rule.[40]

In this way Asante or at least segments of Asante society implicated in the Yaa Asantewaa war represented the last line of sovereign Akan polities and the last of its empires. But that terminal point was unceremonious and its resistive posterchild, Yaa Asantewaa, was, in her own words, not the memorialized icon of rebelliousness against empire. In an letter dated 19 April 1900, dictated to the Basal Mission (BM) catechist J. Akyea during said war, Asantewaa declared, "I have never proposed to fight the Government and will never dare to do so, because it is for the kindness and refuge of the British Government I am living," ending the letter, "I shall continue to serve truly and will never break my agreement made with the British Government."[41] Apparently, through another letter, Asantewaa also requested Governor Hodgon's "protection against the Mampon and other kings who were trying to persuade her to join them against the British." Yaa Asantewaa was not alone, for there were "various Queen mothers who generally were on our side in hope, as for example 'she' of Nkoranza who saved the Brongs [Bono] country and was officially thanked by the Government for it at the end of hostilities."[42] Viewed through these letters, Asante was defeated and subjugated like Takyiman. However, Asante was still viewed with a mixture of awe and suspicion, and so, unlike polities easily seduced by commerce and Christianity, deliberations about the spread of European schooling and religions found little support at the highest level of Asante leadership. These debates, occurring all throughout the nineteenth century, preceded eventual submission to British rule.[43] Whereas the BM only established at mission station in Asante in 1896, a bevy of missionary-run schools, churches, and clinics would establish themselves more firmly in Asante and in the tripartite colony during the early twentieth century.

In the wake of the Yaa Asantewaa war, most of the literate and powerful African voices on the Gold Coast did not view with despair the loss of sovereignty and the inauguration of British colonialism, nor did they live in much anguish. In fact their literacy and perception of power came through their subordination to missionary and commercial institutions—the most important of which was the colonial administration. Those voices emerged principally from the coastal elites and their budding but comparatively small counterparts in Asante. They, like the British who undergirded their importance in the colonial hierarchy, viewed the Yaa Asantewaa war as a "rebellion" against, rather than a war of independence from, British rule. British colonial authorities rewarded these local elites as well as leaders north of Kumase for their nonsupport of Asante role in the war. The British captain D. Stewart wrote, "[the] King of Tekiman has remained loyal all through the rebellion, and kept his people from joining the Ashantis, though threatened several times with destruction if he did not join."[44] The "King of Tekiman" was listed, along with other so-called chiefs, in a table labeled "Rewards to Loyal Chiefs and Others, Ashanti Rising, 1900."[45] Takyimanhene Kwame Boakye was given £75 in cash and gifts of "velveteen, silks, and gold and silver fringes, value £25," for £100 total. On another list dated 28 January 1901, "Kwame Boatchi, King of Tekiman" was granted £50 and £25 in presents.[46] After the Northern Territories and the Crown Colony of Asante became formal colonial holdings in 1901, the Ashanti Administration Ordinance created four administrative districts in 1902, wherein Takyiman was brought under Asante's northwestern district (renamed the Western Province in 1906).[47] This effectively placed Takyiman's richness in cocoa and rubber under Asante overlordship and British colonial control.[48] Those gifts made to the Takyimanhene were intended not simply as reward, but as inducement to sign treaties and make concessions to foreign firms and capitalists well positioned in the global rubber and cocoa trade.

The extraction of rubber and the production of cocoa meant little for local consumption and use; these were integral colonial cash crops, exported raw commodities to be transformed into manufactured products. To get those natural resources from their sites of production to the urbanized port cities for exportation, railways and roadways had to be constructed for transporting goods and passengers by train, car, truck, and modified lorry. In the initial stages export industries and gold mining shaped rail and road construction as well as urban growth. Urbanization and the rampant exploitation of pristine forestlands had clear disease-related consequences, affecting most seriously the poor and children with inadequate nutrition, creating appalling health outcomes. In the new colonial economy, low wages and high food prices meant poor nutritional choices. Child mortality became the colony's most crucial health challenge: infants and toddlers were exposed to a range of infectious diseases—malaria, diarrheal diseases, measles, respiratory tract infections, and whooping cough—during the crucial period of six to eighteen months of age, when a child loses maternal antibodies against malaria and other diseases. Although a child develops antibodies through infections, infectious diseases such as measles or malaria thrive on a weak immune systems and poor nutritional regimens.

These children of the colonial Gold Coast would have experienced during weaning a vital loss of protein and other nutrients, further complicated by the replacement of the mother's milk with starchy gruels or tinned milk. The result was malnutrition and accompanying anemia due to malaria, hookworm, or simply poor diet. Malaria was endemic to the tropical forest and death from it was common during the first five years of life.[49] Beyond the suffering caused by malaria, the disease also crippled long-term economic growth and social capital by killing or disabling masses of people. Statistics for infant mortality caused by malaria were not recorded until 1914, and so we can only understand the number of people harmed or terminated by malaria—much less the human lives themselves—through understanding the efforts to combat a disease expanded by the colonial economy. We know malaria existed before the expansion of the cocoa economy; it had been prevalent for centuries. It is that malaria's geographical reach was increased by a cascading effect of various actions: disturbing forest environs, pulling thousands of laborers from the savanna into these ecosystems, and creating rails and roads in once undisturbed forests that now affected the humans, animals, and spiritual forces that depended on them.[50]

❈

IN THE FIRST DECADE of imperial rule the menace of malaria drove the colonial government to employ fifty-nine medical doctors to join the full-time medical officers at Odumase, Nkoransa, Mampong, Cape Coast, Sekondi, and in the colonial capital of Accra, where the government hospital was equipped with twenty-four beds in the "native ward" and seven beds for Europeans. The apartheid arrangement of the hospital and its delivery of health services flowed from the colonial government's belief in the efficacy of racial segregation as a means of preventing malaria.[51] Quarantine proved futile in the hospital and in the daily extraction of labor because malaria was born not in the hospital but in the agrarian fields where cocoa ruled. In April 1904 a district commissioner wrote, "agriculture in and around Techiman was very good, the country being plentiful in farms," and "the natives of that district were very friendly."[52] That same year cocoa pods were dispatched from Aburi to Asante and on to Takyiman farmers eager to enter the cocoa trade. As cocoa became the major cash crop grown mostly by men—though some women worked cocoa farms alongside them—the virgin forests some distance from the towns were not the only features of the Gold Coast landscape being disturbed.

In 1905–6, the district commissioner reported having difficulty getting markets created for the commerce in colonial crops and in the natural resources of Takyiman, reflecting the growing unimportance of "chiefs" in settling disputes, usually over land and labor. These so-called chiefs might have been exploited by the colonial administration, but they were not members of the club. The district commissioner, under whose administrative authority Takyiman fell, supported the "chiefs" but also subverted chieftaincy, disrupting hierarchies of power and community bonds and making those "chiefs" proxies or the most immediate faces of colonialism.[53] As two earthquakes in 1906 severely damaged many colonial buildings in Accra, seismic social tremors from religious movements devoted to the eradication of "witchcraft" rose to prominence in the Asante heartland. The first recorded wave of "witch-purging shrines," originating in 1906 in the northern savanna, was named Aberewa ("the old woman"), but the movement was suppressed two years later by a partnership between colonial authorities and local, Christianized "chiefs."[54] This would not be the last of these movements. In fact, successive religious movements and disease outbreaks—for example, plague in the colonial capital and commercial hub of Accra, epidemics of sleeping sickness (human African trypanosomiasis) around outstations in the Takyiman region—ran parallel to the socioeconomic transformations wrought by cocoa and colonial rule.[55]

A Sleeping Sickness Bureau of the Colonial Office was established in 1909, and the next year sleeping sickness epidemics broke out in areas nearby Takyiman—more precisely, Kintampo, Wankyi, and Sunyani. These outbreaks were certainly linked to cocoa cultivation and the global demand for it. In 1910 cocoa was the most valuable commodity in the colony, but unlike the Caribbean cocoa used in limited quantities for flavoring, the Gold Coast variety was used in greater quantities.[56] A decade later cocoa accounted for 83 percent of total exports, and it would be the only export to survive the collapse of world trade during the depression years of the 1930s. Many voiced concerns over the production of cocoa and the regulation of the cocoa trade, while local farmers complained of being cheated by buyers who used "compromised" scales to weigh and valuate the crop. But these debates about cocoa were dwarfed by some of the major consequences of large-scale cocoa cultivation. In 1910 and 1912 significant outbreaks of yellow fever and sleeping sickness took over a dozen lives in the colony, and many more were hospitalized.[57] Efforts to halt the spread of sleeping sickness in the Takyiman region stalled because of "the unfortunate invaliding of the Medical Officer at Sunyani," the regional capital.[58] Whereas yellow fever is transmitted by an infected mosquito, sleeping sickness is spread by the tsetse fly; both insects were prevalent in the tropical forest, and as more trees that provided a forest canopy were removed for farming or timber, direct sunlight hitting stagnant water provided near-perfect conditions for the proliferation of these vectors.

In the early twentieth-century Takyiman was a forested area with thick undergrowth in the south and open orchard forest to the north, where "belts of forests are met along the water-courses" and where "towns and villages are situated in small clearings in the forest and in the open country, generally near the forest belts and water-courses."[59] Mosquitoes and tsetse flies were rarely seen during the arid months of December to March, but the relatively few found in April would rapidly multiply and become troublesome in May and throughout the rainy season. Eyewitnesses reported that sleeping sickness followed "the main trade routes and traffic, and that residents becoming infected in these villages on the main roads act as reservoirs for disseminating the disease to susceptible persons in neighboring villages."[60] Horses procured from the northern savanna region "never last long in this Province." Northern migrant laborers fared much better, though, like the ubiquitous diseases, they were quarantined in living quarters called *zongos*, yet sought after for their "witch-catching shrines" and talismans against the insecurity (coded in the idiom of "witchcraft") triggered by the cocoa boom.[61]

Cocoa production had brought thousands of migrant laborers from the northern savanna, politically classified the Northern Territories. In 1912 Takyiman was reported to "have had their [supplies] of north country slaves" (i.e., captives or laborers originating in the north), adding to an estimated population of 7,016. Of 6,046 persons examined by colonial medicinal staff, twelve new cases of sleeping sickness were discovered in Takyiman, including its zongo area (der. Hausa: *zango*). Four additional cases were found in the town of Akomadan on the main Takyiman-Kumase road. The medical examiner, Dr. Kinghorn, noted, "Eight of the sixteen persons found are north country natives; two gave a history of north country slave ancestors. One was a native of Sierra Leone, who was also affected with leprosy, and five were natives of Tekiman." Dr. Kinghorn concluded,

> This increase in the number of affected people found in Tekiman is due, I believe, to the large zongo which is rapidly springing up in Tekiman situated 600 yards from Tekiman, and, consequently, the larger number of north country natives to be found in the division than heretofore. Herds of Gaman [Gyaman] cattle are a frequent sight in the Tekiman villages. Tsetse flies are found all over the division, palpalis

[i.e., the tsetse fly] in the neighborhood of the forest belts, therefore, near the towns and villages.... The division, like the others, has had its supply of north country slaves.[62]

The zongo settlements became notorious "strangers' quarters" of "principally north country people," and "as a rule these people live in zongos when not traveling; there are four such settlements in the Province ... situated on the main trade routes and in open country.... Around these zongos the residents make their farms." The Takyiman zongo was "situated in open country and surround by farms."[63]

According to the district commissioner's reports, the Takyimanhene (called the "head chief") and lower-ranking officials defined a "stranger" as "a native who is not by native customary law a member of the said [Takyiman] division, and who does not serve the Head Chief." Such strangers were required to pay an annual tribute to the Takyiman stool, which held custodianship rights over lands used for cocoa farming, that is, "the sum of one penny in respect of each cocoa tree bearing fruit on all land lying within the said division and farmed or occupying [sic] by him; the said payment to be payable on the first day of January in each year commencing with the first day of January next following the expiration of five years from the date of the planting of the cocoa tree." The colonial authorities decreed that any "stranger" farming or occupying land within the colonial division of Takyiman must pay the "head chief." Defaulted sums would be doubled in cases of nonpayment, wherein "Moneys due and payable under these bye-laws shall be recoverable by suit instituted in the Court."[64] The zongo population was estimated at 130, and the 3 cases of known sleeping sickness represented the kind of cultural groups that made the zongo their transient or permanent home: "one was a Hausa, one a Moshi [Mossi], and one a Sierra Leone native." Except for these confirmed cases, Takyiman's "open country" made it so that "tsetse flies [did] not appear to be so numerous," sparing the township some of the epidemiological harm brought on by successive waves of sleeping sickness.[65]

By 1912–13 the aforementioned disease, migration, and colonial administrative patterns were directly linked to sociopolitical and even ecological transformations around land ownership, authority, and concessions. Because concessions went through local leadership, the Native Jurisdiction Ordinance and Bill ensured that the judicial powers of local leaders remained relatively intact by incorporating them into the colonial administration through an "indirect rule" policy, but made it so that their authority derived from the British crown, not their ancestral custodianship of land. Town councils were established in Accra and Cape Coast, and efforts were under way to halt the individual ownership of the colony's public lands. The creation of "customary laws" and judiciaries; the subsequent advent of "native" lawyers and "chiefs" to arbitrate matters of land and labor; the competing interests of colonists, capitalists, and local proxies; and the missionary jurisdiction over belief, health care, and schooling all formed the sociopolitical world into which Kofi Dɔnkɔ was born. Indeed, a substitution in imperial rule—an African empire in Asante replaced by a European one in Britain—occurred at the abstract level of politics and regulations. On the ground and in the interior corridors of the peoples' lives, centuries of homegrown sociocultural development made it so that each local society interpreted these vicissitudes and their prospects vis-à-vis colonialism in different ways. This broader, emergent colonial context, foregrounded by centuries of specific histories and cultural norms molded in the Takyiman region, formed a more proximate temporal and spiritual milieu for Kofi Dɔnkɔ. Perhaps no other time and place were more favorable for the birth of a healer.

❈

KOFI DƆNKƆ'S PATH AS a healer was carved out in the very circumstances of his birth. All accounts of his early life are unanimous on these circumstances, though the finer details are circumstantial, deduced from a combination of oral and archival print sources. After his two elder sisters were born, the next five children died during infancy. This successive and painful turn of events troubled his parents Yaw Badu (Kwao) and Akosua Toa. While Akosua Toa was pregnant with Kofi Dɔnkɔ, she and her husband consulted the family ɔbosom, Asubɔnten Kwabena, in Yaw's natal town of Nkoransa, hoping a spiritual intervention would ensure the eighth child's safe passage. Both parents made several ritual sacrifices and probably were provided "staying" medicine to help their child survive. Around 1913 Yaw Badu and Akosua Toa welcomed the birth of Kofi Sakyi (paternal name). Popularly remembered as Kofi Dɔnkɔ, the newborn entered the world through the matrilineal Aduana clan and through the spiritual intervention of the family ɔbosom.[66]

As soon as Kofi Dɔnkɔ was born, he was taken to Asubɔnten Kwabena to petition for what would be Kofi Dɔnkɔ's temporal life. Appropriate rituals were performed and spiritually charged objects (*asuman*) were placed on his body to safeguard his life. A large variety of asuman were carefully placed at his joints and on his extremities. A special fiber from the *bofo* plant was used in preparation of some asuman. These asuman affixed to Kofi Dɔnkɔ made it difficult for malicious forces—human or otherwise—to harm him. These assortment of asuman would remain on Kofi Dɔnkɔ for two and a half years or until they simply deteriorated. It was in this ritual context he received the name Dɔnkɔ (ɔdɔnkɔ, "love does not go"), which followed the practice of providing a derogatory name to a child who survived immediately after the death of preceding infant siblings.[67] The praise name (*mmrane*) for those given the name Dɔnkɔ was *bagyina*. If these names indicated a "special" child, they were ascribed during a common birthing and naming ceremony, observed by Basel missionaries and distilled by the recollections of kin and community folk who knew Kofi Dɔnkɔ.

Kofi Dɔnkɔ was both *abagyina ba* ("come-and-stay child") and *ɔbosom ba* ("child of an ɔbosom").[68] Protection given by and a temporal life made possible through an ɔbosom meant Kofi Dɔnkɔ was distinguished by the *mpɛsɛmpɛsɛ* hairstyle he wore and the ritual ceremonies he underwent before elders could cut off this hair at an older age. After Akosua gave birth to each child, her succeeding pregnancies would have occurred in two-year intervals; she would have abstained from sexual intercourse for at least six months after the first child and at least forty-two days after each subsequent child.[69] Viewed from this perspective and considering the premature deaths of Akosua's children, Kofi Dɔnkɔ's birth provided some consolation to those grieving the children who passed during infancy, in addition to the one-week Faa ceremony performed for the first death among children born to the same parents.

If any of those siblings were a year or so old when they transitioned, each would have been buried in the town cemetery or in a small box without ceremony. Those who transitioned during infancy were wrapped in cloth and buried perfunctorily in the forest by an elder. Basel missionaries observed that one might also wrap "the infant into cut grass and bur[y] it in the garbage dump outside of the town," which, the reasoning went, "in such a case the spirit mother [of the child] had perhaps gone on a journey and ... had sent it to earth for the time being and had called it back after her return." Indeed, the belief "that when a child is born here, a mother mourns a child in the realm of the spirits" reinforces the "great disgrace" accorded to mothers who die during childbirth and a naming ceremony based on waiting "the first 8 days with distrust," not knowing "whether the 'spirt child' intends to stay on earth for a longer time."[70]

During the birth of Kofi Dɔnkɔ, the presence of Yaw Badu would have been disallowed while Akosua remained under the care of midwives. Only after the birth would Yaw Badu be summoned. The afterbirth would then be placed in a calabash or clay pot with a lid, and Yaw Badu—or the father or brother of Akosua Toa or an elder woman of the house—would bury it in the forest near the family abode. After Kofi Dɔnkɔ was born, an elder woman would have cleaned the baby's body with either palm oil (a rich source of vitamin A) or water to prevent excessive body odor in later years—profuse sweating in a tropical climate was the norm. "After the newborn has been bathed," BM sources tell us, "one welcomes it by proclaiming: '[Kofi] has arrived, may he stay with us!'"[71] On the eighth day of Kofi Dɔnkɔ's life, an elaborate naming ceremony (*abadintoɔ* or *adintoɔ*) would have been performed, marking his transition from "stranger" to community member.[72] As we have already seen, the eight days' wait—that is, counting the initial day of the seven-day week twice—ensured a child came to stay on this earth and would not prematurely return to his or her spiritual mother in *asamandoɔ*. The "child [who] remained alive … receives after those 8 days a family name at a special celebration."[73] But until the Friday after his birth, Kofi Dɔnkɔ was still regarded as a stranger and thus greeted with *woaba a tena aseɛ* ("now that you have come, sit down [and stay]") to wish him a long life.

Kofi Dɔnkɔ's adintoɔ took place at Yaw Badu's house on the eighth day of his life—on a specific Friday. Before the scheduled day of the adintoɔ ceremony, items such as palm wine or another intoxicating drink, cups, water, mat, calabash, and a cutlass were gathered for the boy child. By then, Yaw Badu had likely provided money and cloth for the child and mother, and the mat and a toilet-pot for his son. Early in the morning, two elders of high character from Yaw Badu's family were sent to retrieve Kofi and his mother from Akosua Toa's house. Kofi's mother then bathed the infant, and both dressed in white cloth and remained indoors until the ceremony began. Certain sacred beads were placed on the child, and marks made with white clay (*hyire*) and specific to this ceremony were likely drawn on the child and mother. Just before daybreak, close relatives and friends of Akosua Toa helped with preparations. The adintoɔ ceremony opened with a ritual libation poured by an elder, perhaps the child's grandfather.[74]

The family of Kofi's mother provided the drink used for the opening libation, which was poured at every doorstep and the main entrance to the house. Because Kofi belonged to the Aduana clan, he was matrilineally associated with the basic clan qualities of sharpness, quickness, and wisdom, but the dog and frog were sacred clan animals (*akraboa*) and thus taboo.[75] Yaw Badu's family provided the drink for the second libation. After this libation Kofi was taken out of the house, stripped naked, and then placed on a prepared area of the ground, a comfortable cushion, or a mat. Once all guests arrived an elder of Yaw Badu's family placed Kofi on their lap and both the water and the alcoholic beverage was poured into separate cups. The officiating elder would have spoken something to this effect: *yɛbefrɛ wo Kofi ne asekyerɛ din yɛ yɛwoo wo ɛfiada* ("we will call you Kofi and this name means your soul [ɔkra] decided to come to this earth on a Friday").[76] The Friday-born is an adventurer (*ntefo-a-ɔkyin*, "stubborn one born to be a traveler") and indecisive and thus takes time to settle, but is highly motivated and competent. The praise name *ɔkyin* (itinerant, adventurer) functioned as shorthand for Kofi Dɔnkɔ's basic temperament during childhood and in his adult life.

After he received the *kradin* "Kofi," the elder dipped their forefinger into the alcoholic beverage or used a leaf, and then placed droplets on Kofi's tongue, uttering three times, *sɛ yɛka se nsa a ka se nsa* ("when we say that it is intoxicating drink [symbolic of untruth], say that it is intoxicating drink"). The elder did the same with the water: *sɛ yɛka se nsuo a ka se nsuo* ("when we say that it is water [symbolic of truth], say that it is water"). Both of these tastings advised Kofi to seek and tell the truth and to distinguish it from falsehood as he strived to live a righteous and ethical life.[77] Because naming the child was the responsibility of the father's family, Kofi's family name (*agyadin*, literally "father name") was provided by his father or grandfather. The family name derived from the father's patrilineal clan (*ntorɔ/ntɔn*), itself complemented by numerous matrilineal clans (*mmusua*) and subclans. Each ntorɔ/ntɔn had its own day of observance, when members ritually cleansed their soul near a specific body of water. Members of an ntorɔ/ntɔn exchanged greetings with specific responses, upheld a set of taboos or avoidances, respected a sacred animal that members tabooed, shared basic characteristics, and assumed one of several patrilineal clan names.[78] Apparently, Kofi Dɔnkɔ belonged to the ntorɔ/ntɔn of Bosomdwerɛbe (a cave and a family *ɔbosom*), responded to others sharing this ntorɔ/ntɔn with "Yaa ahenewa," and learned to bathe his soul on Sundays. As a member of this ntorɔ/ntɔn, Kofi Dɔnkɔ also learned to avoid spotted animals, palm wine, tortoises, and snails on Sundays, but regarded the leopard as sacred and not to be harmed or killed. Kofi Dɔnkɔ was believed to possess some eccentricity and jitteriness about him—basic characteristics of the Bosomdwerɛbe ntorɔ/ntɔn—and was appropriately given the family name Sakyi. Individuals sharing the family names Ampɔnsa, Otieku, Aboagye, Sɛkyerɛ, Ataara, Antwi, and Akuamoa were Kofi Dɔnkɔ's patrilineal kin and ones with whom he shared the aforementioned greetings, taboos, and obligations.

After the naming of Kofi Sakyi, he would have been elevated three times, placed on a mat naked and with a cutlass in his hand, and then covered with a calabash, which would be removed after a few seconds. The cutlass symbolized the ethic of hard work, providing for and protecting his family, and working with his future wife. Kofi would then have been presented to his community, hence the popular translation of the naming ceremony as "outdooring," since this would have been the first time Kofi was taken out of the house. A final libation would consecrate the ceremony, and blessings for the child and his family would be articulated along with requests for the child to be an obedient, truthful, and righteous community member. Thereafter Kofi would be addressed by his name and his ears would receive what family and community members expected of him. Those in attendance bearing gifts such as money or clothing would offer them to the family of the newborn, while Yaw Badu presented gifts to the mother and child.

Although it is not clear whether feasting with singing and dancing followed Kofi's adintoɔ, this was usually the case. Such a festive end, in whatever way Kofi's parents choose to have it, provided joyful closure to the adintoɔ ceremony and welcomed Kofi Sakyi/Dɔnkɔ to his new social world. Male children born in Takyiman before the 1960s, such as Kofi Dɔnkɔ, received no circumcision.[79] After the 1960s most boys were circumcised either at home or at a mission hospital. Kofi Dɔnkɔ, like most children, would have been breastfed for several years. Like most children around five or six months old, he was likely vaccinated and naturalized through a ritual called *aniasetwa* ("cut beneath the eye"), where a horizontal inch-wide incision was made with a razor blade and a composite herbal medicine (*mɔtɔ*) was rubbed into the incision to prevent convulsions (*ɛsoro*). Convulsions had, and still have, a reputation for attacking and killing many children in the Takyiman area.

❋

A CHILD SUCH as Kofi Dɔnkɔ would have then settled in to the patterns of family and community life, with their shared and at times particular sets of routines and expectations. Both children and adults bathed twice a day and periodically sat in water mixed with herbs for good health and strength. As a young child, Kofi Dɔnkɔ was expected to do many household chores: bathing, feeding himself, sweeping and cleaning, trimming weeds and shrubs around the residential compound, and farming. Most of the townspeople woke up between five and six o'clock in the morning, and greetings punctuated the day's beginning and reinforced the age distinctions. After using the restroom, Kofi would have gotten into the routine of fetching water and firewood for various purposes, taking a bath and brushing his teeth, cleaning the compound yard and house with a handheld broom, eating a breakfast of porridge or boiled provisions with a peppered-meat stew, and then traveling to the farm with his parents.

A childhood friend of Kofi Dɔnkɔ recalled, "He never liked carrying firewood for his mother whenever we visited the farm because his mother would never tie the firewood tightly and it would always loosen on the way, and so he never liked carrying firewood tied by his mother."[80] Nonetheless, the adults would have traveled to the farm with their cutlasses and their children. Most townspeople, like much of the world, were full-time farmers, and this meant that lunch was prepared on farmlands some distance from home. Both parents and child(ren) might not be seen until the afternoon or early evening. Evening meals for Kofi's family, prepared by Akosua Toa or her eldest daughters, revolved around the main staple of *fufu* (pounded yams, cassava, or plantain) with a palm nut, groundnut, or cocoyam leaves stew filled with meat or poultry. Some might have had a light soup made of red peppers and broth with fufu or another starch. The Bono were not known for desserts and very few ate sugary foods or uncooked vegetables, which were usually boiled and grounded to a paste and added to a stew or soup. After dinner Kofi would have had an evening bath before retiring to bed.

Kofi Dɔnkɔ's mother had moved from Takyiman to the village of Akumsa Odumase, and so she, like her infant son, had to find her way in a new community. Kofi Dɔnkɔ's elder sister Adwoa Akumsa recalled, "My mother was then very young from Takyiman [and] went into marriage in Nkoransa." Like her younger brother, Adwoa too was born to her "parents through the help of [the ɔbosom] Akumsa as *a tɔ ba* ['bought child']."[81] Adwoa and her sister Afia Asubɔnten would collectively care for Kofi Dɔnkɔ when their parents passed away; in fact, Adwoa carried young Kofi Dɔnkɔ on her back.[82] The community of Akumsa Odumase received its name from Akumsa (*kum*—to kill; *sa*—war) and the Odum tree (*odum*—Odum tree; *ase*—under). "Akumsa under the Odum tree" thus marked the spiritual and spatial foundations of the village, the radius of which extended outward from the spot of the tree (map 2.2). The warrior temperament of Akumsa found its way into spiritual offspring, the eldest of which was Boaboduro ("brave warrior").

Homelands 67

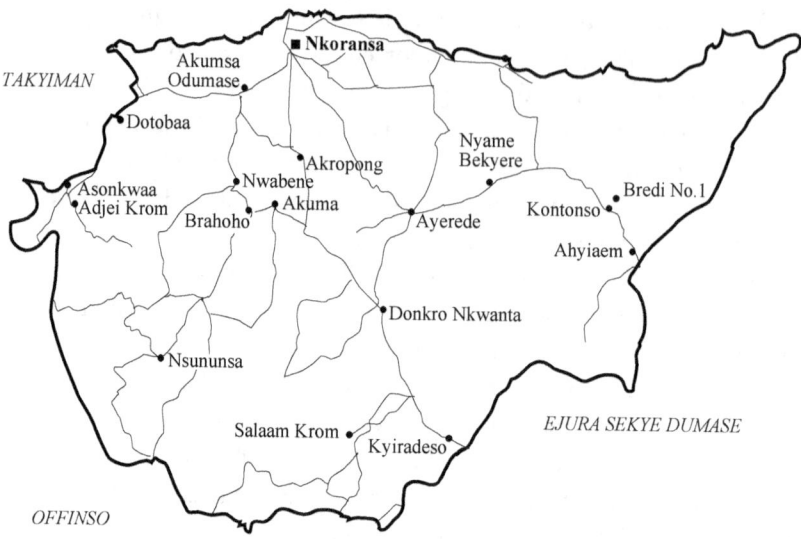

MAP 2.2. Map of Nkoransa. Although Kofi Dɔnkɔ was born in the town of Nkoransa, his specific birthplace and site of his formative years was the village of Akumsa Odumase. Connected by the Takyiman–Nkoransa road, Akumsa Odumase was some twenty-six miles east of Takyiman, the township of Dɔnkɔ's mother and where he lived most of his life. Adapted from Ghana Statistical Service, *2010 Population & Housing Survey: District Analytical Report* (Accra: Ghana Statistical Service, 2014), 2.

Akumsa, like most abosom, had male and female pathways used to engage the spiritual force: whereas ɔkɔmfoɔ Adwoa used "the Nsuo Yaa that is connected to the Akumsa shrine," ɔbosomfoɔ Yaw Bempa carried on his head the *ayawa* containing the physical shrine of Akumsa.[83] Akosua Toa had petitioned Akumsa for the child that became Adwoa, who herself became its ɔkɔmfoɔ during the reign of Takyimanhene Yaw Ameyaw (1927–35). Adwoa's birthdate is uncertain, but about this she had no misgivings: "I can't actually tell you [that I] know my age, since there were no birthdates during our time." During her childhood she played games such as *ampe, adowa,* and *sikyi.* Adwoa, Afia, and Kofi Dɔnkɔ attended neither church nor missionary schools, though a BM station was erected by catechist Godfrid Nyantakyi in Nkoransa around 1911.[84] Besides being the only male child, Kofi Dɔnkɔ was the last born to his parents. More importantly, he and his sisters were molded by an immediate and extended family of well-respected healers and blacksmiths of considerable repute.[85] There is little record that Kofi Dɔnkɔ became seduced by the avaricious and unbridled forces of commerce and Christianization sweeping the tripartite colony. Instead, from an early age he engaged matters of spirituality, culture, and the family crafts.

Although Kofi Dɔnkɔ's mother Akosua Toa and grandfather Kwadwo Owusu passed when he was six or seven years old, the healer-to-be spent his early years with his two elder sisters, Adwoa Asabea and Afia Asubɔnten, and their father Yaw Badu. Yaw Badu was a skilled and reputed herbalist (ɔdunsinni) and blacksmith (ɔtomfoɔ) in Akumsa Odumase. There Kofi Dɔnkɔ began to learn not only the rudiments of the healing arts and a large herbal pharmacopoeia, but also the language of the abosom while actively communicating with family ancestors temporally deceased. That communicative aptitude was further nurtured by a family with a long line of healers, including his grandmother Nana Arku Bagyei (the first ɔkɔmfoɔ for Asubɔnten Kwabena) and his elder sister ɔkɔmfoɔ Adwoa Asabea (also known as Adwoa Akumsa, since her principal ɔbosom was Akumsa) (figure 2.3). On the way to the forest or farm, the adolescent Kofi Dɔnkɔ would appear to talk to himself, laughing as if his friends accompanied him. According to elder family members, Kofi Dɔnkɔ maintained an ongoing dialogue with those in the ancestral sphere of existence, revealing the names of and messages from family members long deceased and whom he never encountered in the flesh.

A childhood friend recalled, "He never had the chance to play much with his peers since he was taken to be an [ɔbosomfoɔ] at a tender age."[86] Others remember, "When he was a child, Nana [Kofi Dɔnkɔ] could foretell something about people and it would come to pass even before he became the ɔbosomfoɔ for Asubɔnten."[87] Those who knew Kofi Dɔnkɔ in his youth underscore his humility, calm, and respect for ancestry, culture, and community at a young age. During his adolescent years, Kofi Dɔnkɔ might have poorly understood the rapid societal changes around him and his community but would have been very much aware of them through overheard adult conversations, passing by newly established shops, and watching the traffic along feeder and main roads while traveling to and from the farm. Although this would have been especially true in the crossroads town of Takyiman, it is tempting to conclude he might have also known very little about life in the urbanized parts of the tripartite colony.

Up until his birth and first years of life, matters of schooling, religion, health care, and governance affected the tripartite colony, but in different ways. In the first place, schooling was principally under the auspices of

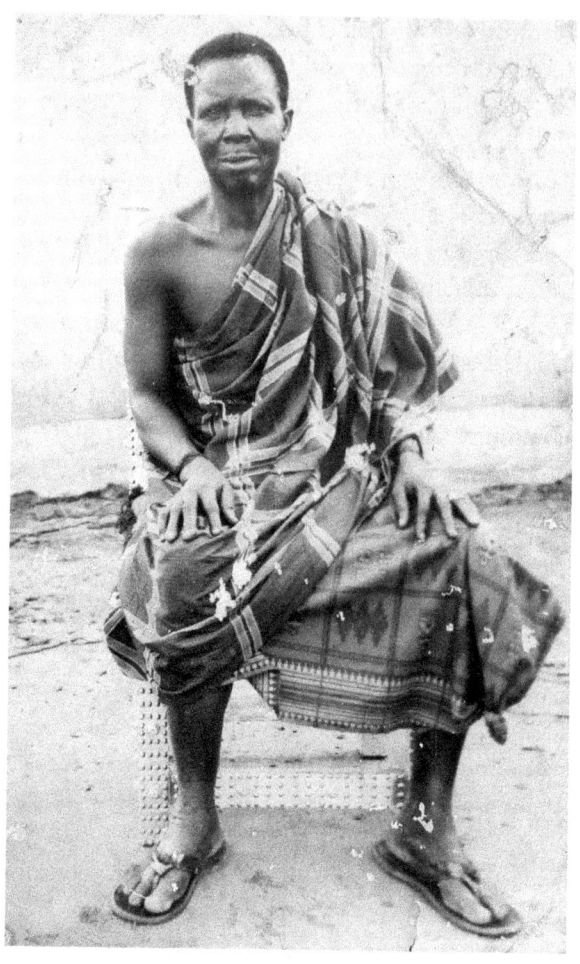

FIGURE 2.3. Adwoa Akumsa, n.d. Nana Kofi Dɔnkɔ Collection, in private hands, Takyiman, Ghana. Used courtesy of Kofi Sakyi Sapɔn.

various missions between 1895 and 1915, reaching twenty thousand pupils among 3 million people through some four hundred noncompulsory primary schools attentive to "literary education" via the English language and industrial and "plantation" work whereby "profitable" cocoa, coffee, kola nut, hemp, cassava, cotton, and rubber were cultivated.[88] In 1900 "the number of children attending school [was] thus barely one percent of the established population of the [Gold Coast] Colony."[89] Although this number would rise to 20 percent, there remained a problem finding qualified teachers, there was little to no provision for secondary or girls' schooling, males dominated the staff and students in the mission and few government schools, and every effort was made "to teach the rising generation their privileges and duties as citizens of the British Empire," where "lectures on the Empire were given by head teachers, patriotic songs sung and the flag was saluted."[90]

In the second place, "the large majority still resort to the 'Native Medicine Man'" in spite of increased numbers of European and African hospitals, rural clinics, and nursing corps and improved sanitation in major towns, especially where the three thousand Europeans in the colony resided.[91] Meanwhile, malaria, yellow fever, smallpox, and sleeping sickness remained the most troublesome of diseases for both European and African medicinal systems. Finally, while cocoa financed the peace and prosperity of the tripartite colony, the process of creating the colony's infrastructure and buy-in from "citizens" of the empire was no clearer than in the Northern Territories. At the end of the nineteenth century, government stores were established there "to give the people a taste for articles of merchandise, and also to accustom them to the use of money as the medium of exchange and to pave the way for the establishment of trading houses by mercantile firms." This "successful experiment" was preceded by military force, occupation, and treaties but followed by mission schools and government officials to manage the territory.[92]

The Northern Territories had the fewest mission schools, perhaps owing to the presence of Islam and indigenous spiritualities, and the fewest resources—"not an integral part of His Majesty's dominions"—and thus was hardest hit by the influenza epidemic.[93] Locally known as "Africa," the epidemic swept through the colony in 1918–19, destroying many lives. In the previous year fear that an outbreak of smallpox might spread to Takyiman was a harbinger of things to come. The district commissioner requested the Takyimanhene to keep "a sharp look out for any strangers who may arrive in your villages with this disease. If any cases arise they should at once be placed in a hut outside the town and looked after by those persons who have already had small pox, and the matter reported to me immediately."[94] Whatever the effect of this strategy, such precautionary measures had mixed results against the scourge of influenza. In the outlying Takyiman village of Asueyi, villagers recalled that the Tanɔ ɔbosom Twumpoduo protected them from the influenza epidemic; Twumpoduo was thanked with two sheep and bottles of schnapps.[95] Others such as ɔbosomfoɔ Kwasi Badu, who became a healer during the epidemic, died from the disease.[96]

The disease was introduced by shipping lines along the southern coast and over land across the northern frontier—all facilitated by the new transportation networks.[97] As the disease reached Takyiman and still farther north, perhaps this was Kofi Dɔnkɔ's first real encounter with the structural transformations to his colony of birth and the disease and health costs of rapid colonial exploitation of the very ecologies he farmed and the medicinal source of his healing. Perhaps the case of Asueyi was more than an isolated one. Overall, however, the records suggest preventive action and quarantine were futile and that both African therapeutics and European biomedicine only alleviated symptoms. This global influenza epidemic struck most of the tripartite colony and the world, infecting some half a billion and killing between 20 and 50 million people worldwide. In the Gold Coast more than 100,000 were killed in fewer than six months, and most of these fatalities occurred in the northern regions where new roads opened the savanna country to the south and where northerners flooded the southern reaches of the colony through the crossroads town of Takyiman. Those beautiful forest rivers now laid next to roads, rails, and footpaths that closed the distance between the multiple lands Kofi Dɔnkɔ now called home—Nkoransa, Takyiman, the tripartite colony, and the world outside it.

CHAPTER 3. **TOOLS OF THE TRADE**

"I was a Blacksmith ... Before I Became [a Healer]"

What really is a healer's work? You may say it's seeing ...
[but no] one sees without preparation.
—AYI KWEI ARMAH, *The Healers*

As Takyiman stood at the crossroads between the northern and southern regions, Kofi Dɔnkɔ would have been in a privileged position to notice the oscillating flow of migrants, materials, and therapeutic responses to social change along the new roads connecting the two regions. In fact, although the Wesleyan school muddled along with seventy-seven pupils, many new buildings in progress and the cocoa market's multiplying effect on the traffic through Takyiman made its ruler even more pleased at the prospect of a motor road from Kumase through his town.[1] Although Takyiman possessed good roads and well-kept *zongo* quarters, it would have to wait until the 1920s, when Kofi Dɔnkɔ was in his early adolescence, for the construction of the first motor road, linking Takyiman with Kumase to the south, and additional roads connecting it to Sunyani in the southwest and Wankyi in the northwest.[2] Before the 1920s smaller quantities of migrants and raw materials moved out to the south, and even fewer medicinal and missionary schooling facilities moved to the interior parts of the tripartite colony. Although much of the material and human resources devoted to medical care, schooling, and commerce targeted the coastal districts where Europeans and their colonial proxies resided, this predisposition did not inhibit these sectors from reaching the interior corridors of the colony.³ Quite the opposite. Certainly, Wesleyan mission schools in Takyiman and Nkoransa would suggest as much. Indeed, the homelands of Kofi Dɔnkɔ provide two of the most poignant cases of the ways in which the emergent themes of religion/spirituality, schooling, health, and family took shape in Nkoransa, Takyiman, and the broader colony during the adolescence and early adulthood of Kofi Dɔnkɔ. This chapter takes up these themes, beginning with Nkoransa.

※

ONLY FIFTEEN MILES separated Nkoransa from Takyiman, but a simmering bitterness—exorcised at each *Apoɔ* festival—existed between the two. Much of this might have been historic, memorialized in Baafo Pim's treachery or the centuries-old actions of pro-Asante Nkoransa versus anti-Asante Takyiman. In either case the marriage that produced Kofi Dɔnkɔ brought these two rivals together, and regardless of our impression, he belonged to both. Indeed, through his and his family's histories Nkoransa and Takyiman shared more in common by way of the themes set out for this chapter, and especially after both rejected Asante overlordship toward the end of the nineteenth century. When Asante's imperial rule over Nkoransa and Takyiman terminated with the British occupation of Kumase in 1896, the Basel mission (BM) established its first mission station in Kumase. In 1899 catechist Hanson Aye traveled to Nkoransa, presumably with the intent to establish an outstation, but returned to Abetifi after eight months because of the "Ashante rising" in 1900.⁴ Ten years passed until Rev. Nicholas Timothy Clerk (ca. 1862–1961), whose father, Alexander Worthy Clerk, was brought from Jamaica to the Gold Coast by the BM in 1843, visited Nkoransa in 1910. Nkoransa's leadership, in turn, requested "a teacher from the missionaries who were in Coomasie [Kumase]." In January 1911 the "Queen of Nkoranza Afua Dapa and elders" also petitioned the BM local committee in Akuapem for a teacher, promising in return to provide said teacher with one hundred boys, land for the outstation, a built school and teacher's house, temporary housing for the teacher, and support for teacher and pupils.⁵ The school soon opened in March with ten boys and one girl under the leadership of teacher-catechist Godfrid Nyantakyi. The missionary outstation claimed one adult candidate for baptism and ten pupils at the end of year, pleading with the town's leadership to return "the fugitive pupils" who ran away and were thus not counted.⁶

By 1912 the BM station in Kumase had twenty-two outstations, its northernmost one in Nkoransa but none in Takyiman. The only BM document that exists for the Nkoransa outstation is the "Chronicle of the Basel Mission out-station in Nkoransa"; entries were kept consecutively by four catechists between 1911 and 1920, and Christian convictions shaped "all important events regarding the mission work [that were] to be entered into this book."[7] The scope of the document and its qualifier—"all important events regarding the mission work"—make this source, on its face, limited and insular. Yet counterintuitively, the chronicle offers several meaningful events that adhere to larger societal themes. It therefore contributes to the conditions in which Kofi Dɔnkɔ was born and reared, and to an understanding of his and his family's choices in the early decades of the twentieth century. That the school had, and would continue to have, a difficult time attracting, coercing, and keeping students is an understatement. The school's low enrollment and the advice from the governor of the Gold Coast, upon his visit and inspection of the school, to the Nkoransahene Kwadwo Faa "to supply more children to such school," suggest that the decision of Kofi Dɔnkɔ's family not to send him or his sisters to a school less than two miles away applied to a much-wider field of local peoples.[8] The outstation-cum-school's acute minority position in Nkoransa and how this frustrated its catechists, perhaps driving the founding catechist Godfrid Nyantakyi to madness and an early departure in July 1913, adheres very closely to thematic events in Takyiman and in the broader tripartite colony.[9]

Several poignant events in the nine-year record for the outstation stand out as representative of both the mundane and the sketchiness that typifies some of the chronicle, but also of seminal matters that pivoted around religion, marriage, cultural practice, and schooling, which resonated with most if not all in the colony. Along with destoolment cases, where litigants fought over who should keep or stay in power, oath cases in which litigants brought charges under "customary law" to "native" courts were equally, if not more, widespread. Unsuccessful parties were usually responsible for the court fees. On 12 April 1912, "A certain man from Nkwabene," some six miles south of Nkoransa township, "came to me [i.e., Nyantakyi]. His object of conversation was to escape an oath matter. . . . I plainly told him to have his matter settled before his name can be admitted to candidates of baptism. He went away" and never returned.[10] Claims to church membership could be used to circumvent "customary" fees and rituals associated with oath-making, especially in unfavorable cases. The next month, "a fetish priest by the name of [Kofi] Nnuma came and enrolled his name in the list of candidates for baptism," but on July 14 Nyantakyi was "sorry to report that . . . I have to cancel the name of Kofi Nnuama (a candidate) by his order."[11] And individuals removing themselves or being removed from consideration for baptism continued into the next year. In October Akosua Boahen, "[the first] candidate [of the outstation] and wife of S. Gyan, consulted the fetish and her name was cancelled according to her order," and "Kwaku Fua swore to his father (a fetish priest) that he is no longer a Christian [and] his name was cancelled."[12] Finally, at the beginning of 1913, four young men from Tadeeso enlisted their names for baptism, but the Nkoransahene and his elders came to the outstation to have their names removed, having agreed only to provide schoolchildren. The catechist refused and no clear resolution was recorded.[13]

In these instances and others it was not that missions made no progress. They did. For instance, annual subscription fees to support the missions were collected from the Nkoransahene, his elders, and subjects by one Mr. Wesley, a Wesleyan mission agent, and a new BM outstation was established in the provincial headquarters of Kintampo at the end of 1912.[14] But the troubles that enveloped the outstation practices, and the weight of local ideas, especially in matters of marriage and culture, seemed to overwhelm them. In the marriage between Kwaku Kokor and Akosua Bema, the "latter being a heathen," it was Nyantakyi who certified the "marriage according to native custom." After two years Yaw Fei had not settled his "marriage-palaver," stopped attending church services, and was planning to marry a second wife. Reverend Yost, who visited the Nkoransa mission in 1914, believed this "gives confusion and a stumbling block to the heathens." Fei was removed from the congregation after he confessed "he cannot do away with his two wives," Yaa Manu and Amma Takyiwaa.[15] Two individuals requested the name of a married woman named Amma Gya be cancelled and the new catechist William Opare, a former middle school student from Aburi and cocoa farmer in Kintampo, refused.

Opare was then given a letter from Gya, explaining that "as her husband do not like her to be Christian, saying she had committed adultery," her name was removed four months later.[16] As the outstation only "baptized the first adults (3)" in August 1915, hoping "more will follow them," marriage remained a challenge. Although the marriage between "a Mohammedan (kramoni)" named Boakye and Akosua Bagyei was "well-arranged," this union was "against church regulations." It seemed Akosua was "not yet of age" and was forcibly married to Boakye by her relatives. And yet these seemed ancillary compared to the specter of Islam. Congregation member Joseph Badu, who had a "new heathen wife," was the uncle of Akosua and was told to settle the case to the mission's satisfaction or he and Akosua would be "excluded from the congregation." A year passed. Badu did nothing and Akosua remained married. Both were then excluded. The apparent ban on Muslim-Christian unions, however, extended to intra-Christian marriages, as church members were "not entitled to marry a Roman Catholic."[17] Despite whether this was official policy, the outstation interpreted regulations this way.

Beyond the veiled threats to leave if the escaped pupils were not returned by the Nkoransahene and elders, the outstation was more concerned with the risk posed by the very people they hoped to bring into their theology and congregation. And the terrain of engagement was cultural forms and practices. By the latter part of 1915, William Opare concluded that the Nkoransahene and his elders, besides their inaction on the "fugitive" pupils, told "their people not to join the Christianity and all this shows me that they don't like school or Christianity."[18] And there were reasons for this unease. In December 1914 four men dug "a hole, put something in it, pour[ed] a pot of palm wine on it, turn[ed] their face to the mission house and fired three shots." The pupils in the house asked them what they were doing; the men responded by flogging the boys and then "they ran away."[19] If indirect recourse with the Nkoransahene was useless, so too were direct approaches.

In February 1917 Nkoransa was set to have a great "fetish" festival—that is, Apoɔ—near the outstation's ground, but Opare objected and the Nkoransahene agreed to "simply pass quietly... without the noise and drumming." But he and the townspeople passed "with drumming and a great noise." Opare tried to stop them, but they refused and returned again "with their noise headed by Queen-mother. Not knowing she was among, I told them to stop. The Queen-mother began to insulted [sic] me, saying, 'woye apō papa ntrā me sre so nsām me [wɔyɛ apoɔ papa ntira, me srɛ so nsam me (because they do good apoɔ, I request/beg you not scatter me)].' Seconded by her daughter Ya[a] Nsia. She again said this land is mine. I will never stop passing with my fetishes with their drums and the noise, whether you are in church or not."[20] Although the matter was escalated to BM and colonial officials, resulting in some compromise, the outstation's challenges also stemmed from within the congregation. Kwaku Koko was one such example. In short, he was accused of drinking gin, playing Ashiko (Aṣíkò) music, engaging in funerary customs, dancing, visiting the "fetish Brekimi at Kranka" and "fetish Tanno," ordering his brother to "kill a [sheep] for his ancestors," and possessing *asuman* in his house. Kwaku conceded only to drinking, funerary rituals, and consulting "Brekimi" and Tanɔ. Outstation leaders decided to not accept him until they had "proper proof of his conversion."[21] As for the outstation in Kintampo, its "few members" did nothing, having "no prayer meeting or even services," and thus was written off.

The outstation received a new catechist, S. Ammiah Atta, in February 1818, just after "the first motor-car arrived at Nkoransa" but two only months before he traveled to Odumase, most likely Akumsa Odumase, "to preach the gospel."[22] Although we do not know exactly what Kofi Dɔnkɔ, five years old at the time, might have thought about Atta's message, we can surmise that he and his community remained less than convinced, with perhaps the same kind of bravado exhibited by the Nkoransahemma Afua Dapa. It does not take a great leap to conclude the matters that challenged the Nkoransa outstation also affected large swaths of Africans in the colony. As the Nkoransa chronicle ended, so did the outstation. At the end of 1918 catechist S. Ammiah Atta was "severally attacked by influenza" so much so he was "near the grave," then replaced by or shared the post with Henry Dokyi. By May 1919 the facility was now the "Scottish mission school at Nkoransa," because British colonists on the Gold Coast expelled European staff of BM institutions and transferred them, including those at the Ewe mission, to the United Free Church of Scotland.[23] The BM would return in the 1920s, but by then their former institutions had been folded under the tent of the Presbyterian Church of the Gold Coast. Like the Wesleyan mission, the Presbyterians began to be managed by "native" leadership, including the second generation of diasporic Africans who originated in Jamaica but laid the foundation of the BM enterprise on the Gold Coast/Ghana. The diaspora would also cross paths with Kofi Dɔnkɔ, but for this moment, what featured prominently in the 1920s were issues that also mattered to the "Scottish mission school": obtaining and training students to serve in the colony and empire, marshaling funds derived from cocoa, and continually working away at the challenges that beset the Nkoransa outstation but that existed at multiple levels in the tripartite colony (map 3.1).[24]

❄

BY 1919–20 COLONIAL officials announced the use of indigenous languages and English among lower standard students in the nineteen govern-

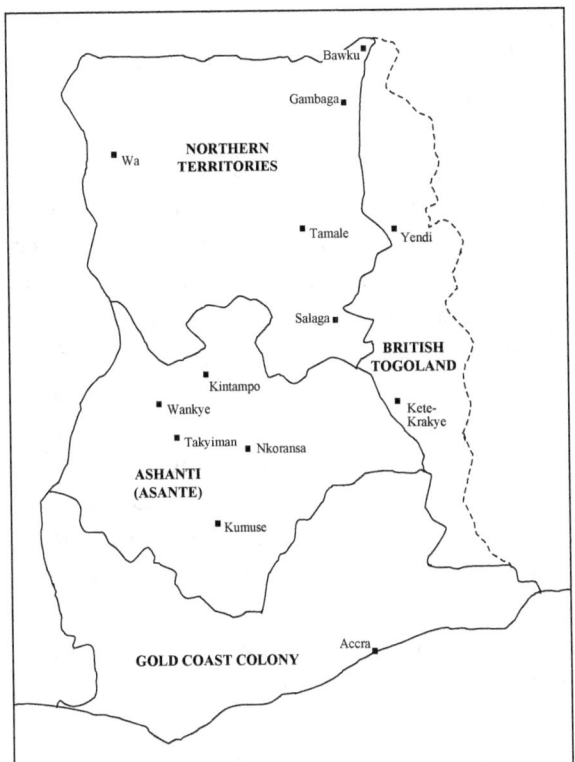

MAP 3.1. Map of the tripartite colony. British Togoland was later added to the tripartite colony to create modern Ghana.

ment schools and fewer than three hundred mission schools it inspected and funded. The principal indigenous languages were Akan/Twi, Fante, and Gã. If language was a conduit of culture, then officials understood language policy, where "English is the language mainly used," to mean an effective colonial strategy aimed at creating bicultural subjects at once appreciative of what colonists deemed "traditional" and worth preserving, and steeped in Christianity and British values, while staffing the colony and empire.[25] Plans were made in 1922 to create the first government-funded secondary school, merged with its Training College, at Achimota. In the spirit of training an elite cadre of Africans to be "black Englishmen" in the service of empire, the Prince of Wales School and College, or Achimota College, opened in January 1927. Instructing mostly males removed from natal culture and community and aged between six and their early twenties, Achimota College sought to create brokers of European ideas who were conversant with—rather than practitioners of—their culture. These individuals were also bred to replace "chiefs" and intellectuals, run local

Tools of the Trade 79

councils, and fill intermediate posts in the colonial administration.²⁶ A notable example of such "black Englishmen" was James Kwegyir Aggrey, cofounder of Achimota College.

Aggrey became a most celebrated product of missionary schooling, having been brought to the United States through A. M. E. Zion missionaries in 1898. Some Africans viewed him as a "European lackey," and he was caricatured as one of the notable characters in Kobina Sekyi's comical satire *The Blinkards*; others, including his daughter, Abena Aggrey Lancaster, shared Christian optics and saw him as a pioneer who acted as "a mediator between the government and the natives."²⁷ Unlike Aggrey, whose father was a Christian with three wives, many male missionary schoolers chose technical training to work in agriculture, mining, and other fields.²⁸ Most became caught up in the "great cocoa rush" of the early 1920s, a majority of whom the colonial governor described in his 1921 annual address as having "lost their heads." Professionals, clerks, and artisans who were literate in the colonial language deserted their work: "It was impossible," the governor lamented, "to get labor." Farmers and capitalists got on board with the new labor imperative and obtained as many cheap laborers as possible to meet the demand for cocoa. The new source of labor was the northern region and, not surprisingly, the main road south went through Takyiman. There is no way to tell whether Kofi Dɔnkɔ and his parents farmed cocoa, but it is hard to imagine they did not have a cocoa farm or two worked by the same migrant labors who first settled the zongo quarters of Takyiman.

Some pulled out when cocoa prices fell from £122 to £39 per ton in May 1920, but most remained, including hundreds of "educated young Africans" who left colonial service jobs for cocoa fields and markets and who the government scorned.²⁹ The monies they earned were used to feed the alluring, anti-communitarian values of self-interest, individualism, and accumulation through the purchase of European cars, cigars, and clothes. For this ethic, colonial officials reviled them as regarding "proficiency in reading and writing as the hall mark of a native gentleman," and among whom luxuries "had become almost necessities" with the "introduction of paper currency" and "European stores in every village of importance."³⁰ Monies earned from an export tax on cocoa financed the construction of roads and railways so that more cocoa could efficiently reach the coastal ports and the world market. In this way the rails and roads were infrastructural means to underwrite the cocoa industry, and that industry ensured the future of rails and roads that transported more than just cocoa. On his 1926 trip to the Gold Coast, William G. A. Ormsby-Gore of the Colonial

Office proclaimed, "Cocoa, and cocoa alone, at present enables the railway to pay its way."[31] The potential profit from cocoa led, on one hand, to fierce competition and problems of coordination between the owners of rail and motor transport over the conveyance of cocoa, and on the other, to the construction of new roads by members and leaders of local communities, who used their own initiative and resources to traverse hills and cut through dense tropical forest.

In 1923 the colonial government affirmed the right of every individual to cultivate as much cocoa as his or her land could produce. This license only unleashed a tidal wave of societal forces—human, insectile, and spiritual. Between 1910 and 1925 cocoa became the principal commodity, but on a parallel track the growth of cocoa matched industrious cocoa farmers—who rarely invested their wealth in raising living standards but rather on funerals, cars, business start-ups, litigation, and consultations with "protection-shrines"—as societal safeguards gave way.[32] If the scourge of yellow fever, which killed a researcher from the Rockefeller Institute invited to study it, was a disease that profited from the commercial opening of the forest, so too can the "protection-shrines" or *abosommerafoɔ* from the north be considered homeopathic.[33] Homeopathic in the sense that forces from an untamed wilderness could potentially eradicate equally violent forces of chaos and anxiety, triggered even more by "the tendency of immigration from the north being unchecked."[34] Yet counterintuitively, abosommerafoɔ such as Tigare made firm ethical demands—no adultery, poisoning, stealing, envy, cursing—and would not support the avaricious and antisocial forces embodied by farmer-capitalists and local elite, whereas churches' memberships grew because they demanded only that their delinquency remain concealed.[35] That the "protection-shrines" were individually owned, in sharp contrast to the family-owned and collective prosperity outlook of Tanɔ *abosom*, should not surprise us. If anything, the volcanic rise in the abosommerafoɔ's popularity correlated with the rise in social anxiety and cocoa expansion. Rather than cluster for group protection, many collapsed under the weight of individual gain against the interests of kin and community.

Throughout the 1920s religious movements such as the ones built around Aberewa/Ablewa decades earlier were followed up by Hwemeso.[36] Although Hwemeso too was outlawed in the colony, waves of similar movements succeeded it in the interwar years, featuring central abosommerafoɔ figures such as Tigare and Kukuro.[37] Christian missions operating in Kumase decried, "[Kukuro] has seized on the people in a frantic way . . . [and]

most of the Chiefs are supporting and promoting it." In sum, "this frenzy is breaking down what the Missions have built up these last 8 years."[38] Kukuro originated in a Takyiman village near the Tanɔ River, but its reach exceeded that village to its base in Nkyeraa to "all over Ashanti and even in the Colony."[39] Although many abosommerafoɔ would decline in popularity or find themselves replaced by "prophetic" Christian churches offering similar services in the 1940s and 1950s, Tigare would achieve a greater staying power, spreading west into present-day Ivory Coast and east into Togo, Benin, and Nigeria.[40]

Once again, Takyiman was vital in the Akanization of forces such as the well-known Tigare and the lesser-known Kalasi (Akan: Boame) in Togo, and in their distribution across diverse colonial landscapes.[41] Tigare originated in the northern town of Yipala and entered the forest region through the Takyiman village of Aboabo, and its transformation from *suman* to *ɔbosommerafoɔ* came courtesy of the Tanɔ River. Tigare accompanied travelers and their share of diseases through Takyiman into the Asante heartland, to the coastline, and onto lands east and west of the colony. Indeed, itinerant traders, children, and the outbreak of disease were often linked, for officials believed northerners and children were carriers of several diseases.[42] When meningitis, for instance, appeared in 1906 in the Northern Territories and in Kintampo, officials selected Takyiman as a detaining site for travelers diverted from the Kintampo-Nkoransa and Wankyi roads to be examined by "a Medical Officer with a military guard."[43] Those meningitis cases introduced in 1920 came through trade routes used by northerners traveling "to Coomassie [Kumase] and elsewhere." Most of the three thousand deaths from meningitis occurred in the northern provinces of Asante, while in Asante proper, "infants and young children seemed to be comparatively immune, [though] the proportion of women attacked was high."[44] In 1921 a meningitis epidemic broke out in the colony, triggering biomedical and religious responses.

In more than one way, Asante's immune system had been weakened by British rule and found itself entangled in the widely used abosommerafoɔ and associated religious movements.[45] Asante was also leaderless, as evidenced by the defilement and looting of the Golden Stool by a group of young men in the 1920s and the emergence of radical individuals. These individuals had acquired private wealth and Christian values by brokering for Europeans on the coast and had returned to occupy an intermediary position between Asante officeholders and nonofficeholders. In 1924 the exiled Agyeman Perempe I and some senior officeholders also returned to

Asante, but as private citizens. When Perempe I became Kumasehene in 1926, he was supported by conservative Kumase officeholders who sought their historic powers, as well as the radicals who saw in Perempe—a man now "civilized" and Christianized like themselves—the chance for a liberal regime that would eliminate those officeholders' power. The hopes of the radicals were misplaced. Governor Gordon Guggisburg's 1924 constitution created provincial councils of chiefs and expanded their representation in the colonial legislative council, thus enlarging, rather than reducing, their powers.

The increased judicial powers of officeholders in much of the colony led to a multitude of legal disputes, such as the ongoing ones between Takyiman and Asante over the jurisdiction of the nine villages placed under the authority of Kumase officeholders and the allegiance of those villages to Asante rather than Takyiman. This protracted dispute over the villages would boil over into nationalist struggles in the coming decades. The dispute would remain not only a divisive issue between Takyiman and Asante but also a substantial divide between the elders and the youth of Takyiman; the latter, however, seemed less caught up in the capitalist and Christianizing verve in much of the colony. Between 1923 and 1927 Governor Guggisburg commissioned the construction of the Korle Bu Hospital and Achimota College in Accra, while the BM built the first mission hospital in the Asante town of Agogo.[46] Insofar as "native Africans" saw their entrance into Achimota College as a mark of civilization and modernity, the ruler of Agogo viewed the mission hospital as a symbol of "development."[47] Interior and rural communities such as Takyiman and Nkoransa received no such edifices of "development," and a hospital would have to wait until the 1950s, leaving the provision of primary health care and combating the forces that plagued the colony squarely in the hands of healers.

✻

IN THE LATE 1920s Kofi Dɔnkɔ and Kofi Kyereme underwent their training to become Tanɔ *abosomfoɔ*—Kyereme for Taa Kwasi, Dɔnkɔ for Asubɔnten Kwabena.[48] Kofi Kyereme was born between 1912 and 1914 to Kwabena Kyereme of Wankyi and Afia Gyamea of Takyiman, and thus he and Kofi Dɔnkɔ also had in common mothers born in Takyiman.[49] For Kyereme, his interest in spiritual culture started as a young child in Wankyi, where he "was interested in using palm fronds in making *dɔsɔɔ* ['raffia skirt'] until I became an *ɔbosomfoɔ*. Onyankopɔn actually gave me my heart's desire to become an ɔbosomfoɔ since that was what I always wanted [to be] when

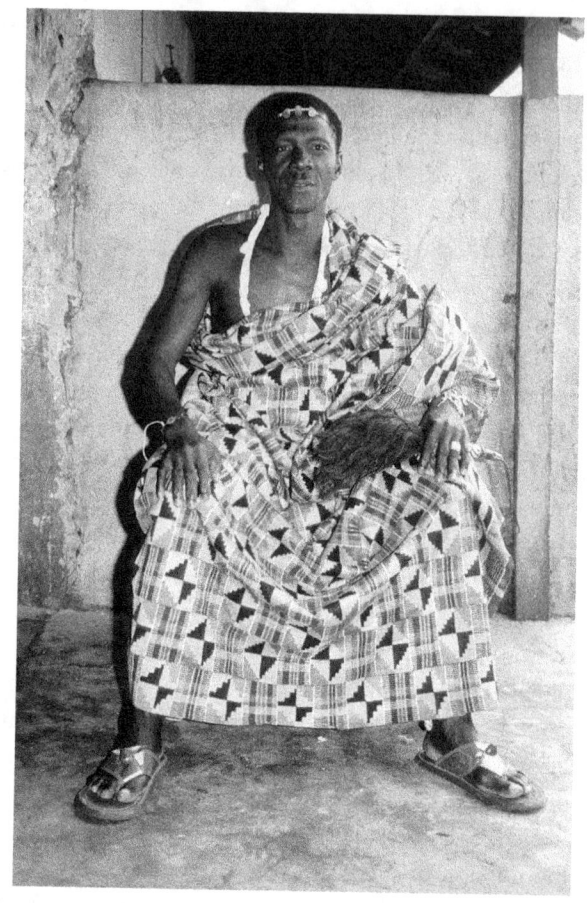

FIGURE 3.1. Taa Kwasi ɔbosomfoɔ Kofi Kyereme, 26 September 1970. From the Dennis Michael Warren Slide Collection, Special Collections Department, University of Iowa Libraries. Used courtesy of Greg Prickman, Head of Special Collections.

I was a child. I never had interest in any game apart from dancing with my dɔsɔɔ by myself, even when I was going to the farm with my parents."⁵⁰ Kofi Kyereme "became the ɔbosomfoɔ of Taa Kwasi," first offspring of Taa Mensa Kwabena, "during the time of Nana Yaw Ameyaw, a year after the revolution in Takyiman" (figure 3.1).⁵¹ This "revolution" refers to the murder of Takyimanhene Yaw Kramo (which I discuss soon) and the consequential beginning of Yaw Ameyaw's reign in 1928. These events suggest that Kofi Kyereme and Kofi Dɔnkɔ were in their adolescence when initiated.

Kyereme studied under Nana Kwadwo Dɔnkɔ (no relation to Kofi Dɔnkɔ), Taa Kofi ɔbosomfoɔ of Twimia. But Nana Kwadwo Dɔnkɔ died and was replaced by Nana Kwaku Badu, Taa Mensa Kwabena ɔbosomfoɔ, who, according to Kyereme, "taught me to finish my training." It was well known that Kofi Kyereme and Kofi Dɔnkɔ began their respective training at relatively early ages, but few knew that Kofi Dɔnkɔ, unlike his colleague and long-time friend Kofi Kyereme, resisted the idea of becoming a healer. Kofi Dɔnkɔ even cried when he had to leave Akumsa Odumase for Takyiman to begin his training.[52] Akosua Antwiwaa, a childhood friend of Kofi Dɔnkɔ from Akumsa Odumase, recalled that at the time of her puberty, Kofi Dɔnkɔ "was a boy . . . between 13 and 15 years old." "He was a boy when I saw him," Akosua continued, "[but during] his childhood, he was very humble and calm. He would gather the children younger than him [and] carry them to the riverside and sometimes bathed them, and so his friends and the children used to call him kɔnkɔnkɔ [i.e., kɔnkɔ, 'large drinking glass'] not Kofi Dɔnkɔ."[53] Those qualities and his love for children would be enduring ones.

While Akosua would have undergone her *bragorɔ* puberty rites after her menses began, Bono/Akan peoples have no formal rites for boys, and so Kofi Dɔnkɔ would have studied the trade of his father or maternal uncle.[54] Kofi's father Yaw Badu was a skilled herbalist and blacksmith, and so naturally Kofi began to learn the craft of blacksmithing and healing through the use of medicinal plants. Blacksmiths collected iron ore or scrap iron and used termite-engineered structures from the earth to make an *abura*. They would pound this termite-designed earth into a mudlike substance and then build the cylindrical abura. An abura was a "shrine" of sorts due to the spiritual considerations implied in blacksmithing: to extract iron from rocks and fashion it into a variety of durable shapes invoked creative forces—or the ability to marshal those forces—by blacksmiths who were guided in their craft by their very own *ɔbosom* called Nyakosaa.

The auspicious color for blacksmiths was black, and accordingly black fowls were sacrificed during the rituals inaugurating the smelting process. In that process the gathered iron ore or scraps were placed into the abura and smelted with the aid of *pontrodom* firewood; bellows were used to sustain the fire. Pontrodom is a huge hardwood commonly found in the semideciduous forest, and its bark has medicinal properties, though it was also poisonous. (Most present-day blacksmiths, however, use charcoal instead of pontrodom.) The heated ore or scraps were transformed into a liquefied iron base, which was then poured into the cast of whatever desired tool, implement, or weapon. Blacksmiths such as Yaw Badu or Kofi Dɔnkɔ's maternal uncle Kwame Ampɔnsa produced farm tools, local firearms, metal traps for animals, iron bracelets, and spears, but not the brass weights reserved for artisans distinct from blacksmiths.[55] Blacksmiths were crucial to the functioning of rural communities, servicing their main clientele of hunters and farmers; in sum, they remained integral suppliers of tools for a people and an economy based on farming.[56]

As a young man, Kofi Dɔnkɔ would have been a full-time farmer, working either on his parent's farmland or on a plot of his own. Whereas most farmers of cocoa and food crops focused on planting and harvesting, Kofi Dɔnkɔ turned his attention to the healing properties of flora in the forest-savanna ecotone, the diseases that affected his community, and the various therapeutic options made available by plant-based medicines. When Kofi Dɔnkɔ was around age 13, the colonial government instituted a plant sanitation campaign in the cocoa industry. The campaign advised farmers like Kofi Dɔnkɔ and his parents about the care of trees, the treatment of various plant-based diseases, the impoverishment of the soil, and deforestation caused by the felling of trees for palm wine and oil (although the palm oil trade declined due to the success of cocoa). During this campaign, Europeans belonging to the BM returned to the colony, but their missionary work was restricted to Asante and constrained by other European missions, such the Anglican mission. Although the Anglican mission had a previous but failed incarnation on the eighteenth-century Gold Coast, the reemergent Anglican Church in the 1920s took root on the coast, in Kumase, and reached Kofi Dɔnkɔ's natal town of Nkoransa in 1926.[57]

The Anglican presence in Nkoransa came through the initiative of teacher-catechist Sydney Andrew Quashie, who established a church school as the "handmaid of mission and evangelism."[58] This Anglican outpost, in what evolved into the parish of Nkoransa, was formerly under the archdeaconry of Kumase. But once the parish was established, other outstations were created, including one in Kofi Dɔnkɔ's natal village of Akumsa Odumase, in Nkoransa. Christian missions might have made significant inroads on the coast and secondarily in the southern half of the colony, but in the Takyiman-Nkoransa region their instruments of proselytization—church and school—failed to convince most indigenes to abandon their cultural cache in favor of a foreign ideology during foreign rule. We do not know whether Kofi Dɔnkɔ saw things this way, but we can surmise he had little interaction with or interest in the missions because his life thus far was brewed in a family of blacksmiths and healers who, like Nananom Mpow among his Fante kinsmen, were less seduced by the Christian and capitalist orthodoxy of the times. His calling anchored him within a genealogy of healers who served their community and who helped to provide security amidst colonially induced anxiety and chaos.

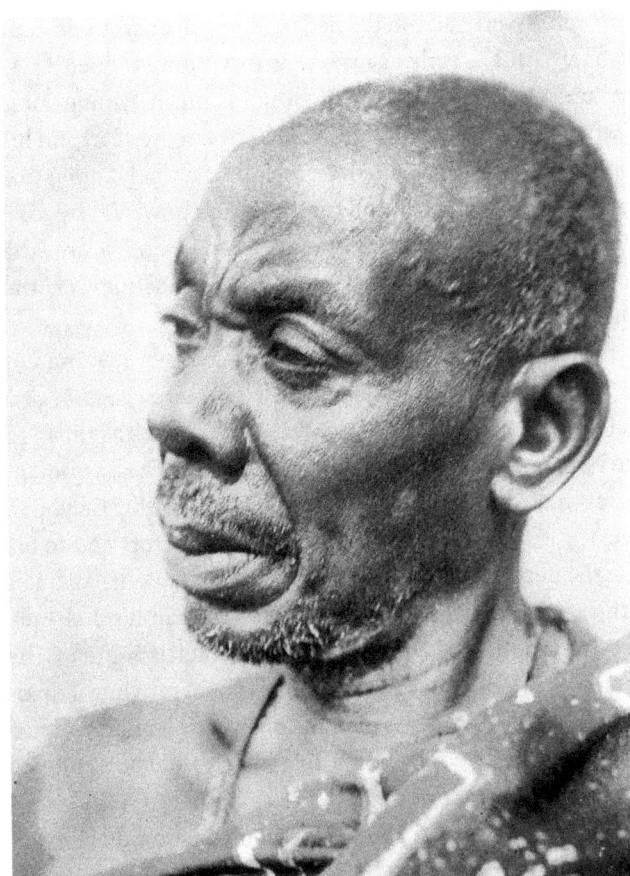

FIGURE 3.2. Yao Kramo, Tekiman Hene. Photographed by Robert Sutherland Rattray, ca. 1920s (MS 445), © Royal Anthropological Institute, London, 300.445–01–097. Used with permission.

Although Kofi Dɔnkɔ cried when he had to leave his family and friends in Akumsa Odumase for his mother's town of Takyiman, he arrived in a Takyiman embroiled in conflicts between elders and young men like himself, and between the constrained authority of local leadership and the real powers of colonial officials. These conflicts took the life of Takyimanhene Yaw Kramo in 1927 (figure 3.2), when Kofi Dɔnkɔ was around 14 years old and most likely in Takyiman to begin his ɔbosomfoɔ training.[59] The murder of Yaw Kramo was rooted in the colonial economy's need for labor and roads—to bring valued natural resources to market—and the colonial use of local "chiefs." These local officeholders operated within the colonial order as salaried individuals working at the behest of the colonial machinery, and thus provided labor through politically powerless young men. Six such young men and one woman had conspired to "riot and destool" Yaw

Kramo in 1919 but were swiftly arrested, tried, and imprisoned to do four months of hard labor.[60] And as early as 1916, District Commissioner Boyle visited Takyiman and observed a "decided progression in 'young men' movement here, which has resulted in a new split between the chief and his people"; he was informed that several people, including a shady individual named Yao Ankama, were "trying to spoil the *omanhin*'s power."[61] By 1927, however, the days of independent "chieftaincy" were over and so was the "contented and prosperous state" of Takyiman, with Kramo's murder "the first sign of any discontent."[62]

At the start of the second rainy season in 1926, the colonial government decided to build a new road from Takyiman to Nkyeraa, because Takyiman was a central node between three provincial roads: from Takyiman to Wankyi (west), to Nkoransa (east), and to Tanɔso (south). The Takyimanhene favored the new road, but the townspeople opposed it. The Takyiman community, especially its young men, opted to hire contractors and to tax themselves to raise the necessary capital to build the road. Colonial officials decided against this, reporting that "the people of Tekiman have already done a good deal of communal road making."[63] These officials argued, "The policy of making natives of a district bear the whole cost of provincial roads in it is also hard to defend." This process of road construction occurred during a reorganization of the districts, in which Takyiman would be a colonial division within the Wankyi-Kintampo district.[64] Nonetheless, officials argued further that "if locals will build roads, Government should use every endeavor to secure efficient contractors to make the road & might properly make a contribution from government funds towards the total costs."[65] The governor noted, "The fact of the young men in this case being willing to engage a contractor at considerable expense appears to indicate that the financial aspect is of little moment in the rich cocoa areas, such as Tekiman." But "native contractors," according to the governor, "[were] of an inferior grade" and their work was of "poor quality."[66] The chief commissioner then advised the Takyimanhene to carry out construction of the Takyiman portion of the road by using communal labor, which the governor preferred over resorting to "native contractors."[67]

The Takyimanhene and his elders, however, favored the use of "native contractors" and they estimated it would take two years to complete their portion by using such contractors. A survey for the new road was completed on 23 August 1926, with an estimated cost of £450 for twenty-one miles of new road. Construction was postponed until end of the cocoa season. On November 15 the Takyimanhene indicated that the contractors, led by a Mr. P. R. Cudjoe, were ready to begin work on the new road, and that Cudjoe's fee of £3,400 would be raised from levied taxes. However, "this suggestion received no support from the Government."[68] On 18 February 1927, the Takyimanhene requested a three-year postponement and that funds be raised by taxation, without questioning the discrepancy between Mr. Cudjoe's estimate and the original estimate. Demonstrations against the Takyimanhene erupted soon after, on April 22. The young men working under "subordinate chiefs" on respective parcels of the road made little progress. On May 20, ɔkyeame Kobina Adom, akobeahene Kofi Kyereme, and safohene Kofi Takyi withdrew their young men. Kofi Kyereme was also the uncle of Kofi Dɔnkɔ's first wife, Afia Monofie. In the end, a dispute exploded between the young men and the Takyimanhene.

On Sunday afternoon, May 22, the Takyimanhene was taken by surprise at the village of Agosa and murdered amidst heavy rains that had started the night before. Of the twenty-four accused in the murder, four elders from Takyiman were placed on trial, along with the young men implicated. Kofi Kyereme, the senior brother to Afia Monofie's father Kwabena Takyi, was one of those elders (he should not be confused with Taa Kwasi ɔbosomfoɔ Kofi Kyereme). The elders were sentenced to death, but the governor gave them life imprisonment with hard labor instead. It was determined that these elders had instigated the young men to destool (i.e., remove from office) the Takyimanhene.[69] On September 23, death sentences were handed down for seven (unnamed) prisoners, who were executed by hanging at the coastal town of Sekondi.[70] Three Takyiman elders were present. Six other (unnamed) prisoners received life imprisonment. Somehow, akobeahene Kofi Kyereme was released from prison a decade or so later. The governor wrote, "The [Takyimanhene's] murder and the lawlessness which resulted therefrom have been vindicated by the execution of seven men and the life imprisonment of six more, and the Division [of Takyiman] is now quiet."[71] Over the next three decades, those occupying the office of Takyimanhene would be removed one after the other, but without bloodshed or loss of life. In fact, elders and youth would form a close synergic bond in support of the various Takyimanhene, who would rally the townspeople in a nationalist and anti-Asante movement.

The slaying of the Takyimanhene and at least twenty-five dead from a yellow fever outbreak closed the 1920s.[72] Both instances remind us that epidemics can be facilitated by trade, especially the cocoa "prosperity of the Colony," and that sociopolitical transformations do not specifically point to planned progress; serious inadvertent consequences, specifically between the generations, escorted the prosperity sponsored by cocoa. To buoy this prosperity, officials turned to long-standing forms of farm-based organizations to improve the quality of cocoa for export and created the Registrar of Cooperative Societies in 1929. The informal *nnoboa* ("mutual help in weeding") labor exchange system and local credit schemes such as *susu* collectives were incorporated into this formal cooperative movement. Nnoboa was a task-specific system of labor organization, dissolving at the end of each task. Used widely in indigenous farming and on road or water well construction, nnoboa consisted of a group of ten individuals.[73] We have seen how the matter of communal labor for road construction led to the death of Takyimanhene Yaw Kramo.

Although cocoa farming, and agriculture in general, had the greatest pull on labor, cooperative or communal labor systems were geared more toward the cocoa industry. By 1931 the number of farmers had grown to 67,700, from a recorded 4,380 three decades earlier, and cocoa production had also grown from 216,100 to 366,700 tons annually.[74] During the same period the number of blacksmiths increased from 298 in 1911 to 1,179 in 1931. Over the next three decades, the number of documented farmers would swell to some 1.5 million and blacksmiths to 8,620.[75] Kofi Dɔnkɔ belonged to both sectors of skilled workers—producing tools for farmers and harvesting cocoa for cash. He also belonged to a cadre of new healers who were well aware of the fissions caused or aggravated by the rule of cocoa in local societies, the rule of lawyers rather than indigenous forms of law and order, and the aspirations of the young for power when this was reserved for elders. Although Kofi Dɔnkɔ was less concerned with the political aspirations of young men in the colony—which were often squashed, as evidenced when the restored Asante Confederacy abolished young men in leadership positions—the stage was set for a series of protracted clashes between older and younger men, between "chiefs" and British officials, and between missions and those they proselytized.

❈

THE CLASH BETWEEN (male) elders and young men may seem to have been ubiquitous in the southern half of the colony, but the relations between the two unfolded quite differently in Takyiman. It is not that conflict did not exist; the murder of Takyimanhene Yaw Kramo is a poignant reminder that it did. But writ large, the fault lines of power and authority ran through Taa Mensa Kwabena and its ɔbosomfoɔ Nana Kwaku Badu, who once again wielded more authority than the Takyimanhene and his council of elders. Moreover, Asubɔnten Kwabena and Taa Mensa Kwabena had worked in partnership since Takyiman's self-imposed exile and return in the late nineteenth century, and the two remained preeminent in the ritual obligations the Takyimanhene performed as a function of his office. This contract between officeholders (custodians of land held in trust for the ancestors and spiritual forces) and ritual specialists (custodians of spiritual forces of the land) was consecrated in earlier times as a mandate of sociopolitical leadership. This same social contract remained true in the Takyiman of Kofi Dɔnkɔ, so much so that Christian missions saw this as the greatest roadblock to their evangelical success. In the early 1930s the Wesleyan mission was the only missionary society in Takyiman; it was headquartered in Wankyi but one to three European missionaries were "resident at Wenchi or Tekiman."[76] As the mission correctly saw it, in "the realm of faith, we have three main rivals: (a) the traditional worship of the local deities, such as Ta Kese [Taa Mensa Kwabena] at Tekiman and Tano Obo at Mim; (b) the influence of the newer divinities, such as Kukuro at Nchira ... and (c) the irreligion ... of the educated or semi-educated for whom the old [abosom] are discredited and the claims of the new [Christian] faith too stern."[77] The confluence of these three forces, especially the bipolar profile of the semi-educated, constituted the roots of present-day Christian fanaticism in Ghana. Nonetheless, the mission commented that a belief in spiritual powers caused the "regrettable reluctance of the people to make use of the medical service provided by Government," but hoped to make advances "during the next few years, especially in the Tekiman area."[78]

As in Takyiman, so too did the Wesleyan mission view "Mim" (Mmem) as "probably the most conservative place in which we work," and it was especially troubled by "the worship of Tano Obo."[79] And there was ample reason for their worries. In 1917 W. G. Waterworth of the mission attempted to "impose [restrictions] on the worshippers of the [Tanɔ Obo]," but after local outrage and an inquiry by the provincial commissioner, "the restrictions were removed and the Mission had to compensate Ohine [ɔhene] Yao Bofa, the fetish Chief [i.e., the leader of the town and ɔbosomfoɔ of Tanɔ Obo]."[80] When Waterworth sought permission for fellow evangelist Sampson Opon to visit the town in 1923, "the Chiefs of Mim strongly disapproved of his visit," and the provincial commissioner rejected the request. Another was request was made in 1924 to visit Mim, Takyiman, and elsewhere but with police protection for Opon, given the "trouble [he caused] at Tekiman" in 1921. For the Wesleyan mission, "Sampson Oppon [sic] the evangelist [had ...] been a helping hand in the cause of Christianity," but when "this evangelist came to Tekiman for evangelical work . . . the fetish priests and priestesses together with the Omanhene [Yaw Kramo] were greatly alarmed and reported him to the commissioner at Wenchi as though disturbing their people."[81] Opon had appealed to the Takyimanhene to become a Christian, but the Takyimanhene had to "first ascertain how becoming a Christian would affect his authority and the Stool oath" he took.[82]

The Takyimanhene then rejected Opon's request, and Opon was arrested and ordered to leave Takyiman "before saying anything more." Incensed, Wesleyan officials in Wankyi viewed this outcome "as a triumph for fetishism."[83] If we substituted the caricature "fetishism" for the social contract between officeholders and spiritualists—and the broader agreement between the spiritual forces of nature and the world created by human culture—this statement would remain true. The frustrated attempts at missionary penetration and reports of the Takyimanhene drinking notwithstanding, Takyiman was one of the "cleanest" towns: its population grew from 826 in 1921 to 2,254 in 1931; its tribunal was "working excellently"; and political conflicts had "gone quietly" in the late 1920s and early 1930s.[84] It is this Takyiman polity and its community of healers that welcomed Kofi Dɔnkɔ into their contractual bonds as the next ɔbosomfoɔ for Asubɔnten Kwabena. "I was then very young," Kofi Dɔnkɔ recalled, "when I started my training to become [an ɔbosomfoɔ], I was a little older than this boy (pointing to a boy of about 13 years of age). . . . At that time, I could travel to the north to buy meat."[85] Although Kofi Dɔnkɔ was perhaps the youngest candidate, he was not the first. In fact, it was only after three other candidates failed to grasp the prerequisite skills that Kofi Dɔnkɔ was chosen.

Indeed, the standards were high, for Asubɔnten Kwabena was the second (and sometimes at par with the) most important ɔbosom in the Takyiman polity—Taa Mensa Kwabena. The inability to secure a competent medium led to a slight abeyance until Kofi Dɔnkɔ was trained. But Kofi Dɔnkɔ was not sold on the idea of becoming an ɔbosomfoɔ. As he later explained, "I was a blacksmith at that time. I was about to complete my blacksmith's course when my uncle [Kwame Ampɔnsa] selected me because there was no other suitable boy to be chosen. Many boys were tried but they could not do it and I was the fourth boy to be tried. When he appealed to me . . . I became very unhappy because I [did] not know how I [would] leave my profession to do this kind of work." But as Kofi Dɔnkɔ explained, "I however pitied my uncle because if I did not do the work, he would be compelled to do it himself notwithstanding his old age. As soon as I came, he handed me over to a trainer to train me. As soon as [my trainer Nana Kwaku Badu] completed my training, he died exactly . . . seven years after I finished."[86]

Kwame Ampɔnsa's son Kwasi Ampɔnsa Nkron Amoah knew Kofi Dɔnkɔ "when he was under his *akɔm* training. My father [Kwame] Ampɔnsa actually sent Nana Kofi Dɔnkɔ into the *akɔm* training. [Kofi Dɔnkɔ] also became my father when my real father Amponsa died."[87] Kwame Amponsa was "Fie Panin, the head of the family," an herbalist, and an ɔkɔmfoɔ "to an [ɔbosom] in the north. Amponsa's uncle was the bosomfoɔ, but the bosomfoɔ was not there and Amponsa himself could not do the work. Therefore, he had to get a boy to do it on his behalf. My grandfather," Kofi Dɔnkɔ continued, "the *bosomfoɔ* who died and whom I succeeded, he was called Kwadwo [Owusu]."[88] Kwadwo Owusu died when Kofi Dɔnkɔ was six or seven years old. Although abosomfoɔ Kofi Dɔnkɔ and Kofi Kyereme would have taken a required oath to the colonial division in which they lived—Takyiman—their real allegiance was to their respective abosom and serving their community.[89]

Kofi Dɔnkɔ's childhood friend Akosua Antwiwaa recalled, "[Kwadwo Owusu] was the *ɔbosomfoɔ* of Asubɔnten Kwabena and after his death several *abosomfoɔ* came but none was able to hear and understand the language of the *ɔbosom*. [Kofi Dɔnkɔ] came to inherit it. His uncle Nana [Kwame Amponsa] said to [Kofi Dɔnkɔ's] mother that the unborn child would be the leader and without him there will be no improvement in the house [i.e., the family] though some will come and go."[90] Akosua also remembered Kofi Dɔnkɔ "crying the day they came to take him from Akumsa Odumase to be the *ɔbosomfoɔ* because he never wanted to leave his mother and cousins. [But,] Asubɔnten said he was his 'wife' even when he was in his mother's womb. [Asubɔnten Kwabena] knew [Kofi Dɔnkɔ] before he was born." From Akosua's recollection, Kofi Dɔnkɔ "never had the chance to play much with his peers since he was taken to become an *ɔbosomfoɔ* at a tender age."[91] Kofi Dɔnkɔ was certainly not as enthusiastic as Kofi Kyereme about his calling, but once he arrived in Takyiman and began to train under Nana Kwaku Badu, he excelled at the healing arts, prepared in some ways by years of farming, learning the local pharmacopeia, communicating with ancestors, and blacksmithing.

Those skills, especially the last, took shape in Tunsuase, the blacksmith ward where Kofi Dɔnkɔ lived with his uncle and relatives. Tunsuase was a ward long known for its blacksmithing families, where lineages lived in houses built in contiguous quarters.[92] We lack earlier statistics for Tunsuase, but we can still get a sense of the ward from data collected in the early 1960s and 1970s (map 3.2). In 1961 Tunsuase had forty-one inhabited and eight unfinished houses, growing to fifty-eight inhabited and ten unfinished houses a decade later. By 1971 there was one public latrine, two to four schools, two public water taps, and three to five churches but no mosques.[93] Few livestock lived there, though for the period of Kofi Dɔnkɔ's youth the Takyiman township possessed 1 horse, 4 cattle, 72 donkeys, 846 pigs, and 1,192 sheep and goats.[94] The tsetse fly, the principal vector for sleeping sickness, killed horses and cattle throughout the entire Takyiman region, ensuring their near invisibility in any census of livestock. Asubɔnten Kwabena tabooed cattle and did not ritually consume goat; these and other ritual obligations and avoidances Kofi Dɔnkɔ would have learned during his training, along with translating that groundwork into social use, much like his skill at blacksmithing.[95]

The new healer did not fully relinquish his blacksmithing trade, though farming and healing would come to occupy much of his adult life and livelihood. "I was a blacksmith," he exclaimed, before he was selected by his uncle to become the next ɔbosomfoɔ for Asubɔnten Kwabena. In fact, he "was about to complete [his] blacksmith's course." And it seems he did complete his apprenticeship and became quite respected among other blacksmiths. Kofi Dɔnkɔ put it this way: "My grandfather [Kwadwo Owusu] who put me in this [ɔbosomfoɔ] position was a blacksmith and was the most senior son of the Adontenhene. I am the supervisor of all the other blacksmiths because my grandfather taught me the work and I know I can provide food for him—i.e., I know how to serve him better."[96] And there is reason to believe Kofi Dɔnkɔ would have continued to do some blacksmithing after he became an ɔbosomfoɔ. For one, blacksmiths were well-respected artisans, memorialized in folk consciousness. Among the people of the colony, and later the nation, that respect and the blacksmith's self-appraisal were archived in songs. Three songs should suffice to demonstrate:

Yɛnim atono oo.
Atomfoɔ yɛnim atono
Nnadeɛ yi so.
Wonim atono na wo nnadeɛ wɔ he?
Yɛnim atono oo.
Atomfoɔ yɛnim atono
Nnadeɛ yi so oo.

Asafo Akwawua kodɔ kum no
nana e,

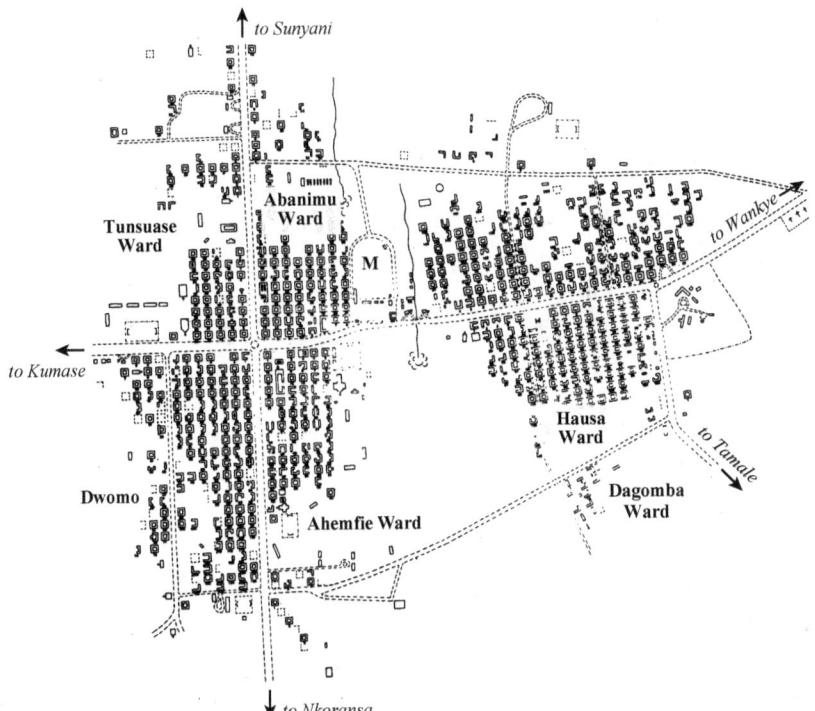

MAP 3.2. Map of Takyiman township, ca. 1971. As much as the five "roads" criss-crossing Takyiman made the area a crossroads town for trade and migrants, five "wards" or quarters where specific lineages lived demarcated the town's settled population and its demography. Kofi Dɔnkɔ lived with his uncle and relatives in the Tunsuase or blacksmith's ward, where he learned the art of blacksmithing and the healing arts. Adapted from Dennis M. Warren, "Disease, Medicine, and Religion Among the Techiman-Bono of Ghana: A Study in Culture Change" (PhD diss., Indiana University, 1974), 175.

Yɛnim atono oo.
Atomfoɔ yɛnim atono
Nnadeɛ yi so oo.

Yee Asam Kurotwianoma e,
Yɛnim atono oo.
Atomfoɔ yɛnim atono
Nnadeɛ yi so oo.

We know our craft.
Blacksmiths, we can forge

> These pieces of iron.
> You know the craft, where are your tools?
> We know our craft.
> Blacksmiths, we can forge
> These pieces of iron.
>
> Grandchild of Akwawua of Asafo killed by
> love of war,
> We know our craft.
> Blacksmiths, we can forge
> These pieces of iron.
>
> Weaver bird, the bird that stirs up the town,
> We know our craft.
> Blacksmiths, we can forge
> These pieces of iron.[97]

In the same way a blacksmith transformed "pieces of iron" into tools, a healer too learned during their training the innerworkings of their craft and were equipped with the tools of the trade. Kofi Dɔnkɔ's training in blacksmithing increased his value as a healer-to-be. But training for either blacksmithing or healing was a sacred process, packed with rituals, knowledge unknown to others outside the fraternity, and specific techniques shrouded in some secrecy. During Kofi Dɔnkɔ's training, colonial anthropologist Robert Rattray traveled to Takyiman and devoted some attention to Bono spiritual culture, but his and Kofi Dɔnkɔ's paths never crossed. Kofi Dɔnkɔ would have been in the earlier stages of his six and a half years of training and was a very young trainee, not the old "grey-beards" Rattray preferred. Using his experiences in Takyiman, Rattray regarded the polity as "the ideal ground upon which to study Akan customs and beliefs."[98] In *Religion & Art in Ashanti* published in 1927, Rattray revealed some of the curriculum for healers in training, but his passing insights were no stand-in for the healer's coveted yet almost inaccessible experiential knowledge.[99] The lid sealing that knowledge was a sacred oath of confidentiality—consecrated by rituals—which all abosomfoɔ and akɔmfoɔ make. Guided by that covenant between Kofi Dɔnkɔ and Nana Kwaku Badu, we can do no more than provide a general sense of Kofi Dɔnkɔ's training.

When Kofi Dɔnkɔ was chosen by his family to become the next ɔbosomfoɔ, he was adorned with white cloth and white clay markings on his body, and then he, an alcoholic drink, and a chicken were presented to

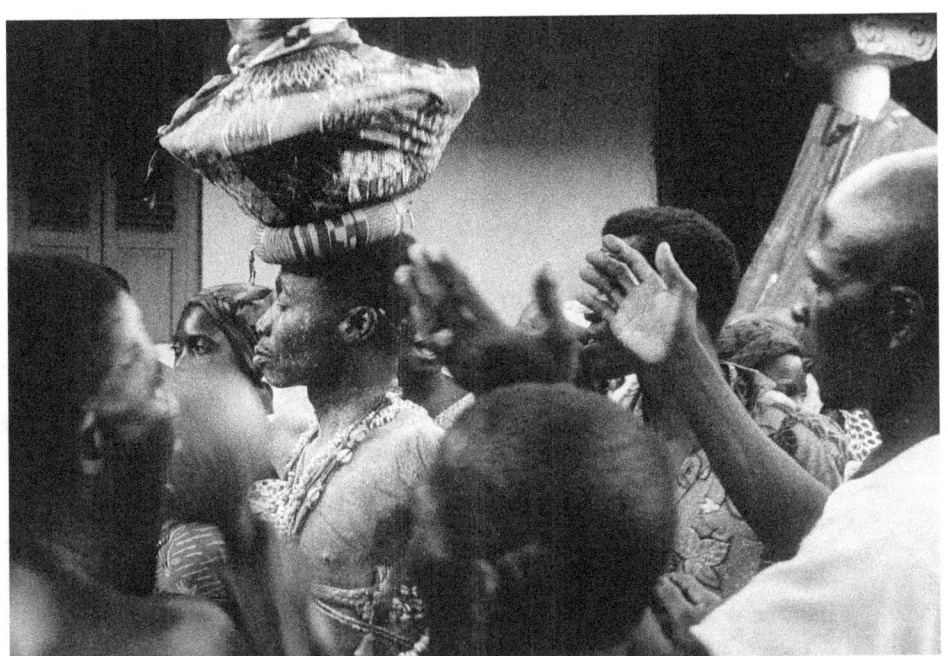

FIGURE 3.3. Kofi Dɔnkɔ carrying the Asubɔnten Kwabena shrine at the Takyiman Fofie Festival, 6 October 1970. From the Dennis Michael Warren Slide Collection, Special Collections Department, University of Iowa Libraries. Used courtesy of Greg Prickman, Head of Special Collections.

Asubɔnten Kwabena. Afterward the ɔbosom was asked to go into spiritual communion ("trance") with Kofi Dɔnkɔ when he carried the *ayawa* containing the "shrine" on his head. After the ritual sacrifice of the chicken, a special day was set aside where shrine elders invited singers and drummers, and a senior ɔbosomfoɔ of another ɔbosom (in this case Taa Mensa Kwabena), to pour libation on the *kahyire* (*kente* cloth pad) that sat on Kofi Dɔnkɔ's head beneath the ayawa, amidst singing and drumming (figure 3.3). Listen to a number of those songs:

1 *Yee yee, mɛkɔ ne nsamanfoɔ agoro, kyerɛ sɛ mehunu wiem oo*
 Sakyi Akomea akaneho, ɔbɛkɔ akɔne samanfoɔ agoro, kyerɛ sɛ ɔbɛhunu wiem oo
 I will go and play with the ancestors so I will be able to see through the skies
 Sakyi Akomea has received the spirit, he will go and play with the ancestors so he can see through the skies

Tools of the Trade 97

2 ɔhene ayowa a, akɔmmere wɔ no,
  Nana ee, hyira makɔm so oo
  The town leader's wife who deserves red beads
  Nana, bless my akɔm initiation training

3 Gya ne awuroko oo, Sakyi awurokoo.
  Akɔm suman awuroko gya ne wu oo
  Yɛhunu bi yɛwu oo, yɛhunu bi yɛ nya kwa oo
  Fire and beads, Sakyi beads (specific type of bead)
  Akɔm talisman bead has been administered on you
  We see some and we die, and some we see, we live.

4 Ee, bɛhyɛ den oo anowa hunu yɛ oo
  ɔbɛyɛ dɛn na me bɛyɛ den na wahunu yɛ oo
  Wo bɛyɛ den na wahunu yɛ oo, tete akomfoɔ ɔbɛyɛ dɛn na wahunu akɔm yi oo
  He came to be made strong and great
  What did he come to learn and see?
  How is he going to learn this akɔm training from the ancient akɔm practitioners?

5 Nkɔmmoa hena ɛna oo, nkɔmmoa hena ne gye mene muo mesoa gya mentumi
  Ee osono agya kokroko
  Osono agya Takora
  A good akɔm dance is not easy to dance for it is like carrying a load of firewood which you are unable to carry
  The biggest elephant of all
  Taa Kora (Tanɔ), the father of elephants

6 otonsi ampono oo, ɔbosom na mane wɔ bɛ, ɔbosom na mane wɔ bɛ, ɔbɔ ɔbosom na mane wɔ bɛ oo
  Totonsi ampono oo, Tano na mane wɔ bɛ, Tano na mane wɔ bɛ
  Kwabena Asubonten na mane wɔ bɛ oo
  Asuotipa na mane wɔ no oo
  ɔbosom na mane wɔ bɛ
  The abosom are the custodians and keepers of the land, the owner will not leave you
  A custodian, Tanɔ is the custodian and keeper of the land
  Kwabena Asubɔnten is the owner of the land

Asuotipa is the custodian of the land
The abosom are the custodians/keepers of the land.

These songs need little interpretation considering Kofi Dɔnkɔ's ontological world outlined in the first chapter. But if we look beyond their face value, each song reveals something about the training of healers, not in their exactness but in the inevitability of the journey—"How is he going to learn this akɔm training from the ancient akɔm practitioners?" As we have already seen, "The abosom are the custodians and keepers of the land," and they, "the owner" of the land, "will not leave" the trainee—*Akomea* was shorthand for trainee. Such affirmation, however, was often spiced with soberness: "A good akɔm dance is not easy to dance for it is like carrying a load of firewood which you are unable to carry." For the ɔbosomfoɔ, who had to literally carry the ayawa on his head to go into spiritual communion with his ɔbosom, that message was not only a truism for his lifelong practice but also for the very beginning of his training. Once the ɔbosom goes into spiritual communion with the candidate, the ayawa is removed from his head. This step is repeated three times, followed by a final removal of the kahyire, which signals the ɔbosom's acceptance of the candidate. According to BM observers, "he is on the day of his consecration shaved from head to toe, bathed completely, oiled, and dressed in a white gown. When he is thus prepared, the rest of the priests arrive and lead him to the fetish stool and let him quickly sit down on it three times."[100] Once accepted, Kofi Dɔnkɔ was placed under the care of Taa Mensa Kwabena ɔbosomfoɔ Kwaku Badu for training (figure 3.4). Kofi Dɔnkɔ would have been inundated with medicines in the first year—drinking, bathing, incisions, and for the eyes and ears—and then taken to a graveyard where other medicines were prepared for him to bathe with during the second year.

Most training ends in year three, but as BM observers noted, "if the person in question is acceptable to the council of fetish priests, the person has to apprentice with one of them for two years or also longer."[101] Kofi Dɔnkɔ's training lasted six years and seven months, receiving his graduation ritual—called *kumkuma*—much later than the average trainee. The length of Kofi Dɔnkɔ's understudy confirms his youth; young or immature candidates averaged six to seven years of training. Kofi Dɔnkɔ's family and other healers assembled for the kumkuma ceremony. Dɔnkɔ's family, in consultation with Nana Kwaku Badu, would have gathered the following items: two black chickens (one for Onyame, the other for Asase Yaa), a

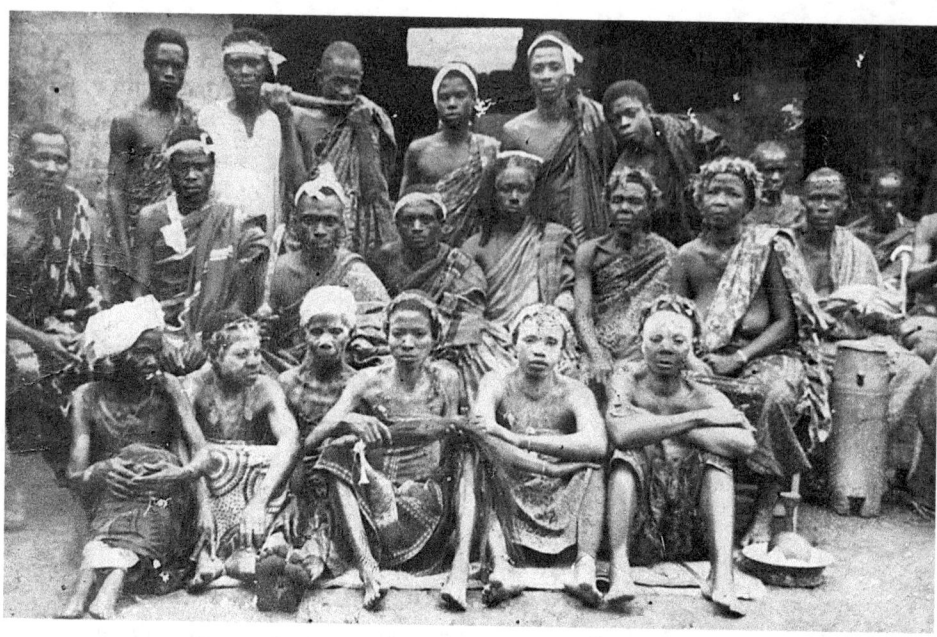

FIGURE 3.4. Group photo of healers and trainees during the funeral of Nana Kwasi Yankam, Boonin ɔbosomfoɔ of Sansama, Taa Mensa Kwabena *bosomfie*, Takyiman, ca. 1967–68. First row, left to right: Kɔmfo Abena of Tuobodom (middle), Adwoa Akumsa, Akumsa ɔkɔmfoɔ (end). Second row, left to right: Kofi Mosi, Taa Mensa Kwabena ɔbosomfoɔ; Kofi Kyereme, Taa Kwasi ɔbosomfoɔ (middle); Adwoa Fodwoɔ, *sodohemaa* (end). From Nana Kofi Dɔnkɔ Collection, in private hands, Takyiman, Ghana. Used courtesy of Kofi Sakyi Sapɔn.

new pot, a knife, plant medicines (e.g., *adubrafo, humatre, ɔde, ɔdwannkyene, akokɔduru*), hair, raffia (from the dɔsoɔ worn during training), black powdered composite medicine (*mɔtɔ*), feathers from the chickens, thirty eggs (cooked with mɔtɔ), green plantain and roasted corn (for eating), and scissors to cut the candidate's *mpɛsɛmpɛsɛ* hairstyle.

If the sacrificed chickens were accepted, this meant Kofi Dɔnkɔ had not broken any of his taboos; if they were not accepted, he would retrain for three more years and pay a fine of one sheep, cash, and alcoholic drinks. All went well, and thus Kofi Dɔnkɔ's mpɛsɛmpɛsɛ hairstyle was cut, giving him the short, almost bald hairstyle typical of the Tanɔ ɔbosomfoɔ.[102] The herbs were cooked to make mɔtɔ and the chickens were cooked with mɔtɔ. The raffia was added to the pot: because Kofi Dɔnkɔ bathed frequently using many "powerful" plants while training, the power (*tumi*) absorbed by the raffia would make an equally powerful mɔtɔ. Before the chickens are fully cooked, the candidate and those who helped in his training walk around the pot seven times, patting the pot and dipping their fingers into the pot to taste the broth each time.[103] Having successfully completed his atypically long training, he assumed the title "Nana" and henceforth became Nana Kofi Dɔnkɔ. Sometime during his early to mid-twenties, Kofi Dɔnkɔ set out to serve his community and the ɔbosom that knew him before birth but that had a history bound to Takyiman long before Kofi Dɔnkɔ was born.

❃

AS NOTED IN chapter 1, there are competing stories about the identity and source of Kofi Dɔnkɔ's Asubɔnten Kwabena. According to Dɔnkɔ's family, Asubɔnten Kwabena is the second iteration of an Asubɔnten associated with a river in present-day Nkoransa but that was part of old Nyafoman in the Bono kingdom. The compound term *asubɔnten* refers to a "river created to run straight/long," or as Rattray defined it, a "street river," deduced from a combination of *asu* (river) and *abɔntén* (main street).[104] Whatever the actual etymology, it is clear the subject is a river. But what kind of river? The Asubɔnten Kwabena in question is recognized by multiple praise names that qualify it: Asubɔnten Kafena, Kwabena Tenten, Kwabena Asuo, Kwabena Bɛte Kwane Mu, and Bediako Te Kwane Mu.[105] When was Asubɔnten Kwabena created? Kofi Dɔnkɔ conceded it was "difficult to know; likewise the events which led to the creation of the [ɔbosom] were hidden by the ancestors."[106] We know Asubɔnten Kwabena revealed itself on a Tuesday (Kwabena) and was as old as the Bono kingdom, be it Nyafoman or Tanɔso. Sometime during the nineteenth century Kofi Dɔnkɔ's grandmother Nana Arku Bagyei brought the ɔbosom or an iteration of it from Nkoransa to Takyiman. According to Kofi Dɔnkɔ, "My grandmother and the then Takyimanhene had one father. For that reason, she came to greet her brother, and he gave her somewhere to stay. It was through that that she went back and brought [Asubɔnten] here [i.e., Takyiman]." A war erupted between Takyiman and Asante a year and half later, in 1875. "When the war broke out," Kofi Dɔnkɔ continued, "[Asubɔnten] Kwabena decided to take the people to Gyama [ca. 1877].... [From Takyiman to Baafi, Kranka, and Wankyi and across the Tain River to Gyaman Asubɔnten] Kwabena alone had his own township like this place [called Badu Akura].... Each of the [abosom] had his own town."[107]

Upon their return from Gyaman,

we stayed at the other side of the Tano River. After that, Abanem Tano [Taa Mensa Kwabena] showed us a place under that Dadeɛ tree [...] for us to go and stay. [Taa Mensa Kwabena] was the owner of the land and therefore asked us to stay there.... At the end of each year, we had to go to Nkoransa to perform the necessary customary rites [for Asubɔnten.... Asubɔnten] stayed at Akumsa Odumase [for some years...] during the reign of Takyimanhene Nana Konkroma. He made an effort to have [Asubɔnten] back here. He had to slaughter about seven sheep before it returned. When it came back its landlord was the Adontenhene.[108]

Although Asubɔnten Kwabena is linked to a Tanɔ pedigree, as perhaps all significant rivers ultimately are, it is genealogically viewed as the second-born offspring of Akumsa and thus called Asubɔnten Manu (second-born child), but also the offspring of Taa Kora and Kranka Afua.[109] It is certainly plausible to have two Asubɔnten Kwabena from the same polity and kingdom—or two polities under the same kingdom—but if we use the metric of seniority, it bears to reason Asubɔnten Kwabena is a "child" of Taa Kora, and that offspring could have had iterations at Tanɔso and in Nkoransa, made intelligible by the same (praise) name, as in the case of multitudes of Taa Kofi or Taa Kwabena. Assuming Tanɔboase, the locus of Taa Kora, is the source, there is an equal twenty-six-mile distance between the Tanɔso and Nkoransa and between Nkoransa and Tanɔboase. That Takyiman sits perpendicular to all three sites—Tanɔboase (north), Tanɔso (south), and Nkoransa (east)—suggests a triangular radius for the diffusion of Asubɔnten Kwabena and strengthens the claim for a Tanɔ River provenance (figure 3.5).

As Nana Amea Ampromfi was the town founder and first custodian for Asubɔnten Kwabena at Tanɔso, so too was Nana Arku Bagyei the founder and first ɔkɔmfoɔ for Asubɔnten Kwabena at Akumsa Odumase. Arku Bagyei not only brought the shrine from Akumsa Odumase to Takyiman, she also procured and acted as custodian for the abosom Akumsa and Pro Kwasi. "Since she was a woman," Kofi Dɔnkɔ reasoned, "she never ate any food sacrificed to Asubɔnten. She never ate any meat or drank any wine offered to the [ɔbosom]; she could only accept money. She could, however, eat animals sacrificed to the [abosom] Akumsa and Pro [Kwasi]. Little is known of the origin of these [abosom], except that it was [Arku Bagyei] who brought the [ɔbosom] Asubɔnten [and] who gave birth to them. The woman took Asubɔnten and the other [abosom] to Gyama during the war [with Asante].

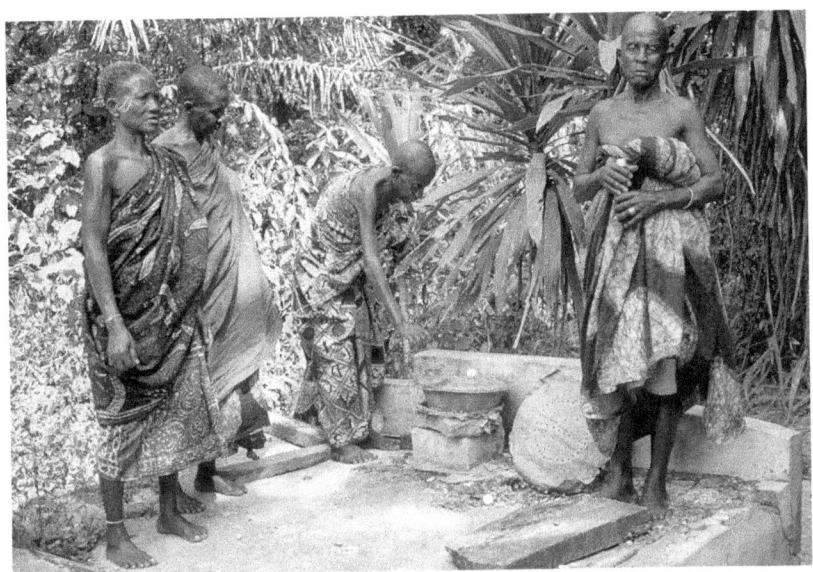

FIGURE 3.5. Tanɔso Asubɔnten at the Tanɔ River. Abena Tutu (far left) and her *akyeame* Kwadwo Amoa (center) and Kwadwo Dakrobo (right), 24 January 1971. From the Dennis Michael Warren Slide Collection, Special Collections Department, University of Iowa Libraries. Used courtesy of Greg Prickman, Head of Special Collections.

All these [abosom] accompanied Taa Mensah." Further, Kofi Dɔnkɔ indicated that "anyone who becomes [ɔbosomfoɔ] for Asubɔnten is also responsible for Akumsa and Pro [Kwasi, and thus . . .] Akumsa and Pro [Kwasi] celebrate their yam festival on Kwabena together with Asubɔnten."[110]

Kofi Dɔnkɔ recounted during an interview a remarkable family history, charting how his family and Asubɔnten Kwabena migrated from Akumsa Odumase to Takyiman; his elder sister Adwoa Akumsa related a similar story written on a single five-by-eight sheet of paper. We start with Kofi Dɔnkɔ's account, beginning with Nana Arku Bagyei:

> Obaa [Arku Bagyei] was a paternal sister to the Omanhene of Techiman. When she came to Techiman to visit him, she decided to stay permanently as he was very hospitable. Later, she made love to the Adontenhene of Techiman, Nana Diaka Owusu. The Omanhene, her brother, was very pleased and gave her to Nana Diaka Owusu to marry. When Diaka Owusu died, he was succeeded by Nana Otomfo ["blacksmith"] Kwabena Kera. He married his predecessor's wife,

the priestess [Arku Bagyei], and they had a son called Okomfo Kofi Dua. Asubonten was taken from Nkoranza and brought to Techiman where the priestess had taken up her abode. When Okomfo Kofi Dua grew up, he took over his mother's work and became the first [male] priest for Asubonten. A few years elapsed and the second battle between Asante and Techiman ensued. Both armies fought well but the Asante were more powerful; they overcame Techiman and the Techiman people sought refuge at Gyama [Gyaman]. Taa Mensah and Asubonten took the people to Gyama. The Omanhene who took Techiman to Gyama was Nana Kwabena Fofie. He died before he could come back to Techiman. His successor, Nana Gyako, brought the people back from exile. Techiman started a new life. All their houses and farms had been destroyed by the Asante army. People started to build new houses and gradually the town began to develop again.[111]

Though attributed to Adwoa Akumsa, the following account was recorded by a scribe of the family. Much of the account is intelligible, but a few areas are marked *torn* (indicating where the paper was torn and where words are illegible).

Madam Adwoa Akumsa told us, how we came from our town Akumsa Domasi to Techiman. Nana Domasihene whose time our grandfathers and mothers were referred to Techiman was Bodee Dwaa. Nana Komfour [ɔkɔmfoɔ] Dabia, Akumsa Fetish Priest said that war would come. So Nana Domasihene Bodee Dwaa send [sic] our grandmothers named Nana Arku Bagyei, [Afia] Asubonteng and Asuabea [i.e., Adwoa Akumsa] to Techiman to be kept because maybe the war would come. Techiman chief of that time was Ohene Ameyaw. Secondly, Nana Bodee Dwaa sent Ama Asubonteng and Arku Bagyei to Nana Takra who was Ankobeahene at Techiman but he refused to get them. So Nana Bodee rather referred them to Adontenhene who was called Nana Kwao Boraa [a.k.a. Diaka Owusu?]. He was called Atomfohene. Fetish Asubonteng [i.e., Asubɔnten Kwabena] changed [*torn*] from Atomfohene to Adontenhene, [*torn*] they were led to war at Germa [Gyaman]. [*Torn*] they were going to face the war, [*torn*] Ofuma. There Asubonteng Fetish said to Nana Kwao Boraa that he should take thirty three (33) people to return back to face the war. They returned and met . . . [*the writing abruptly ends here*][112]

In all available accounts of Takyiman's nineteenth-century exile and return the two principal abosom of the polity—Taa Mensa Kwabena and Asubɔnten Kwabena—were central, nonhuman figures. Among the custodians for Asubɔnten Kwabena missing from the above accounts were those that followed Kofi Dua: Nana Kwadwo Ampɔnsa, Kwadwo Owusu (a.k.a. Kwadwo Asubɔnten), ɔkɔmfoɔ Gyapon (who "could not do the work"), Kwadwo Aboagye (who "was not able to do the work"), and once more ɔkɔmfoɔ Gyapon, who "came back to do the work again."[113] Nana Gyapon, like Nana Aboagye, "could not understand the language for the [ɔbosom] and therefore he was destooled." Kofi Dɔnkɔ succeeded him during the second reign of Takyimanhene Yaw Ameyaw in the 1930s, but Gyapon's nephew Kofi Ɔboɔ and his niece Akua Anane (Asantewaa) would later become the ɔkyeame and an ɔkɔmfoɔ for Asubɔnten Kwabena, respectively.[114] Born to Kwaku Owusu and Afia Fofie (Gyapon's sister), Akua and Kofi were Kofi Dɔnkɔ's niece and nephew. These family ties have been central since at least the time of Nana Arku Bagyei, and the prominence of Asubɔnten Kwabena in their lives and in the life of Takyiman has been equally significant. So much so that the Takyimanhene remained in "close communication with the [ɔbosom] and pays his contribution to the [ɔbosom's] festivals on Kwabena" (Tuesday) during the "new year" period, occasioned by the appearance of new yams around August or September.

The role taken on by the Takyimanhene was one the Odumasehene Bodee Dwaa played while Asubɔnten Kwabena was in Akumsa Odumase. The Odumasehene, according to Adwoa Akumsa, "would have to provide the yam that will be used to make the *etɔ* (mashed yam) for the *abosom* and ancestors on the Kwabena day. The mashed yam is made without palm oil. The next day Monowukuo is used as purely for drumming and dancing by the male and female *akɔmfoɔ* who might attend the festival. We kill the sheep, the blood is sprinkled on the shrines of the *abosom*, and the meat is distributed among the elders of the Akumsa shrine."[115] The communal significance of Asubɔnten Kwabena was encoded in two major festivals in which the entire Takyiman polity participated—the Apoɔ festival in March or April and Asubɔnten Kwabena's annual festival "celebrated on a Tuesday (Kwabena), five days after the Fofie (the yam festival day for the [Takyimanhene] of Techiman). The ɔbosomfoɔ gives the [ɔbosom] a sheep, some yams and eggs. The [Takyimanhene] also sends the [ɔbosom] yams, oil, salt and wine for the important day, since the [ɔbosom] is his sister's. The Adontenhene also sends the [ɔbosom] yams and wine since it is his wife's [ɔbosom]. The Krontihene and the [ɔbosomfoɔ] of Taa Mensah also send yams. The yams are cooked and the sheep is slaughtered as a sacrifice to the [ɔbosom]. A libation is also poured for the long life and prosperity of the town and her people."[116] The major themes of religion/spirituality, health, and family would take more intimate shape as Kofi Dɔnkɔ and a new class of healers worked for the "prosperity of the town and her people," and as Kofi Dɔnkɔ grew into a life of medicine, of marriage, and of navigating the politics of a colonial territory.

CHAPTER 4. **MEDICINE, MARRIAGE, AND POLITICS**

"Assist this State to have Progress"

Men walk through the forest.... They see many things. But they see little.
They hear many forest sounds. But they hear little.... A healer sees differently.
He hears differently.
—AYI KWEI ARMAH, *The Healers*

Through Asubɔnten Kwabena, Kofi Dɔnkɔ grew to be a most effective healer, evidenced by records he and observers left between the late 1960s and early 1990s. Although we have no more than anecdotal impressions before the 1960s, evidence for a remarkably productive Kofi Dɔnkɔ in his elderly years firmly suggests that a younger Kofi Dɔnkɔ would have been equally if not more prodigious from the late 1930s to the early 1960s (figure 4.1). During these years, by necessity he not only focused on maladies traumatizing the colony—malaria, yellow fever, sleeping sickness—but also paid specialized attention to barrenness, tuberculosis, cancers, stomachaches, coughs, heart diseases, and mental diseases, the latter of which his sister Adwoa Akumsa avoided because she was admittedly "afraid of mad people."[1] The healer also helped individuals obtain jobs and extend their temporal lives, and he generally made concrete progress possible in the life of Takyiman residents, in his words propelling "this state to have progress."[2] One of the most significant facets of Kofi Dɔnkɔ's approach to his craft was an enduring quest for knowledge. He acquired the whereabouts, types, preparations,

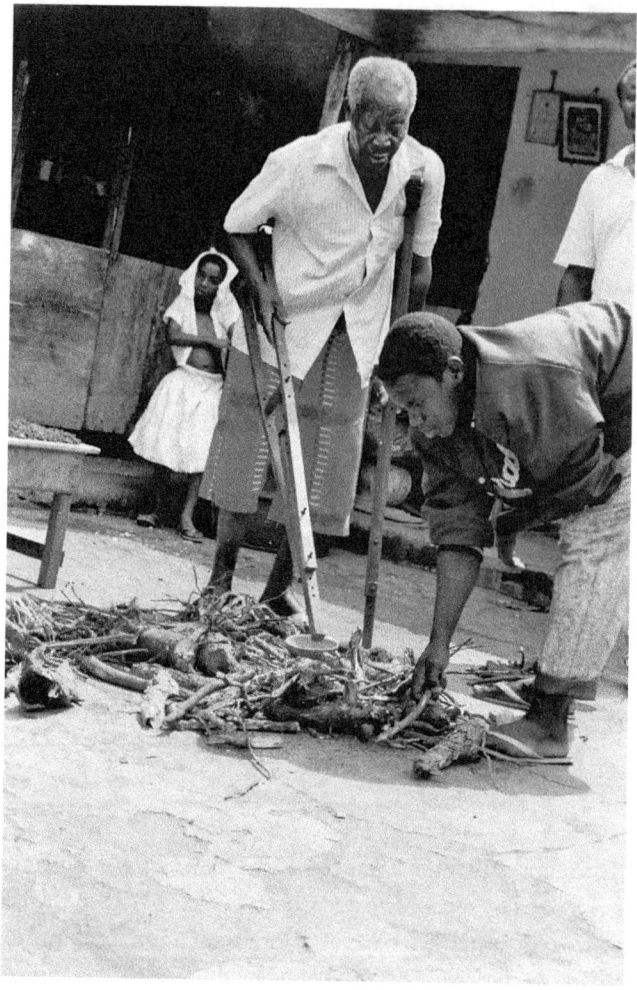

FIGURE 4.1. Kofi Dɔnkɔ preparing an herbal medicine with the help of a young man, ca. 1991. From Nana Kofi Dɔnkɔ Collection, in private hands, Takyiman, Ghana. Used courtesy of Kofi Sakyi Sapɔn.

and uses of a vast library of medicines through Asubɔnten Kwabena, other healers, gifts, and travel, especially to northern Gold Coast/Ghana. Nana Kwaku Sakyi, a former trainee and adopted son from the Caribbean, recalled, "I did hear that he traveled far to acquire knowledge and *asuman*. [Afia Monofie] said he left children wherever he traveled. I know he went north and pretended to be a Muslim so as not to endanger his life since he was a traditional practitioner."[3] He translated that evolving knowledge into therapeutic use, and he did not charge "very much when he cured diseases. At times, he used to charge nine pence or one shilling and sixpence, a pot of palm wine, a chicken and some eggs."[4] The kind of "payments" he received ensured those excluded from or who rejected the colonial cash economy could be treated in exchange for the cultural currency of sheep, fowl, eggs, palm wine, or alcoholic drinks. These items of giving thanks signified a feedback loop wherein patients communicated their illness and history, healers consulted spiritual forces to guide the procurement and use of suitable medicine, patients received treatment, and if treatment was efficacious the *abosom* and their caretakers received payment (in cases of unsuccessful remedy, patients would either seek another healer or medical facility).

The blacksmith, farmer, and healer in Kofi Dɔnkɔ constituted a skill set parlayed into a decent livelihood, all made possible by producing tools and implements for farmers and metal wares and bracelets for healers. He and his first wife, Afia Monofie, would invest time and energy in his healing vocation and in their cocoa, yam, plantain, cassava, and cocoyam farms. Whereas starches from cassava and yam were for local consumption, the most prosperous cash crop was cocoa, the "staple product" of most people who lived "in small villages and are engaged in farming."[5] And so, Kofi Dɔnkɔ and his wife placed their farming energies into cocoa (figure 4.2). Cocoa farms were established in a year, with one-fourth of one's time and labor devoted to planting and harvesting the major shade crop (plantain) and other food items. The major task of weeding consumed much time on a full, bearing farm. Then land was cleared, cocoa harvested, maintenance performed, and cocoa dried.[6] Extracting cocoa meant opening the pods and fermenting and drying the beans—farmers hired laborers called *nkokouano* to extract cocoa for a fixed price, but these nkokouano had no duty to help with food crops.[7] Stranger-farmers who were not members of a stool (symbol of custodianship) were granted farming rights in exchange for giving one-third of cocoa produced to local rulers who, as land custodians, used the *abusa* system whenever gold, rubber, or cocoa were extracted on their lands. This practice was exploited by private farmers, and Kofi Dɔnkɔ did the same.[8] After working on Nana Kwaku Badu's farm, Kofi Dɔnkɔ and Afia Monofie started a cocoa farm at Dumasum on the Takyiman-Nkoransa road, but then relinquished management of and laboring on the farm to Kwadwo Mensa of Oforikrom under the abusa system. This chapter focuses on the politics of and competing claims to land, religious authority, and decolonization during Kofi Dɔnkɔ's adulthood, as cocoa and other natural resources buoyed the colony, and pays specific attention to his layered role as blacksmith, healer, farmer, husband, and father.

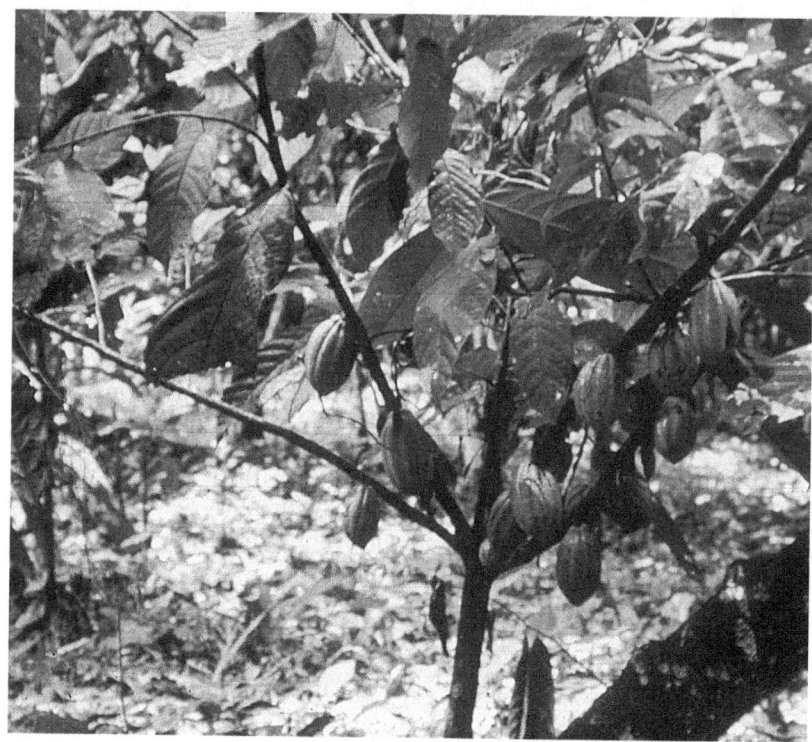

FIGURE 4.2. Cocoa trees in Takyiman, July 1974. From the Dennis Michael Warren Slide Collection, Special Collections Department, University of Iowa Libraries. Used courtesy of Greg Prickman, Head of Special Collections.

AROUND 22 YEARS OF AGE in 1935, Kofi Dɔnkɔ witnessed yet another twist in the fight for Takyiman lands between the Takyimanhene, the Asante leadership, and the colonial administration. We have already seen how the nine villages belonging to Takyiman were captured and placed under Asante officeholders in the wake of the Takyiman-Asante war of 1877. At the end of the nineteenth century, Takyiman convinced the colonial government to return the nine villages by seizing on Asante capitulation to British overlordship, Agyeman Perempe's exile to the Seychelles, British anti-Asante sentiments, and Britain's interest in the northeast trade once controlled by Asante. A colonial court ruling in 1935, however, overturned the previous decision to revert the villages to Takyiman. Now, these villages of agrarian and spiritual importance were incorporated into Asante's territory under the auspices of the Asante Confederacy, which was reinaugurated in 1935. Prompted by a crisis of "indirect rule" in the 1920s, the

Asante Confederacy was restored along "traditional" lines through colonial officials who used a blueprint outlined in Rattray's *Ashanti Law and Constitution* (1929).[9] By colonial necessity, however, "indirect rule" also subverted indigenous bases and structures of authority, contributing significantly to the morass of succession disputes and cases of destoolment (i.e., removal from indigenous office).[10] In these instances and others, constant destoolment became the norm, and Takyiman was not spared. Takyimanhene Kwasi Twi conceded to his destoolment in 1936 after providing an impetus for the Bonokyɛmpem movement that defined Bono identity in opposition to political allegiance to the Asantehene and the Asante Confederacy a year earlier.[11] Ironically, only a few years earlier, the Takyimanhene had received an Asante Loyalty Medal for "those Chiefs who have proved their loyalty."[12] Nonetheless, Nana Kwaku Kyereme (r. 1937–41) became the new Takyimanhene and continued the struggle to reclaim the nine villages, but he was also destooled. Nana Kwaku Gyako III (r. 1941–44) succumbed to the same fate as his immediate predecessor.

A common denominator in these destoolment cases was the claims of political aspirants who viewed themselves as more "civilized" and "modern" during an era of renewed cocoa cultivation, social anxiety, and culturally ambiguous responses to the tidal waves of commercialism and Christian missions. For Takyiman, commerce came through the town without leaving a trail of great prosperity; only the Wesleyan mission had a presence, yet even then, and into the 1930s, its activities were significantly constrained. In 1936 the Roman Catholic mission established a parish some miles from the sacred Tanɔ cave and grove in Tanɔboase, soon erecting a monastery on disputed lands belonging to Takyiman but claimed or controlled by Asante. In fact, the Catholic parish was the evangelical extension of the diocese in Kumase, under which it and the village of Tanɔboase was subordinate. During the next decade Roman Catholic schools were established in the Takyiman villages of Aworowa and Taakofiano (in 1942–43) by teacher-catechist Sidney Andrew Quashie. Readers will recall from chapter 3 that Quashie was also responsible for an Anglican school in Nkoransa some two decades earlier. While Quashie remained the head teacher at Aworowa for only two years, his successor, Yaw Effa, lasted one year and was followed by J. A. Asamoah in 1945. The school reopened in 1946 with students being sent to the Taakofiano site. Averaging twenty-five to thirty-five students during its years in operation, Asamoah pleaded with the Takyimanhene to "ask his people to send in more children."[13] The school at Taakofiano opened an infant school in 1945 with some thirty-seven children, but it, too, under teacher Amadu Hakeen, was "strongly fighting for more children to fill the school."[14] Except for modest gains in the Gold Coast colony, that is, the coastal region and its hinterlands, the number of mission schools and attending students throughout the tripartite colony was as impactful as these schools in Takyiman or the Basel mission school in Nkoransa (table 4.1).

As Christian missions began to break evangelical ground in Takyiman, the importation of these church-schools literally followed the rapid expansion of road construction and transport made possible by cocoa. While missions were given some liberty to proliferate, cocoa was kept under tight colonial control. The Carriage of Goods Road Ordinance passed in 1937 prohibited the transport of cocoa to the coast by road. The roads were equipped with barriers and police that inspected vehicles, and this lasted until the 1940s. Given the centrality of cocoa within the colony's economy, the West African Produce Control Board standardized the buying prices of cocoa, which gave producers the same price in upcountry locales such as Takyiman as in the coastal port areas, to mitigate the inducement to send cocoa by road, guaranteeing railways the ability to transport cocoa unfettered. In this instance Kofi Dɔnkɔ would have enjoyed some relative success from cocoa farming but would have been cautious of the Christian missions and the new diseases that followed the roads paved by the cocoa and timber industries. But he would have been doubly concerned by a smallpox outbreak in Takyiman traced to an infected thirteen-year-old from Ivory Coast and the vaccination campaign to eradicate it, as well as the "swollen shoot" disease that severely affected the prized cocoa trees.[15] The disease was first identified in 1936, and it was spread from tree to tree by a bug that fed on the sap of infected trees; a diseased tree died within sixteen to twenty-four months.[16] Much was at stake because the cocoa industry remained in the hands of independent farmers of small plots, who competed with multiple and absentee property owners, employed migrant laborers, and dealt with violent price fluctuations. A buying agreement to purchase the bulk of cocoa by twelve firms led to a five-month "holdup" and a boycott of European goods, creating a popular grassroots movement, led by farmers such as Kofi Dɔnkɔ, that suspended the agreement.[17] As the holdup and boycott shook the entire cocoa industry, so did the most destructive earthquake in the colony's history. The 6.5-magnitude earthquake affected all, killing seventeen and injuring hundreds within thirty seconds.[18]

LESS SEISMIC BUT equally significant in Kofi Dɔnkɔ's life was family. Toward the end of the 1930s and into the next decade, Kofi Dɔnkɔ found himself with several wives, a growing family, and children of his own.[19] He first married Afia Monofie (Kwaa), but under uncommon circumstances. Afia Monofie's parents, Abena Adomaa and Kwabena Takyi, had difficulty having a female child and petitioned Asubɔnten Kwabena for a spiritual intervention. Kofi Dɔnkɔ and his sister Adwoa Akumsa were the beneficiaries of this common practice. Afia's parents agreed to a cultural stipulation: if a female child were conceived, she would be given as a "wife" to the *ɔbosomfoɔ* who succeeded the elderly Kwadwo Owusu. Once Kofi Dɔnkɔ became the next ɔbosomfoɔ, he was scheduled to marry Afia Monofie when she came of age. When Afia was an adolescent, Kofi Dɔnkɔ's father, Yaw Badu, arranged an *asiwa awadeɛ* (marriage between a [unborn] girl child and a suitor who provides for the child's family until her puberty) and informed his family, who began to provide food and money to Afia Monofie's family.[20] From expressions of interest to consummation, the hands-on process of Akan marriages flowed through the suitor's maternal uncle, who functioned as representative of and liaison for the suitor and his family in all interactions with the bride's lineage head.[21] Kofi Dɔnkɔ's maternal uncle Kwame Ampɔnsa performed this role by presenting alcoholic drinks for libations and thank-you gifts to Afia Monofie's father, lineage head, and matrilineal kin.[22]

Certainly, Afia Monofie could have withdrawn from the *asiwa* marriage agreement between her parents and Kofi Dɔnkɔ's family, but she and her family would then have to repay all the money, gifts, and expenses incurred by Kofi Dɔnkɔ's family. Until then she was not free to remarry, as it were. In the early 1940s the teenaged Afia Monofie had her first menstrual discharge (*kyima*), which announced sexual maturity and the biological beginnings of womanhood. Soon thereafter, Afia underwent her public *bragorɔ* rites of passage, with the requisite supplies and gifts provided by Kofi Dɔnkɔ and his family. Basel missionaries described bragorɔ this way: "If a daughter has her first menstrual period, her mother ... runs around in the city and announces the happy news ... [Then] the daughter is made beautiful by having her hair shaved off around her head, having her neck, arms and legs being adorned with clumps of gold 'soul gold' and strings of pearls and being draped with precious cloths. ... Thereby the women are singing: 'She did it, she did it. Our sister has accomplished it!' ... Now the girl is led in a solemn procession by women ... to the waters and is bathed by her mother."[23] Afia Asubɔnten, the other elder sister of Kofi Dɔnkɔ, procured

TABLE 4.1. Schools Inspected and Assisted by the Gold Coast Board of Education*

	Basel Mission	Wesleyan Mission	Roman Catholic Mission	Islamic	Bremen Mission
1898	47	54	11		
1899	60	50	12	1	
1900	61	55	12	2	
1901	61	49	12	3	3
1902	57	43	10	1	6
1903	55	41	12	1	7
1904					
1905					
1906	58	52	14	1	11
1907	61	48	18	1	10
1908	60	49	19	1	11
1909	65	49	21		12
1910	63	48	23		13
1911	62	46	22		15
1912	69	32	22		16
1913	64	31	26		15
1914	67	31	28		15
1915	67	34	29		15
1916	68	39	32		15
1917	76	39	32		24
1918	80[a]	40	31		25
1919	83	42	32		25
1920	88	31	41		27
1921	94	46	34		27
1922–23	93	48	34		23
1923–24	95	55	33		23[b]
1924–25					
1925–26					
1926–27	46	47	29	1[c]	
1927–28	89	49	38	1	
1928–29	103	51	35	1	
1929–30	107	55	42	1	65
1930–31	111	58	45	1	69

	A.M.E. Zion Mission	Church of England S.P.G.	Government schools	Total mission schools	Total students
1898			7	112	11,181
1899			7	123	12,240
1900	1		7	131	11,996
1901			7	128	12,018
1902			7	117	12,136
1903	1		7	117	12,803
1904			7	132	13,955
1905			7	136	14,370
1906	2		7	138	14,780
1907	1	2	7	141	14,046
1908	1	4	7	145	14,889
1909	3	3	9	153	16,711
1910	4	3	9	154	17,570
1911	4	3	9	152	18,680
1912	5	3	11	147	18,524
1913	3	3	11	142	18,609
1914	3	3	12	147	20,246
1915	4	4	13	153	120,68
1916	4	4	14	162	22,456
1917	5	4	16	180	24,724
1918	5	4	18	185	26,496
1919	6	5	19	193	27,318
1920	5	5	19	197	28,580
1921	6	6	20	213	31,089
1922–23	7	6	20	211	33,353
1923–24	7	6	21	219	35,408
1924–25					
1925–26					32,827
1926–27	7	7	17	137	32,461
1927–28	7	7	17	191	
1928–29	7	9	18	206	
1929–30	7	12	19	289	
1930–31	7	16	19	307	

	Basel Mission	Wesleyan Mission	Roman Catholic Mission	Islamic	Bremen Mission
1931–32	117	62	46	1	74
1932–33	118	66[d]	48	1	76
1933–34					
1934–35	116	67	58	1	81
1935–36	113	65	58	1	82
1936–37	110	63	60	1	84
1937–38	107	72	79	4	86
1938–39	105	72	80	4	83

[a] Basel mission schools fell under the Free Church of Scotland between 1918 and 1922–23. Thereafter, these schools were folded under the Presbyterian Church of the Gold Coast.

[b] These schools were brought under the Ewe Mission in 1923–24 and then the Ewe Presbyterian Church from 1929–30.

[c] This Islamic school was attributed to the Ahmadiyya mission in Saltpond from 1926 to 1927 and onward.

[d] These schools were brought under the Methodist Church from 1932–33.

for Afia Monofie such items associated with menstruation as a gateway to motherhood (*asakyima*, "flowered [and able to bear fruit]").²⁴ Menstruating women were considered, especially by healers, to be ritually unclean and during their menses were secluded in a menstrual dwelling away from the family house. "Before a woman returns to her house after her menses, the head of the household sprinkles her with purified water from a pot sitting on a Nyamedua tree (*Alstonia boonei*) to cleanse her and make her acceptable once again in her home."²⁵ Afia Monofie would have been taught this practice, and the items and advice Afia Asubɔnten gave her were preconditions for sexual intercourse with her proposed husband.

Afia Monofie was born in 1927, the year Takyimanhene Yaw Kramo was assassinated at the village of Agosa, making Kofi Dɔnkɔ fourteen years her senior. But Kofi Dɔnkɔ's family and hers had much in common, perhaps more than the families of any of his other wives. Afia Monofie was born on a "new Friday" (*monofie*) during the "yam festival" for the Takyimanhemma (female leader of the polity), in a part of the Tunsuase blacksmiths' ward called Bansiase. Kofi Dɔnkɔ lived with his uncle Kwame Ampɔnsa in Tunsuase. In the year of Afia's birth, her father, Kwabena Takyi, became the *akobeahene* because his senior brother, Kofi Kyereme (then the akobeahene, and not to be confused with Taa Kwasi ɔbosomfoɔ Kofi Kyereme), was

	A.M.E. Zion Mission	Church of England S.P.G.	Government schools	Total mission schools	Total students
1931–32	7	16	19	323	
1932–33	7	18	20	334	
1933–34				361	
1934–35	7	19	19	349	
1935–36	7	19	19	345	
1936–37	7	19	19	344	
1937–38	8	24	19	380	
1938–39	6	24	19	374	90,000

Note: Data are number values. Although the colonial government tried to "exercise a closer supervision over the non-assisted schools," such schools were excluded from government aid because their daily attendances averaged less than twenty students. There were 129 such schools in 1902 and 360 in 1938–39.

Source: Colonial Reports—Annual. Nos. 271–1919. Gold Coast. Reports for 1898–1939 (London: Her Majesty's Stationery Office, 1899–1939).

arrested and imprisoned regarding Yaw Kramo's assassination. Kwabena Takyi was also an herbalist who farmed cocoa and other crops. As herbalists tend to possess, he had a *suman* called Pennsari, which was procured from part of the northern region populated by Dagarti peoples. He is remembered for healing multiple diseases, especially those in children.

Upon Kyereme's release from prison, Kwabena Takyi did not relinquish the akobeahene position to his elder brother. Eventually, however, Kwabena abdicated himself from the akobeahene stool, fearing reprisal from less-than-supportive family members. Within Kwabena's own family there was enough discord to prompt a divorce between him and his wife, Abena Adomaa. But Abena was more than capable of rearing her daughter; she and her brother, for instance, had established the village of Kanigoro ("if you have debt, you cannot stay"). Now left primarily under her mother's care, Afia did not attend missionary schools. Rather, her mother decided Afia should learn to bake as an apprentice under a woman named Asantewaa from the Asante village of Abofo. Afia showed little interest in baking and began selling locally produced gin (Gã: *akpeteshie*) instead. Afia also acquired over time some trading experience from friends and relatives, becoming a commercial broker in yam, akpeteshie, cooking utensils, and other commodities. Part of these trading commodities was supplied by yams, peppers, cassava, and plantain from her farming. Her plans to buy materials and hire laborers to build her own house, however, were deferred to her husband, who promised to build her the house soon.

While compelling oral sources tell us something about Kofi Dɔnkɔ's early adult life, unfortunately they do not dance to the rhythm of chronology, leaving a frustrating sequence of life events without the kind of order we prefer. From what we know about the life of his natal family, this much is clear: At some point during his early ɔbosomfoɔ practice, a woman named Afia Tɛbua visited Asubɔnten Kwabena to request a "permanent husband" for her daughter Adwoa Opokuaa, who had already divorced four husbands. Asubɔnten Kwabena was carried by Kofi Dɔnkɔ. During the state of spiritual communion, Kofi Dɔnkɔ was told by the ɔbosom to marry Adwoa Opokuaa. Once the ritual sacrifices were completed for Afia Tɛbua's petition, and once Kofi Dɔnkɔ resumed his consciousness, he requested to marry Adwoa Opokuaa. Kofi Dɔnkɔ kept this matter private and did not share it with his intended wife, Afia Monofie, until Adwoa Opokuaa became pregnant with his first child. At that point Kofi Dɔnkɔ followed cultural communicative protocol and sent his apology to Afia Monofie through Akua Ampɔnsaa, a fellow resident of Tunsuase and a "shrine" cook. If Kofi Dɔnkɔ was married to Afia Monofie under normal circumstances and he desired an additional wife, he would have had to pay her a compensation fee (*mpata*). The first wife's acceptance of the money served as formal permission for the husband to marry another, but if she refused, she was entitled to a divorce. A man who proceeded without this permission did so at his own peril. A first or senior wife might grant permission for additional wives in order to lighten the total labor needed for farming and trading, for nursing and rearing children, for cooking and performing household chores in general and during menstrual cycles, and in carrying out important social obligations. But Afia Monofie did not figure into this equation. And the reasons for this situation may have been the conditions under which her marriage was based or the devotion of her husband to his "shrine" and its directives, or a combination of the two. In addition to Afia Monofie and Adwoa Opokuaa, Kofi Dɔnkɔ would have (at least from what we know) three additional wives, who, like the others, became so under circumstances that typify the range of culturally permissible marriages.

In the end, Kofi Dɔnkɔ had several wives and many of the personal difficulties that flowed from the conflicts between co-wives. The third wife, Akosua Dɔnkɔ, was an "inherited wife" from his deceased uncle Kwame

Amponsa. In matrilineal Akan societies, inheritance and leadership ran through the mother's lineage and from uncle to nephew. This largely explains the "widowhood marriage" of Kofi Dɔnkɔ to his maternal uncle's wife. For Akosua, Kofi Dɔnkɔ was more caretaker and companion, though they would have two children—Afua Kwafie and Kwasi Nsowa—in the early 1950s.[26] The fourth wife was Akosua Buruwaa of Gyaman in the Ivory Coast. They had no children, and she terminated the marriage and returned to her hometown of Mori, a village near the current Ghana–Ivory Coast border at Sampa. The names of a few other wives have been floated—Ama Fosuaa, Yaa Owusuaa, Adwoa Asamoaa—but only the latter, with whom Kofi Dɔnkɔ had two children and whose marriage ended in divorce, seems credible. Adwoa Asamoaa recalled, "Nana Kofi Dɔnkɔ was an elder when I first saw him and he was not all that old but because of sickness, he became old prematurely.... I came to meet Afia Monofie as his wife and so I was the second wife."[27]

Adwoa Asamoaa's place as "second wife" is questionable, but perhaps she was either unaware or did not care to know about the other wives. Be that as it may, at some point a serious conflict erupted between Akosua Dɔnkɔ and Adwoa Opokuaa over the wifely care of Kofi Dɔnkɔ. Although the details are murky, Adwoa seemed to protest her unmarried state by refusing to provide bathwater and food for Kofi Dɔnkɔ; Akosua sought to put her "rival" Adwoa in her place. Kofi Dɔnkɔ was displeased, but in Adwoa Opokuaa's favor. When Akosua apologized and insisted on maintaining her widowhood marriage, Kofi Dɔnkɔ rejected her plea and perhaps the marriage. Kofi Dɔnkɔ eventually traveled to Adwoa's father's town of Gyaakyi in the Asante region to perform the marriage rites and pay the requisite "customary" fees. By then, however, Afia Monofie had about six children with Kofi Dɔnkɔ and Adwoa Opokuaa had two children. Adwoa had given birth to Kofi Dɔnkɔ's first child, Yaw Akɔm. The name Akɔm was given to the first male child of a healer, but Yaw Akɔm died during infancy—a pain Kofi Dɔnkɔ and his mother knew all too well. Their next and last child was Amma Kɔmfo, who was born when her father finally performed the long overdue marriage rituals. Of all his wives, real and suspected, only three remained connected to him through the children of each union, and only one—Afia Monofie—lived with him, partnered with him, and had the greatest impact on him and his life's work (figure 4.3).

Together, Afia Monofie and Kofi Dɔnkɔ would have eight children: Kwame Ampɔnsa, Kwasi Amoako, Afia Serwaa, Kofi Effa, Kwabena Takyi, Afia Adomaa, Yaa Badu, and Kofi Sakyi Sapɔn. His other children included

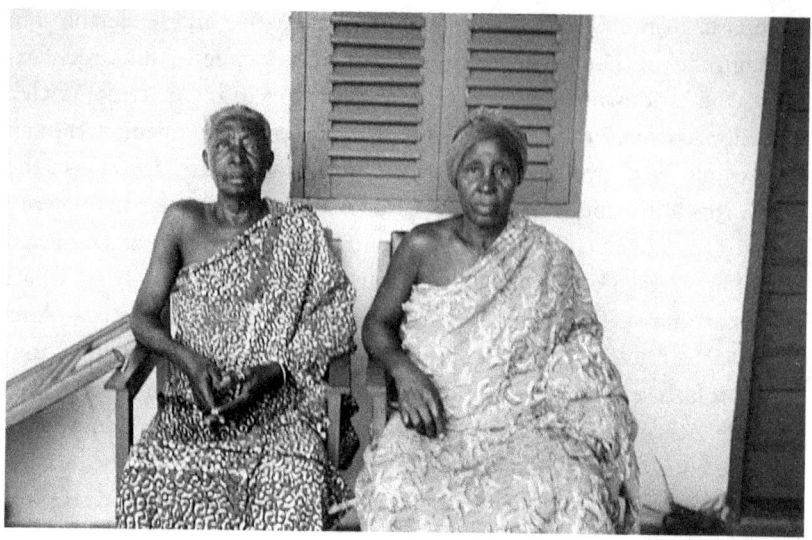

FIGURE 4.3. Kofi Dɔnkɔ and wife Afia Monofie, 1994. From Nana Kwaku Sakyi Collection, in private hands, Miami, Florida. Used courtesy of Nana Kwaku Sakyi, photographer.

Yaw Akɔm (deceased) and Amma Kɔmfo with Adwoa Opokuaa; Afua Kwafie and Kwasi Nsowa with Akosua Dɔnkɔ; and Kofi Kune, Yaw Anane, Afua Owusuaa, Kwasi Adow, Kwaku Adamu, Adwoa Badu, and Yaw Poku. In the early twentieth century, "the parents of numerous children [were] highly revered."[28] Most of Kofi Dɔnkɔ's children were born outside of Holy Family Hospital, a facility erected in 1954 through a partnership between the Takyimanhene and the Medical Mission Sisters, a Catholic organization. A few were born in the Sunyani General Hospital (SGH), which was established as a regional hospital in 1929.[29] One encounter with SGH was a harbinger of things to come and in some ways distinguished Kofi Dɔnkɔ from his peers. In 1965 Afia Monofie took Kofi Dɔnkɔ to SGH for treatment. He was operated on by an "old white woman" doctor. A week after the operation, Afia went into labor while visiting her husband. The nurses and that doctor rushed to attend to Afia.

Early on a Friday morning, their son Kofi Sakyi Sapɔn was born. The doctor asked Kofi Dɔnkɔ whether she could suggest a name for the child. Apparently elated by a male child born on his soul day—Friday—Kofi Dɔnkɔ agreed to add the name Daniel to his child's legal name—Kofi Sakyi Daniel. Kofi Dɔnkɔ's healing colleague Kofi Kyereme would have done differently, filled as he was with a deep sense of pride in the efficacy of indigenous institutions and therapeutics. When asked whether any of his children were born in the hospital, Kofi Kyereme replied, "Only two were born at the hospital in my absence. If I were there, I would not allow them to take them to the hospital."[30] Hospitals represented foreign institutions that competed with and also undermined healers, and so Kofi Kyereme preferred "self-medication," and after a car accident and an offer for prescribed medications he indicated, "I finally had to take care of myself with herbs."[31] Although both had a deep respect for each other and their craft, Kofi Dɔnkɔ took a slightly different approach to European institutions and as a result became one of the foremost healers to collaborate with European/white doctors, anthropologists, and researchers in the academic coming-of-age of African studies.

For Afia Monofie's part, she too joined the healing work of Kofi Dɔnkɔ and his extended family by acquiring her own healing knowledge from her grandmother, who she lived within a large family compound in Tunsuase. Her paternal grandmother, Nana Yaa, taught her medicines for prenatal and postnatal care, making her a "traditional birth attendant" (minus the formal hospital training). Afia also specialized in curing stomach pains and childhood diseases. Between Afia and Kofi, healers among their offspring were a natural outcome. One of their sons, Kofi Effa, became a sought-after healer through his principal ɔbosombrafoɔ named Asutipa (figure 4.4). Kofi Effa's ɔbosom was part of that historic *abosommerafoɔ* wave from the northern region. The Tanɔ abosom that Kofi Dɔnkɔ and Kofi Kyereme possessed kept a stable but threatened following.

This historical moment, like other transformations of the late nineteenth and early twentieth centuries, had roots in the social instability occasioned by colonial rule and by farmers withholding their cocoa to raise prices during an upsurge in the cocoa industry, facilitating the rise of abosommerafoɔ. It is not surprising that the majority of abosommerafoɔ came with the expansion of migrant workers from the north, as southerners hoped these "wild" spiritual powers packaged into asuman and shrines would know how best to deal with the antisocial forces in their otherwise "civilized" lands. The anxieties released by the cocoa boom and recovery were also at the center of rural, labor, and youth movements politicized by the quandary created by "indirect" rule. Colonial society writ large was riddled by a dependency on, but a frustration with, "native" institutions, as evidenced by voluminous destoolment and succession disputes brought by a range of litigants, including women and cocoa farmers. The need to heal a people could not have been greater, and who better qualified and less seduced

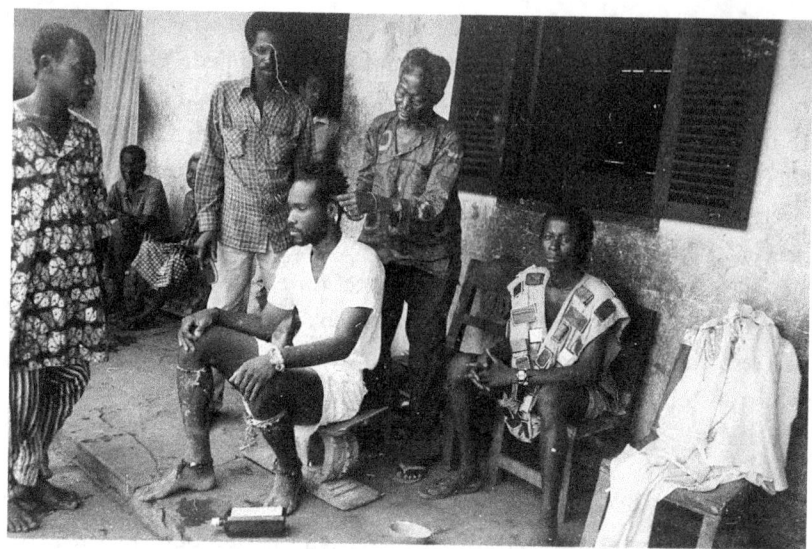

FIGURE 4.4. Nana Kofi Effa (left), Nana Kofi Ɔboɔ (center), and Nana Kofi Dɔnkɔ (right) cutting Nana Kwaku Sakyi's hair at graduation, 1989. From Nana Kwaku Sakyi Collection, in private hands, Miami, Florida. Used courtesy of Nana Kwaku Sakyi, photographer.

by the fashions of the times than the likes of Kofi Dɔnkɔ and his healing family?

❋

KOFI DƆNKƆ AND AFIA Monofie entered the cocoa-farming business in search of financial prosperity and were thus no different from other rural dwellers who seized a historic opportunity. And why not? Most people in the colony were farmers, and cocoa was the crop with the greatest monetary yield. As the colony became a world leader in cocoa production, however, the cocoa economy transformed indigenous understandings and laws regulating land ownership and property inheritance. These transformations brought to the fore the rivalry between local elites baptized by religious orthodoxy, on the one hand, and "paramount chiefs" and their divisional subordinates, on the other hand. Conflicts between these colonial subjects were no clearer than in the decade and a half of legal disputes over control of the mineral- and cocoa-rich lands of Asamankese.[32] Whether diamonds, gold, or cocoa, the Asamankese case was symptomatic of the legion of litigation and conflicts brought on by the commercialization of communal land.³³ For the cocoa industry, its ascension not only led to sharp declines in palm and coffee products, but allowed thousands of farmers to become prosperous, creating tremendous income gaps between themselves, urban professionals, subsistence farmers, and underemployed migrant laborers.

Riots erupted in 1930 when Governor Alexander Ransford Slater introduced income tax in the colony; cocoa farmers organized the first significant cocoa protest by withholding their crops to raise prices. A second holdup in 1937 after efforts to curb dissent in the colony through the enactment of "Obnoxious Ordinances" were also met with protest. At the end of the 1930s, a restored Asante Confederacy, a newly enstooled Asantehene, and the heavily revised Native Administration Ordinance guided by Ofori Atta I of Akyem Abuakwa did not end but rather intensified conflicts over land and the litigation surrounding them. For cocoa farmers in Takyiman and elsewhere, the spread of swollen shoot disease and land disputes gravely affected the cocoa crop and its benefit to the broader community, whereas the indirect rule policy seriously undermined "traditional" institutions but propped up or "reinvented" others when it served British interests in producing and trading cash crops or minerals. These battles over land and the oral traditions the litigants marshaled to prove their claim were fought in the colonial courtroom.

The colonial judiciary vacillated between English common law and "traditional law," confusing rather than resolving the conflicts over property ownership and the multiple versions of one "traditional" account or another underpinning custodianship.³⁴ Colonial rule and its imperial policies also vacillated between a hostile posture toward "chiefs" in favor of direct rule and a penchant for indirect rule through "paramount chiefs" and their divisional subordinates.³⁵ The shifting and unsettled nature of colonial rule underscored the ubiquitous litigations. Such disputes bankrupted some stools as a result of the heavy litigation fees, ushering in the widespread role and rule of local lawyers. Descriptions of two cases should suffice—one in a small village of little commercial importance, the other in a large tract of land with minerals and cocoa. In the 1930s or early 1940s, Kwaku Owusu and Kwasi Mensa of Berekum came to farm cocoa on unclaimed lands and founded a village called Amangoase. Kwaku became the village's first leader (*odikuro*), but both men returned to Berekum. Wankyihene Kwame Yoguo (a.k.a. Kwame Abrefa) and Takyimanhene Akumfi Ameyaw III both claimed Amangoase for their respective stools, and people from each township were dispatched to farm there.³⁶ The Takyiman contingent soon formed a majority of the farming population, whereas relatively few individuals came from

Wankyi. This demographic imbalance morphed into claims and counterclaims over ownership, leading to litigation.

The Takyimanhene and Wankyihene litigated the matter at the principal court in the regional capital of Sunyani. This "boundary of land" case would reach the West African Court of Appeal and the Privy Council, where it was "dismissed with costs."[37] The Takyimanhene had also been unsuccessful in an earlier case that reached the Privy Council and where the "Courts had to consider native customs and to hear evidence as to tradition" concerning one Kwame Safo, who wanted to sell land claimed by Takyiman. This case was dismissed and Takyimanhene Akumfi Ameyaw III had to pay Safo's legal costs.[38] Farmers on both sides of the divide in Amangoase fought among themselves but found a resolution, albeit on the ground rather than in the courtroom, for the founders of the village had appointed Kofi Amankwa of Takyiman to manage the affairs of the village. Kofi Amankwa was succeeded by Kwadwo Aning, the nephew of later Takyimanhene Kwakye Ameyaw II. Peace resumed and villagers paid the appropriate land usage tax to the Takyimanhene, who was victorious on behalf of his townspeople, with relatively few legal fees involved.[39]

The case of Asamankese town and its subordinate village of Akwatia was quite the opposite, though it shares the same stubborn theme. As colonists understood it, each polity (ɔman) was headed by an ɔmanhene, subordinate leaders (ahene; sg. ɔhene) of its territorial divisions or towns, and leaders of subdivisions or villages (adikuro; sg. odikuro). Asamankese was one of the fourteen divisions of and Akwatia was a village under Asamankese within the Akyem Abuakwa polity, headed by Akyemhene Ofori Atta I. Following a long history of both ahene and adikuro pursuing their own interests and selling communal land to migrant farmers and concessionaires independent of the ɔmanhene, Ofori Atta I began to enforce his overarching authority and demand his "traditional" one-third of all revenue once gold and diamonds—in addition to timber and cocoa—were discovered in Asamankese and Akwatia.[40] For almost a decade and a half a protracted and costly legal battle ensued, amounting to over £160,000 in legal fees on both sides and forever fracturing the hierarchy of power exercised in the "traditional" polity.[41] Local lawyers such as K. A. Korsah, W. E. Sekyi, and J. B. Danquah seized on the land conflicts and succession disputes that plagued the colony, representing both amanhene who wanted to strengthen their positions and recalcitrant ahene who wanted to assert their independence from the "paramount" stool and profit from their land's natural resources.[42] In fact, Sekyi and Danquah were opposing counsel in the legal fight between Danquah's older brother, Ofori Atta I, and Kwaku Amoah, ɔhene of Asamankese, and Kwasi Kuma, odikuro of Akwatia.[43] Eventually, Ofori Atta I would use his influence as the colonial spokesperson for all Akan "chiefs" and framed his quest for power in terms of British interests. Ofori Atta I also shaped the very ordinances that quelled the unrest in Asamankese and dashed Amoah and Kuma's hopes.[44] Moreover, Amoah and Kuma had their petitions dismissed in the West African Court of Appeal and the Privy Council, retaining responsibility for the legal costs.[45] Undaunted, they rejected the Privy Council's decision. Although Amoah's successor, Kofi Adom, continued the fight against Ofori Atta I, he was removed from office by authorities after losing in court and after a failed petition for secession.[46]

In the immediate wake of the Asamankese case, one Privy Council member lamented,

> I found myself growing more and more depressed at the apparent powerlessness of Arbitrators, Courts and Government to put an end to the continuous and ruinous litigation between this paramount and those subordinate stools. Thousands and thousands of pounds have been diverted from the social services to which they should have been devoted and expended on a legal warfare of attrition. Instead of the schools, hospitals, welfare centres, improved sanitary (so badly needed), roads and public buildings which the people of those contending stools might have acquired and enjoyed as a result of the discovery of great mineral wealth beneath their lands, they have had a never ending chain of indecisive legal battles with the prospect of at least two more expensive journeys to the highest Court of Appeal in the British Empire.[47]

By 1935 the colonial administration effectively placed "native courts" under government control and created stool treasuries to control the finances of polities and their territorial divisions through the district commissioner. Such was the case for Asamankese: the authorities argued that its finances had to come under government control because Amoah and the other litigants were poor stewards of their community's resources. In fact, the first of these treasuries was in Akwatia.[48] Both the Amangoase and the Asamankese cases illustrate the broader political consequences of colonial rule and the cocoa boom. Indeed, increased cocoa production triggered an unprecedented increase in land values (and where communal land "sales" were viewed as private transactions), and an equally increased number of conflicts between claimants to the (potential) revenues of valuable lands. But these political outcomes were matched or surpassed by social and cultural consequences, measured by the sharp rise in the use of spiritual interventions to address the anxiety and transformations diffused across the colony.

In the 1930s colonial anthropologist Margaret Field became intrigued by the new abosommerafoɔ movement and its psychological implications, and she began to conduct research on a "witch-catching shrine" akin to Kofi Effa's at the village of Mframaso, twenty miles north of Takyiman. She concluded the social tensions and insecurity found among those interviewed (through an interpreter) were rarely attributed to causative factors such as stress and worry but rather to "witchcraft."[49] What Field perhaps failed to realize was that the colonial order that sponsored her research and made available colonial subjects and Christianized interpreters lay at the root of the tensions and anxieties she falsely understood as "witchcraft." Colonialism was both an inquisition where indigenous cultures remained on trial and a particular "witchcraft" that unleashed anti-communitarian forces for which most indigenes had no ready answer in their cultural toolkit. This, in part, explains why the clear majority of abosommerafoɔ originated from *outside* Akan societies, but also why Field and colonists alike failed to grasp the virus indirect rule unleashed and how that malignant virus left little of indigenous societies untouched. The volcanic rise in abosommerafoɔ use was conterminous with the equally and socially disruptive land disputes, claims and counterclaims for cocoa and mineral revenue, and bankrupting litigations and destoolment cases.

At the time of Field's research, Kwaku Kyereme (r. 1937–41) became the new Takyimanhene. He continued the struggle to reclaim the nine villages that were home to eminent Tanɔ abosom and prime farming lands, but he was destooled. Kwaku Gyako III (r. 1941–44) was then installed. A colonial official visiting Takyiman in 1942 estimated its population at three thousand or more, described its market as "primitive" and its water supplied by streams, but was troubled by "much of the sanitation of the village," stating "that unless ... the people ... cooperate with the village overseer I would not consider giving them any further help. [The] chief [Kwaku Gyako III] said he wanted a midwife. I told him a midwife took several years to train & that the supply was short [and] I was providing only the better villages with them so that if he wanted his village put on that list he would have to improve conditions."[50] Although Gyako III's successor claimed that nine sanitary laborers paid with money collected from townspeople kept the town clean, Gyako III "promised [the official] cooperation in [the] future."⁵¹ That future never came, as Gyako III's reign prematurely ended with his destoolment. The next Takyimanhene, Akumfi Ameyaw III (r. 1944–61), whose uncle was the slain Yaw Kramo, resumed the fight for the nine villages. In this moment the youth and elders worked together to support the struggle marshaled by Ameyaw III.⁵² Their collective meetings produced several petitions that were then dispatched to the Gold Coast government and the British parliament. These petitions unequivocally declared Takyiman's withdrawal from the Asante Confederacy because of the disputed nine villages, Asante's mistreatment of its officials, unfair tax collection practices, and lack of enforcement of the treaty signed with the government assuring the return of those villages.⁵³ Despite Ameyaw III's best efforts to reclaim those villages or to unify the Bono, the townspeople rebelled against him seven times and he was forced to abdicate the stool.⁵⁴ His successor, Kwakye Ameyaw II, also faced rebellion and attempts to oust him a month after his enstoolment. It would take more than eight years of litigation to destool him.

During the uncharacteristically long reign of Takyimanhene Akumfi Ameyaw III, several Christian missions sought to establish a foothold during a relatively calm period of Takyiman politics, using the church-school as its chief "tool for the Christianization" of a community.⁵⁵ Seventh-Day Adventists founded a church in the 1940s and then a school with nineteen students in 1952; the Catholics established a primary school in 1944, followed by a middle school a decade later. Catechists from the coast opened a Methodist middle school and a Presbyterian church in 1945 (figure 4.5).⁵⁶ These missionary efforts can be collectively measured by the conflict in culture that erupted in 1950 around the Seventh-Day Adventists in the Takyiman village of Oforikrom, which also had a school with twenty-seven students under the leadership of headmaster R. E. Kwaku.⁵⁷ In a series of letters between the Takyimanhene, Seventh-Day Adventist church members, and the Benkumhene and Oforikrom stool elders, this much is clear: conflict arose concerning the cultural prohibitions placed on farming and collecting water. These universally understood norms predated the Christian orthodoxy in the colony, but in this instance they offer a window into the tensions wrought by empire and its missionary reach into subjugated peoples' lives. The letters framed the conflict as one between "Christians" and the "Fetish people" who preserved a sacred Friday for abosom named Bote Kofi and Fia Kofi, the Kwamene festival held on a sacred Saturday for the Oforikrom stool, and the festival for the ɔbosom Akumsa celebrated on Tuesday each year.

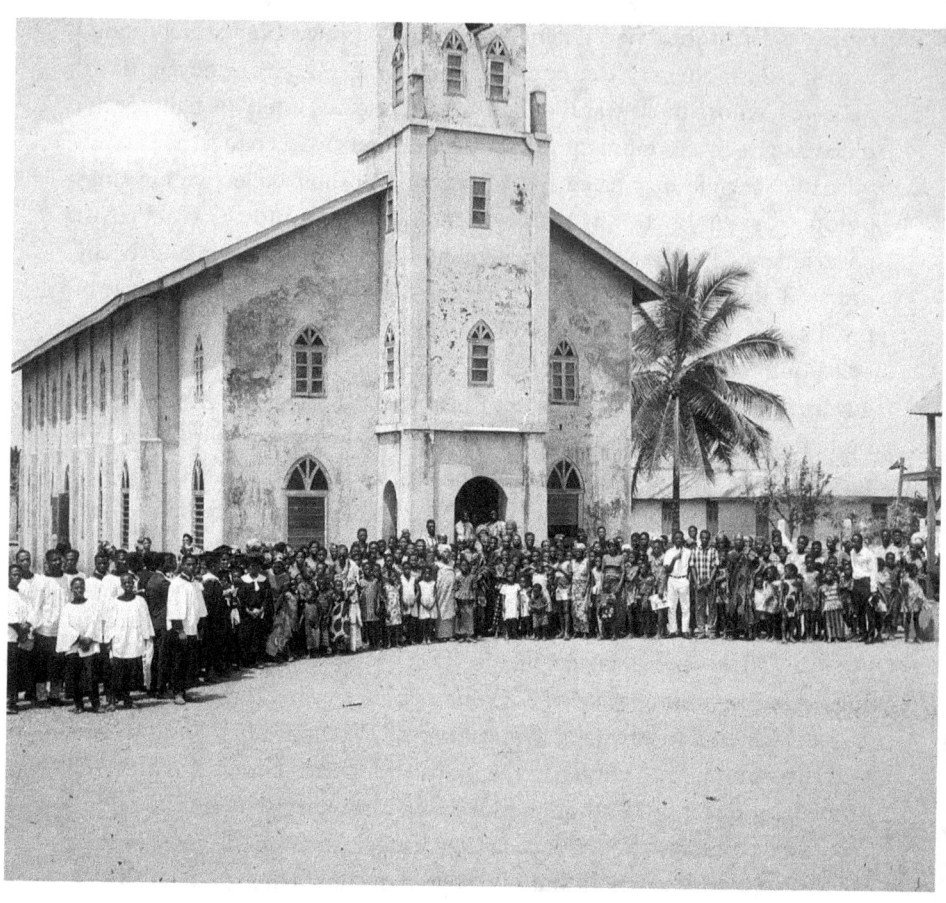

FIGURE 4.5. Methodist church, 1970. From the Dennis Michael Warren Slide Collection, Special Collections Department, University of Iowa Libraries. Used courtesy of Greg Prickman, Head of Special Collections.

The Oforikrom church members argued for exemption from "fetish" practices and their ecologically protective guidelines, claiming "no public place for collecting water is ever dedicated as sacred, for the reason that all common people and strangers resort to and have the benefit of using it freely." For annual purifications, the Takyimanhene selected the Adaa stream, source of the Atwereda that flows into the Tanɔ River. Church members suggested that the Asukatia Abena stream in Oforikrom should be moved to a private place in conformity to the stream chosen by the Takyimanhene.[58] The churchgoers further complained they should not be asked to offer an egg or a chicken to purify the Asukatia Abena stream on sacred Tuesdays, nor should they be only allowed to work two days on their farms—Tuesday was reserved for the veneration of Asukatia Abena, Wednesday for Nyanhu Kwaku, Thursday for Akagyensu Yaa, and Friday for Bote Kofi and Fia Kofi. They balked against such "Fetish Practice" and attempted to sway indigenous authorities to see things their way: "We think Nana [Benkumhene] would admit that our ancestors from time immemorial knew the worship of God and therefore gave their allegiance to Him." Fighting a losing battle, church members conceded that neither the prohibited days nor "chieftaincy" should be abolished, but that they "be given liberty to separate from Fetish practices."[59] Success remained elusive for the missions and their converts, as Seventh-Day Adventist efforts waned and would have to await a resurrection in 1965.

In the larger scheme of things, the missions wished they had the kind of success cocoa enjoyed in the colony. The value of cocoa rose between 1945 and 1959, but because the colonial administration depended on cocoa revenue for its financing, it could not impose effective control over cocoa producers.[60] As the price of cocoa recovered from the depression years, cocoa farmers dealt with swollen shoot disease by leaving infected farms, scattered throughout the forest, to recuperate by themselves. Of the approximately 400 million cocoa trees, some 50 million were infected, spreading at a rate of 15 million a year and with no cure for the disease. Against this tide, periodic abandonment was a natural remedy for disease- and pest-ridden farms. The devotion of both colonists and local farmers to cocoa, however, was not without peril. As farmers neglected basic food crops in favor of cocoa, many Africans were forced to pay higher prices for provisions or essential commodities, creating frustration and social unrest that eventually morphed into boycotts against the purchase of imported goods. The boycotts against European goods were also supported by "chiefs" who, for different reasons, complained about the high prices of imported goods; "hostile" demonstrations erupted in the colonial capital of Accra, followed by strikes in secondary schools.[61] These social upheavals were reminiscent of the successful boycott and cocoa "holdup" of 1937. In January 1948 serious and politically motivated opposition flared up against the Department of Agriculture for cutting diseased trees without the owners' consent. After some instances of violence, the colonial secretary met with local officeholders in February; the cutting of diseased cocoa trees was suspended in April and a boycott was called off.

The financial strain high-priced commodities placed on families was not lost on locally recruited service members fighting in World War II. One

Kofi Nsia wrote a letter to Takyimanhene Akumfi Ameyaw III on behalf of young men serving in India and Burma. As part of the South East Asia Command, these men sent with the letter monies to help their wives and children, and they asked the Takyimanhene to pray for their safe return.[62] For Ameyaw III's part, each month he claimed to have met with the wives of soldiers in active service, and advised and encouraged them, asking various village leaders to do likewise for "such wives in their respective villages." He also traveled twice to Accra and spoke to soldiers on the battlefront from the Broadcasting House, established in 1935 or 1940, while contributing yams and palm kernel to the war effort.[63] Not long after his visit to Accra, Ameyaw III received from Osu (Accra) a retinue of two hundred, headlined by Nii Kwabena Bonne III, leader of the Osu Alata quarters in Accra.

On their visit to Takyiman, Ameyaw III remarked, "my subjects who migrated from Techiman to Egyas (Cape Coast) about 200 years ago and thence to Osu (Christiansborg) Accra visited me, and joined up with the Techiman state again." Nii Kwabena Bonne III was installed as "Nana Owusu Akenten III," Oyokohene of Takyiman, because "when they were migrating, they were the Oyokos in rank at Techiman."[64] What stood out from this crowning achievement was not the name or position, but the act itself. It infuriated the chief commissioner based in Kumase and the Asantehene. Whether creating this "Oyokohene" position was a show of power behalf of a Takyiman subservient to Asante and the colonial government, Ameyaw III fired back. He argued that the chief commissioner did not understand clan affiliation and Takyiman's internal politics, for creating or resurrecting an Oyoko stool was "purely an internal matter concerning Techiman alone, and does not affect the external relations of the Techiman Divisions in Ashanti."[65] More than a war of words, the Takyimanhene's act and response following World War II was part of an enlarged moment of defiance from the seemingly powerless against authoritative institutions.

With foreign exchange earnings and purchasing power within the colony dependent principally on cocoa, the state of the colony's economy—the largest producer of cocoa in the world in the 1950s—was intimately linked to sociopolitical unrest. Fluctuating cocoa prices in the world market and poor price control over locally produced foodstuffs or imported goods often led to upheaval and protest, which disrupted the economy and led to more unrest.[66] The Cocoa Marketing Board (CMB) and the United Gold Coast Convention (UGCC) were established in 1947. Founded by J. B. Danquah and other local elites, the UGCC was a political organization that added future prime minister Kwame Nkrumah to its ranks as general secretary and sought to preserve the commercial interests of the elites. The CMB, on the other hand, determined the optimal conditions for cocoa producers, fixed prices locally and for distribution to world markets, and appointed agents who bought cocoa cheaply from farmers. Although the marketing of cocoa stimulated early nationalism, local farmers such as Kofi Dɔnkɔ and his wives felt the exploitative brunt of the CMB agents' actions and the eventual decline of cocoa a decade later. Yet, the decolonization struggle for political independence in the mid-twentieth century would involve the popular revolt of villagers and town dwellers, former servicemen, and cocoa farmers. A peaceful demonstration by former servicemen in Accra in 1948 ended in shootings and riots that left twenty-nine dead, and later in that year, leaders of the UGCC were arrested. Although Danquah was a key factor in the politics that anticipated political independence, Kwame Nkrumah was the one who broke away from the UGCC, formed the Convention People's Party (CPP), and transformed this widespread discontent into a nationalist struggle that extended across the colony.

In the same year the UGCC and the CMB were established, the Asante Youth Association (AYA) was created by a group of young men without the prospect of political office and who were subordinate to chiefly authority. The AYA became the driving force behind the creation of the National Liberation Movement (NLM) launched in Kumase in 1954. The NLM famously struggled with Kwame Nkrumah's CPP. The NLM, under the leadership of Baffour Osei Akoto and future prime minister Kofi Busia, would demand Asante self-determination in the form of an autonomous Asante "nation" within the Gold Coast configuration or Asante secession. This demand clashed with the anticipated blueprint—worked out with the British government—for a politically independent Ghana that would not afford Asante "special" parliamentary consideration.[67] The political clashes over the course of the new republic had less to do with the NLM and Nkrumah's CPP, and more to do with internal Asante politics in terms of protracted conflicts of interest and power between young men, on the one hand, and the established order (notably represented by the Asantehene, officeholders, and intellectuals), on the other hand. Ironically, the established order would usurp the leadership of young men within the NLM and transform it into a parliamentary party. This party would reach a compromise with Nkrumah's CPP, articulate the position of local officeholders in the republic's constitution, and provide Asante with a semblance of regional autonomy. The transformation of the NLM marked a pivotal victory for the established order within Asante, and the voices of workers and farmers who supported the NLM remained muted and without political remedy. In 1949 the colonial government imprisoned Nkrumah and the CPP's leadership. Two years later the CPP won most of the seats in the legislative council, and Nkrumah, released from prison, became the leader of government business. Eventually, in the 1957 election, the CPP won many of the seats against anti-CPP forces, including the reconfigured NLM.

❉

WHILE A RANGE of political actors became embroiled in electoral and mass politics, Takyiman's leadership used these undercurrents for political representation in the colony, as well as a self-proclaimed anthropologist, for its own benefit. A year before Nkrumah and leaders in the CPP were arrested by colonial authorities, Takyiman was allowed to disengage from the Asante Confederacy, along with several other Bono polities that followed Takyiman's lead and helped form the Bono Federation in 1951.[68] The Bono Federation—or Bonokyɛmpem movement, as Takyiman envisioned it—became a call for Bono unification rather than reclamation of the contested nine villages. The focus on unification came, ironically, from British parliamentarian Michael Foot, who received Takyiman's petition through Eva Meyerowitz, a mutual friend of his and Takyimanhene Akumfi Ameyaw III.[69] Instead of real estate, anti-Asante sentiments fueled by centuries of insults and subservience made the Bonokyɛmpem movement relevant to other Bono constituents, and it took on greater meaning on the precipice of the colony moving toward political independence. In the new political configuration that would be the republic of Ghana, Asante had leveraged its former empire status and its subdued hegemonic weight—vis-à-vis other indigenous polities—to carve out a prime space in the new republic.

In this context rejection of a subordinate place in a regionally autonomous Asante by Takyiman and the other Bono polities, and their secession from the Asanteman Council, were met with protracted legal disputes in which the Federation's constitution and a range of legal correspondences were drafted by none other than J. B. Danquah for some £1,000.[70] Even peripheral individuals deemed associates of the "rebelled Takyimanhene" and thus disloyal to the Asantehene were dragged into costly and time-consuming legal battles.[71] Nonetheless, Takyiman, on behalf of the Bono Federation, articulated its position to the Asantehene, head of the Asanteman Council, and appealed to the Gold Coast governor and King George VI of England.[72] Colonial officials reasoned that "the Brong Division [is] not essential to the [Asante] Confederacy. Six out of ten are opposed to restoration [of the Asante Confederacy]." The chief commissioner of Asante advised that the "choice be left solely in their hands to enter [the Confederacy] when they so feel disposed; those not willing should be administered separately as they are today."[73] Knowing the Asantehene was supported by the colonial government, Takyimanhene Akumfi Ameyaw III used all resources at his disposal and appealed to quasi-anthropologist Eva L. R. Meyerowitz of London to advocate for Takyiman's case in the seat of the British empire. In return for her political assistance, Meyerowitz was granted access to "knowledgeable" elites in Takyiman who, through several interpreters, would facilitate her research into and series of books about Akan/Bono cultural histories.

After spending some years in South Africa, Herbert V. Meyerowitz arrived on the Gold Coast with his wife Eva in 1937 to teach art and crafts at Achimota College. Both were sculptors who immediately toured the Gold Coast and greater West Africa to collect data on indigenous art forms. Herbert became an influential advocate for African art and craft production using indigenous traditions and motifs among his students, which included one of Ghana's and Africa's most celebrated painters and sculptors of the twentieth century, Kofi Antubam.[74] The son of the ɔmanhene of Wassa-Amanfi, Kofi Antubam refined his talents by studying abroad and undergoing years of training under Herbert Meyerowitz and others at Achimota. Antubam completed his studies at Achimota in 1946. Herbert died a year later. Although Eva Meyerowitz would continue working at Achimota for a year or so after Herbert's death, she had since 1943 turned her attention to collecting oral histories in the colony and Antubam was her principal interpreter and research associate. Eva Meyerowitz's first and second books—*The Sacred State of the Akan* (1951) and *Akan Traditions of Origin* (1952)—were largely based on research conducted on her behalf by Kofi Antubam, especially in Takyiman between 1947 and 1948.[75] The new Takyimanhene, Akumfi Ameyaw III, saw Antubam's research for Meyerowitz as an opportunity to further Takyiman's political cause. Of interest are a series of letters between Akumfi Ameyaw III and Meyerowitz during 1949, a year after Takyiman officially removed itself from under the historic weight of Asante hegemony. These letters also reveal something of the Takyiman people and their cultural forms as filtered through Ameyaw III and Meyerowitz's interpreters, among whom included Takyiman police chief J. K. Ankomah and Ameyaw III's close kin D. K. Owusu (figure 4.6).

Meyerowitz's relationship with Ameyaw III began around a 1940 petition from then-Takyimanhene Kwaku Kyereme and his elders to Gold Coast

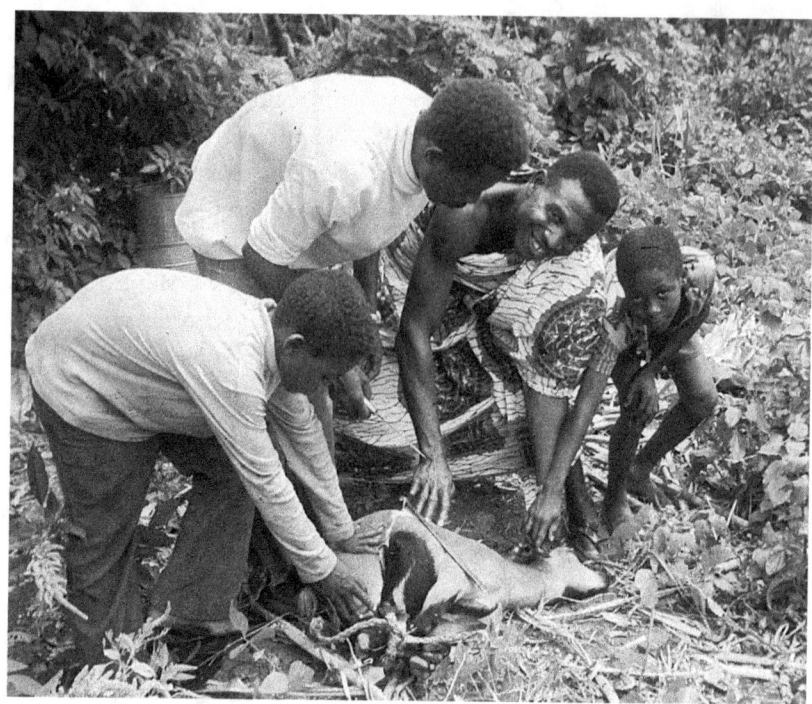

FIGURE 4.6. D. K. Owusu, Takyiman, August 1973. From the Dennis Michael Warren Slide Collection, Special Collections Department, University of Iowa Libraries. Used courtesy of Greg Prickman, Head of Special Collections.

governor Gerald Creasy. Creasy rejected the petition. On Takyiman's behalf, Meyerowitz wrote to the governor to have the petition reconsidered in light of her recent letters from the Takyimanhene and, she claimed, because the townspeople suffered through no fault of their own and should not be punished for a "demand that is legitimate enough."[76] In a series of correspondences between January and February 1949, Ameyaw III agreed with his lawyer J. B. Danquah that "the Committee of Privileges, being purely an advisory body, has not the power to deal with land disputes, and these still have to be settled by the Courts (if necessary)." Meyerowitz replied, "You are very well advised by Dr Danquah to send a supplementary Petition to the Governor, and only should this fail address yourself to the Secretary of State," but informed him, "I still have not received an answer [from the governor]."[77]

The Adontenhene of Takyiman passed away while Ameyaw III was in Accra. When Ameyaw III arrived in Takyiman, he performed the appropriate rituals for the stools and the funeral rites for the Adontenhene. Ritual protocol, as a function of his office, required the Takyimanhene to load the gun fired in the air at state funeral rites. Unbeknownst to Ameyaw III, however, a servant handed him a loaded gun and the gun discharged accidentally, tragically killing his niece and wounding one of his stool carriers. Fearing impending legal troubles for a ritual gone wrong, Ameyaw III retained a lawyer named Koi Larbi, but with the understanding he would not step foot in Asante until a trial.[78] During this debacle, one of the Takyimanhene's wives gave birth to a female child on a Thursday, and thus she was to be named Yaa, but Ameyaw III requested Meyerowitz's permission to name the child Eva "for the fine things you are doing for Techiman." Meyerowitz consented.[79]

Further discussions revolved around an additional petition with a copy of the 1897 "peace treaty" between Takyiman and England, and the Takyiman Traditional Council firmly made their point to Meyerowitz: "You can see from the Treaty that we wish the British Government to protect us from any harm and to support us in times of need but the maltreatment perpetuated to us by the Gold Coast Government makes us feel that the Treaty has been violated. We the people of Techiman embraced the British Flag not through conquest but by our own free will." The council strongly urged Meyerowitz to "impress on the Home Government to see that Justice be done in this case else the consequences might be disastrous with the elimination of Techiman from this Earth." Two high-ranking police officers from Kumase arrested Akumfi Ameyaw III, but council members stood firmly behind him, exclaiming, "Our loyalty to our Omanhene will never be unsavoured [sic], we shall never forsake our dear Omanhene."[80]

At the beginning of June, Meyerowitz wrote to Ameyaw III to assure him "not to worry. Everything will be done to help you and your people." She also announced the completion of her first book, *Sacred State of the Akan*, and requested to use for the book another picture of him "as a great chief" rather than one that might imply an "inferior position."[81] Ameyaw III lamented his legal difficulties, his suspension from office and the restrictions placed on his ritual obligations as Takyimanhene—that is, "periodic observances or propitiation of rituals [for the] stools in Techiman." The colonial government withdrew all grants-in-aid after Ameyaw III's suspension, which crippled Takyiman's fiscal affairs and its ability to dispense medical care, for there were no clinics, nor could the town afford to build and staff one. In turn, a traveling dispenser visited the town on Fridays to treat the sick in the local prison. Suspension or not, Ameyaw III never lost sight of what he called the "cloudy developments in the Gold Coast

Political field" and Takyiman's political cause. He therefore asked Meyerowitz to "be so kind to peruse any of the facts embodied in any document or petition which any of my lawyers might forward to the Secretary of State before it reaches him. This is important."[82] By August, Meyerowitz informed the Takyimanhene of her September visit to Takyiman and made a request for a reliable interpreter. Ameyaw III, in turn, requested that she, "in your usual kindness, communicate with the local Government or the Governor to forward" the petition of Takyiman to the Secretariat in Accra. As for the interpreter, Ameyaw III assured her he had "one who will do the interpretation."[83]

Meyerowitz arrived on the Gold Coast in late September, and while eating lunch in Kumase on 3 October 1949, she was introduced to a young man and her new interpreter, "Mr. D. K. Owusu, grandson of the Tekyiman Stool."[84] Meyerowitz recalled, "My interpreter in 1949–50 was the late J. K. Ankomah, chief of police of the Tekyimin State, who was just as keen and devoted to my work as Kofi Antubam. In the last month of my stay in Tekyiman in 1950 Mr. D. K. Owusu took over from him, and he also interpreted for me on my return to Tekyiman in 1964 and 1967."[85] Because Eva was an absentee researcher who relied on Antubam and others to collect data during her "absence from Tekyiman," it was not surprising that Antubam invented or reinterpreted data to fit Eva's expectations and that "Antubam [was] apparently the only outsider ever to have had access" to the data used to write her books.[86] When anthropologist Dennis M. Warren reviewed Meyerowitz's body of work and interviewed many of the same people Antubam interviewed on her behalf, using D. K. Owusu's son Owusu Brempong as his interpreter, Warren's data explicitly "contradict information written by Mrs. Meyerowitz."[87] Anthropology as an offspring of colonialism and the role of anthropologists in colonial and imperial situations are well known and have been thoroughly critiqued elsewhere.[88] In the end, Meyerowitz brazenly continued to publish on Akan peoples despite damning methodological and analytical flaws, Kofi Antubam emerged as the leading artist and cultural figure in the nationalist fervor engendered by Kwame Nkrumah and his party, and Akumfi Ameyaw III would survive yet another rebellion or threat to his position before abdicating the stool in 1961.[89] Although Meyerowitz, Antubam, Nkrumah, Ameyaw, and Kofi Dɔnkɔ had divergent agendas and constituencies, they all framed their efforts as assisting the "state to have progress."

CHAPTER 5. **INDEPENDENCES**

"Never Mingled Himself in Local Politics"

In the universe there are so many signs. A few we understand, the way farmers know what clouds mean, and fishermen understand stars. But most signs mean nothing to us because we aren't prepared to understand them.
—AYI KWEI ARMAH, *The Healers*

Although Kofi Dɔnkɔ garnered "a great deal of respect from Takyiman people" and "was also admired by various paramount chiefs of Takyiman, including Nana Akumfi Ameyaw [III, he . . .] never mingled himself in local politics." Owusu Brempong, principal research associate to Dennis Warren and paternal kin of Kofi Dɔnkɔ, believed Kofi Dɔnkɔ's strategic distance from politics "was his trump card."[1] During the reign of Akumfi Ameyaw III, those removed from the perch of authority—farmers, craftspeople, merchants, and healers—constituted a clear majority in Takyiman and across the colony. Their optics approximated a people's history. Kofi Dɔnkɔ the healer, blacksmith, woodcarver, farmer, husband, father, and family head functions as an imperfect human prism through which to approach that history. By the 1950s Kofi Dɔnkɔ had grown into his physically small but socially enlarged frame, where "one could hardly tell his age because of his looks, a very handsome man." When Kofi Dɔnkɔ inherited the *ɔbosomfoɔ* position from his maternal grandfather Kwadwo Owusu, he also inherited the social role and responsibility of "grandfather" vis-à-vis Kwadwo's kin relations. Kwadwo Owusu was Owusu Brempong's paternal grandfather. Upon Kwadwo's passing, Kofi Dɔnkɔ assumed the role of paternal grandfather to Owusu Brempong, and since then Kofi Dɔnkɔ referred affectionately to Owusu as *agya* (father) because the latter bore the name of his own paternal grandfather. According Owusu, "I knew [Kofi Dɔnkɔ] since my childhood, because he was my doctor for *asasaboro* (rheumatism), boils, and other childhood illnesses. I grew up to know him better when I worked with him and Mike Warren on traditional medicine."[2]

The person Kofi Dɔnkɔ matured into by age forty was clear to Brempong and others who knew him well:

> He was a very simple, modest, humble and dignified person who always tried to avoid conflicts. He spoke very little sometimes, [especially] when his head was down; but his words were always with substance and we all loved to listen to him and his wisdom. He spoke very little perhaps because he had a [shifting] voice; [his] voice would change from tenor to soprano while talking. He had large [eyes but was] crossed-eyed and occasionally lifted his head for people to see his eyes. When things [did not] turn in his favour, he would always walk to his bedroom, stay there for a while and return with vitality and more ideas. He loved to dress simple but would put on ceremonial wears such as *kente* or white cloth during important occasions. He loved children and often played with them before applying any medicine to them. He was very good with children diseases such as convulsion, boils and others. Several mothers in Takyiman and its surrounding villages loved Nana Kofi Donkor. He was also known in Akomadan, Wenchi, Nkoranza (his ancestry), Kumase and several places in the north and Ivory Coast. He helped several mothers for their children's diseases. The Yoruba mothers who lived in Takyiman loved him because he was always kind and nice to them and their children, especially in times of crises. Indeed, he was a very good traditional pediatrician.[3]

Others who knew Kofi Dɔnkɔ unanimously subscribe to this profile. Beyond his handsome appearance, they all characterized him as "very respectful and humble," "very compassionate," "a good counselor," "very gentle," and "very strong until a [sick] woman from Akomadan came to him and asked Nana [Dɔnkɔ] to carry her and when he tried, he fell down and broke his leg."[4] Although this incident happened later in life, it underscores the qualities ascribed to him. Kofi Dɔnkɔ's efficacy in dispensing health care for little or no compensation was routine, for he "was always interested in the good health of his patients," and many affectionately remember him as a compassionate "giver [who] loves everybody and even accepts mad people at his table and dines with them."⁵ Naturally, when he participated in the first health projects in contemporary Africa geared toward a working relationship between biomedicine and indigenous therapeutics, Kofi Dɔnkɔ strategically incorporated a few biomedical techniques into his practice, creating "a unique form of healing.... He [would] later conform to the modern procedures of accessing health care where patients were given attendance cards with their medical history and herbs given to the patient written [on them]."⁶

His approach to healing, however, flowed from his core values: a deep confidence in the *abosom* and medicines embedded in nature, in family, in a particular love for children (and treating their illnesses), and an abiding respect for culture, for ancestry, and for "people from all walks of life."⁷ Although most patients came to him, he "used to travel to Sunyani, Kumase and the northern part of Ghana to provide services to people who are in need of it," often "attending to patients in critical conditions in different areas like Wankyi and others."⁸ The most common ailments, and the ones for which he was often called on to cure during his healing career, included childhood diseases, tumors, chicken pox, convulsions, guinea worm, stomachaches, cholera, gonorrhea, piles, menstrual pains, and diabetes, which took the lives of many, including family members.⁹ And of course there were "instances where some patients were referred to Nana Dɔnkɔ from the Holy Family Hospital in Takyiman for healing and [there]after the patients are sent back to the doctors to prove his ability in curing such diseases."¹⁰

In the same way that Kofi Dɔnkɔ had grown—and was still growing—into his healing craft and into a reputation for effective therapeutics, so too were Takyiman and the tripartite colony evolving along jagged lines of freedom and interdependence. Between 1950 and 1970, the patterns of life ran on parallel tracks for Kofi Dɔnkɔ, in Takyiman, and in the colony and nation, crisscrossing each other and providing scaled perspectives on some of the same crucial events. Kofi Dɔnkɔ's and his sister's known expertise in their community enabled their family to turn a tragedy into an independent "healer's village," while a Takyiman-led Bonokyɛmpem Federation, a movement that consolidated Bono identity and independence from Asante, partnered with Kwame Nkrumah in forging a nation independent of British colonial rule. The competing national factions and organizations vying for independence reveal similar tensions at the local level, where Kofi

Dɔnkɔ and colleagues formed an autonomous healing association, while he shaped healers' engagement with the new hospital in Takyiman and the contents of new forms of "customary laws" promulgated during the early Ghana republic. The new republic ironically inhibited "traditional" institutions but provided the conditions for "independent" African churches and an Islamic organization (Ahmadiyya) to take root under one-party rule. Rather than become divided along religious and political lines, Kofi Dɔnkɔ remained sought out by Christians and Muslims and avoided much of the conjoined twins of local and national politics that fomented military coups and crises. In this way the chapter narrates a series of relationships, freedoms sought, and twists of fortunes around the evolving story of Kofi Dɔnkɔ, his community, and his nation to be.

❊

THE WORK AND adoration enjoyed by healers such as Kofi Dɔnkɔ grants us some insights into his fellow townspeople and, as principal recipients of his therapeutic care, their self-understandings of healers. By 1948 the township's population had reached 2,581 individuals settled in some 253 households. Because Meyerowitz or her research assistants were only interested in the views of Takyiman's political elites, we are left with the recollections of Kofi Dɔnkɔ's contemporaries and their children for our window into the townspeople's world. In such a relatively close-knit community, however, these specimens of remembrance take on greater meaning and in many ways represent popular views of healers, as each of the 253 households might possess one kind of healer. Healers were undoubtedly viewed as members of "their community with a cultural sensitivity whom they could trust," as "very powerful men [and women] capable of healing all sorts of physical and spiritual diseases," and as "highly respected for the kind of services they provided." Among these general observations, Kofi Dɔnkɔ ranked among "the most powerful healers in the Takyiman district because of the potency of his herbs," while some viewed him as "the most powerful traditional healer in the whole of Takyiman." These emphases on "power" (*tumi*) in ranking Kofi Dɔnkɔ among his peers are deeply significant: tumi is the conductive force through which social relations and hierarchy in Akan societies were determined. View from this perspective, Kofi Dɔnkɔ's prowess was enlarged not simply by his "very potent medicine for curing all sorts of diseases," but also through patients who were referred to him by biomedical experts at the principal hospital in Takyiman and through the wide healing net he cast among a range of individuals, including Christians and "even Muslims."[11] But an even greater measure of Kofi Dɔnkɔ the healer—his principal vocation by the mid-twentieth century—was the colonial setting in which he operated and the increasing weight of colonial policies on the practices of healers.

Prompted by a 1949 incident in the colonial capital of Accra involving the deeds of an alleged "quack doctor," the colonial police force was encouraged to verify healers applying or reapplying for licenses in the various districts and to submit clearance reports to Native Authority officials on the basis of character references from persons in the healer's community. In 1949 ten licensed and registered *abosomfoɔ/akɔmfoɔ* were in Takyiman, whereas neighboring polities such as Dormaa had twenty-five; Nkoransa, twenty-nine; and Wankyi, five.[12] Although no evidence points to Kofi Dɔnkɔ's inclusion among these licensed healers, the extremely low number of registrants, compared with the possible number of healers among a population over 2,500 does not seem to add up. One explanation, however, can be found in the relations between political authority and spiritual authority in Takyiman. Two contemporary cases should suffice. On 3 May 1948, ɔkɔmfoɔ Akosua Pomaa of Bamiri, a village in southeast Takyiman, was tried for violations not mentioned in the records, but for which she was ultimately "deprived of being a priestess [ɔkɔmfoɔ] from this day by the motion of the whole state meeting which consists of all fetish priests of Techiman and the Techiman State."[13] In effect, all the abosomfoɔ/akɔmfoɔ in Takyiman, including Kofi Dɔnkɔ, had ruled with the Takyimanhene and his elders against Akosua Pomaa, who was discharged from her role as ɔkɔmfoɔ. The next case concerned Kofi Mosi, who held the highest-ranking position among all healers in Takyiman (figure 5.1).

In January 1950 Kofi Mosi, *ɔbosomfoɔhene* (head of all abosomfoɔ/ akɔmfoɔ in Takyiman), was destooled from his position. Although politically motivated, his destoolment was likely processed through the same "whole state meeting" that removed Akosua Pomaa from her position.[14] Kofi Mosi and Akosua Pomaa might not have taken this view, but Takyiman was much more favorable to healers than comparable towns of its size, including the future regional capital of Sunyani, where healers had to secure a permit to play drums, dance, sing, and festively fire a gun in association with particular abosom. The owner and custodian of the Horo *ɔbosom*, Kwadwo Boahen ("Kojo Buahin"), for instance, applied for a four-month permit for "worshipping Horo Fetish" in the town of Sunyani and its surrounding forest. The application letter dated 12 April 1949, along with a report on Horo by the criminal investigation unit of the police force, went

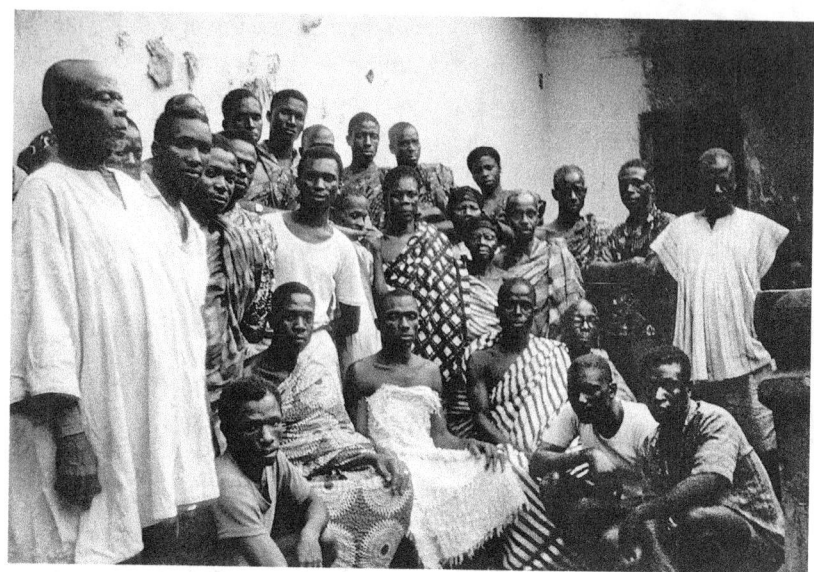

FIGURE 5.1. Taa Mensa Kwabena ɔbosomfoɔ Kofi Mosi, 1965. From the Dennis Michael Warren Slide Collection, Special Collections Department, University of Iowa Libraries. Used courtesy of Greg Prickman, Head of Special Collections.

to the Gold Coast police in Sunyani and then the district commissioner. The report notes, "Since its institution police have kept an open eye over the adherents of this fetish but have in each case failed to secure an order to confiscate it for the simple reason that it does not come under the prohibited fetish list."[15] Drumming, dancing, and singing in town were prohibited without a permit and fines were issued for each infraction. Eventually, on May 10, the district commissioner granted the permit but limited the request to one month, concluding, "you must therefore renew this permit on 12th June, 1949."[16] In Takyiman, such draconian regulations were nonexistent. Instead, the numerous healers, including Kofi Dɔnkɔ, celebrated the festival of their abosom and Takyiman-wide celebrations such as the *Apoɔ* festival, which featured seven days of drumming, dancing, singing, culturally approved insults, and the ridicule of authorities with "a large crowd of visitors and spectators" in April 1948 (figure 5.2).[17]

Because Takyiman was granted permission to leave the Asante Confederacy in 1948, this Apoɔ celebration might have taken on added meaning, especially as an event infused with anti-Asante sentiments. That feeling of autonomy from Asante overlordship and humiliation would have been

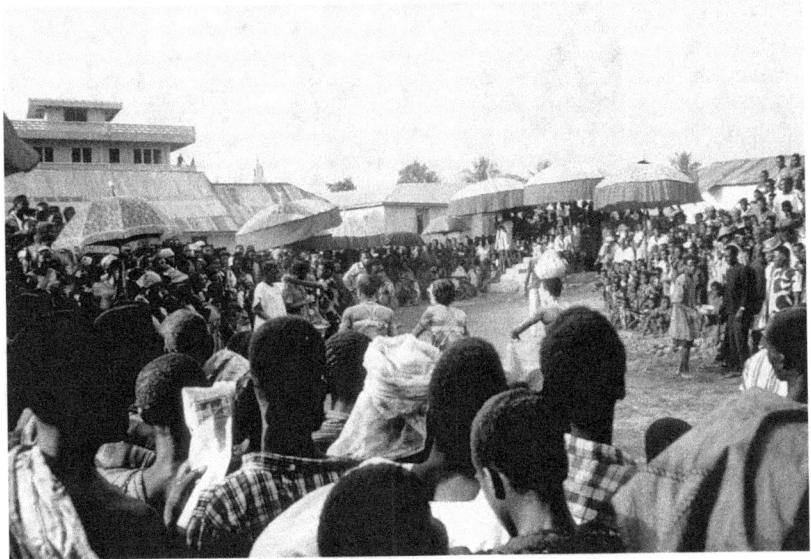

FIGURE 5.2. Takyiman Apoɔ Festival, 1970. From the Dennis Michael Warren Slide Collection, Special Collections Department, University of Iowa Libraries. Used courtesy of Greg Prickman, Head of Special Collections.

cathartic. But this liberating moment was filled with an ironic consequence that would soon become a blessing for Kofi Dɔnkɔ and his family. No sooner than Akumfi Ameyaw III was successful in the fight to secede from the Asante Confederacy and to engineer a movement for Bono unification did he unfortunately kill his niece and wound one of his stool carriers during a ceremonial gun firing at Adontenhene Nana Kasampire's funerary rites. Ameyaw III was soon placed in custody and suspended from carrying out any of his duties as Takyimanhene. For his anti-Asante and pro-Bono position, Ameyaw III drew supporters from the Takyiman Traditional Council and from many among the townspeople. When he traveled to Kumase for his trial, these constituencies in Takyiman were deeply concerned about whether or when he would return. We have already seen how unsuccessful Ameyaw III was in legal disputes involving the Wankyihene and the Privy Council, and so his supporters had good reason to worry while he traveled to the capital of his Asante nemesis.

In the suspense, the townspeople and their leadership turned to several healers. The wise and dynamic Adwoa Akumsa, the elder sister of Kofi Dɔnkɔ, came to the rescue and proved to be more able than other

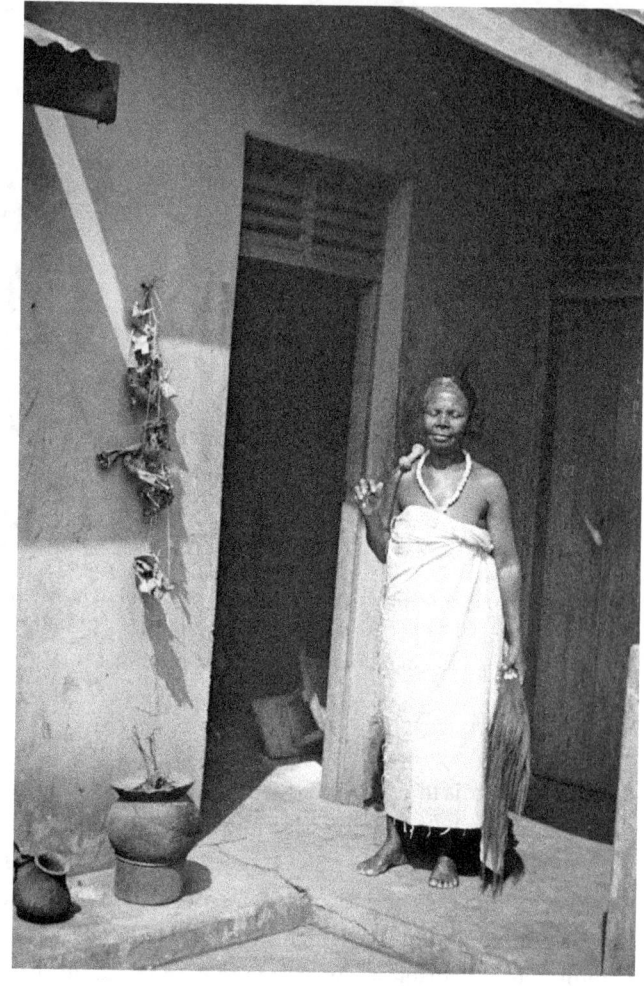

FIGURE 5.3. Kofi Dɔnkɔ's sister, Adowa Akumsa, 1969. From the Dennis Michael Warren Slide Collection, Special Collections Department, University of Iowa Libraries. Used courtesy of Greg Prickman, Head of Special Collections.

healers consulted (figure 5.3). After consulting her principal ɔbosom and performing a few ritual sacrifices, she told everyone that Ameyaw III would return to Takyiman free and safe in three days. As Nana Kofi Ɔboɔ, ɔkyeame for Asubɔnten Kwabena and Kofi Dɔnkɔ's nephew, recalled, "We were initially in Tunsuase and Nana Adwoa Akumsa prophesied [what would happen to] Nana Akumfi Ameyaw [who accidently] shot... the queen mother of Dwomor, a suburb of Takyiman, [who] was hit by [the] stray bullet and died. Because of that, Nana Akumfi Ameyaw, the then Takyimanhene, was to be arrested and [Nana] Akumsa said nothing will happen to Nana Akumfi Ameyaw... and Nana Akumfi Ameyaw was freed."

Because of Nana Akumsa's "prophesy," the Takyimanhene gave her "a vast land" in Takyiman called Nyafoman—reminiscent of a polity bearing the same name during the Bono kingdom era in present-day Nkoransa. A village called kɔmfokrom ("healer's town") was built on this land. According to Nana Kofi Ɔboɔ, Kofi Dɔnkɔ "asked his sister to give him a room for Asubɔnten in [the] Akumsa house in Nyafoman/Kɔmfokrom due to the size [of] and pressure from the family in Tunsuase. Nana Yaw Taahoo, the uncle [or nephew] of Nana Kofi Dɔnkɔ, was about to build a family house in [a] building [with several floors] in Tunsuase [but he] offered the building blocks to be used to construct a house for [the] Asubɔnten shrine here in Kɔmfokrom."[18] Building the new *bosomfie* ("shrine house") for Asubɔnten Kwabena on new land and with the help of kin ran concurrent with Kofi Dɔnkɔ's expansion of his family and his life work.

Kofi Dɔnkɔ's passion for family rather than politics is most evident in the highly fragmented and scant notes he left in what amounts to a diary. Most likely penned by a secretary, possibly his nephew and successor Yaw Mensa, Kofi Dɔnkɔ's diary is a small black book with loose and missing pages, but with entries, typically one-liners, on several pages. Much of the book is blank. Be that as it may, Kofi Dɔnkɔ could have chosen to record anything, so what is remarkable about these first-person fragments is his stubborn focus on the birth and death of kin in the extant entries for the early 1950s. On 27 January 1950, he recorded, "my wife Akosua Donkor delivered female child . . . the child is called Afua Kwafie."[19] On March 3 or 5, Kofi Dɔnkɔ noted, "my wife Effua Murufie [Afia Monofie] delivered a male child on Sunday the 5th March, 1950 (the child's name is Akwesi [Amoako]) (father's name, Kofi Donkor)." On June 23 he tells us, "My sister Abena Nsia died; it was on Tuesday." A few months later, on September 18, he recorded, "My brother Kofi Boo has died."[20] On 15 August 1954, Kofi Dɔnkɔ recorded, "wife Akosua Donkor brought forth a male child by name Kwasi Nsowa," and on 21 February 1955, "my son Yaw Sakyi was born."[21] Kofi Dɔnkɔ intuitively knew these entrances and exits of human life. If celebrations marked these comings and goings, there is no way to tell what emotional impact, if any, they had on Kofi Dɔnkɔ. The diary simply does not give us any latitude either way, though we can suppose joy and other emotional content were interwoven in each life transition. While family was central to the foreground of Kofi Dɔnkɔ's midcentury life, the political background to that existence and the social context in which his children were born revolved around three themes, equally central in the life of Takyiman and the colony: cocoa, colonial politics, and the consolidation of Bono identity.

COCOA REMAINED KING during the 1950s, especially in the "protectorate of Ashanti" and Takyiman, while the anticolonial drive toward political independence led by Nkrumah found support in the Bonokyɛmpem movement based in Takyiman. Nkrumah saw in their struggle a way to advance his party's objectives vis-à-vis the recalcitrant and conservative elements in Asante. In 1951 Nkrumah became the leader of Government Business and the Cooperative Department—essentially, the de facto prime minister. Cooperative unions in the Asante and Bono regions constituted some two-thirds of the total workforce, where cocoa farming was the primary occupation and produced approximately 60 percent of the colony's cocoa.[22] The mixture of cocoa profits and colonial politics in the recent aftermath of World War II provided an opening for the growth in the number of missionary hospitals—and churches and schools—established amid hostility and with a sense of "mission" and zealousness. The three hospitals run by missions in 1951 would increase to thirty in 1960. Although Takyiman was not exempt from the inflow of medical missions or unaware of the positive political implications of its cocoa endowments, the import of missionary institutions was slow in coming and their presence only permissible when the polity's leadership saw them as serving a newly consolidated Bono identity.

The newly crafted constitution of the Bonokyɛmpem Federation (approved 25 March 1951), which I will simply call the Bono Federation, makes abundantly clear the premium placed on that identity. Article 2 the Federation aimed "to raise the socio-economic and educational status of Brong peoples," "maintain complete unity among the peoples of the member states," "serve as a political vanguard for the Brong peoples," "fight relentlessly until the Brong States are redeemed from want, ignorance and tribal inferiority complex," and to "encourage and foster rural development." The governing body of the Federation—the council—also declared the "Brong language" rather than the mutually intelligible Asante language "shall be the medium of speech in the council."[23] Arising out of Takyiman, the Bono nationalistic movement compelled leaders of the contested nine villages to assert their allegiance to Takyiman and not Asante. In a 1953 resolution, these leaders lamented being "tossed between" the two sides and resolved, "We want to make it unequivocally and specifically plain.... We the Brongs of Tuobodom, Ofuman, Tanoso and Ahyiayem (New-Techiman) are subjects of the Techiman Stool and that we or our ancestors had never been Ashantis."[24]

A year before political independence, Nkrumah's Convention People's Party (CPP), Asante and its National Liberation Movement (NLM) party, and the Bono Federation were still enjoined, although Asante and the NLM sought to carve out a space for themselves in the design of the new republic. Nkrumah's plan for a modernized "socialistic society" built around indigenous values required local leaders to buy into his vision of national governance to which "chiefs" would be subordinate and through which they would receive their legitimacy. Nkrumah's CPP had been very much involved in the everyday struggle of folks in the countryside, and in the morass of land and succession disputes, but on the side of opponents to incumbent "chiefs." The CPP, however, needed the rural support central to its nationalist movement, yet that support came through the very institution of "chieftaincy" the party sought to marginalize. The mutually beneficial arrangement between Nkrumah and the Bono Federation was clearly strategic, but it did not sit well with Asante's leadership, the loudest opposition to Nkrumah's attempts to marginalize "chieftaincy," if not replace it with local versions of a central government. Targeting the secession of Takyiman and the question of the nine villages, Asantehene Osei Prempe II charged that the government and the British crown were setting a precedent for secession through a mere resolution, and he regretted that the government had "not kept its hands off the issue." "The present government," Perempe II continued, "appears to favour the secession movement as if it furthers its policy of annihilating Chieftaincy."[25]

The Asantehene was indeed correct that "chieftaincy" was the central problematic for Nkrumah, Asante, Takyiman, and other political actors in the colony's transition from colonial rule to political independence. In fact, the localization of national politics and the institution of "chieftaincy" in the Asante-Bono dispute led to the creation of the Brong-Ahafo region—a confluence of the Bono Federation led by Takyiman and Nkrumah's support of this movement to create regional governmental bodies, including regional houses of chiefs, under which "chiefs" were subordinated. Local courts and matters of local justice under "chiefly" jurisdiction were replaced by paid magistrates. The 1955 Mate Kole Commission, chaired by Nene Azu Mate Kole, was organized by Nkrumah's government to examine the Asante-Bono dispute. Nkrumah endorsed Bono unification, and within two years of political independence in 1957, the Asante Confederacy was reconstituted with reduced powers for the Asantehene and stool revenues placed under the central government, while the Ahafo and Bono/Brong districts were combined to create the Brong-Ahafo region, which was run by government ministers.²⁶ In similar fashion, but on a much broader scale, the Gold Coast Colony and British Togoland were merged on 6 March 1957 to create the politically independent republic of Ghana. As Nkrumah's CPP fought foreign colonial rule and internal "neocolonial" institutions such as "chieftaincy," the party and its leader also had to fight for the new nation's economic survival. Ironically, the anticolonialist government of Nkrumah replaced the cast members but not the colonial instruments of governance and, as in the colonial era, came to anchor the country's economic development on cocoa.

The United Ghana Farmers' Council (UGFC), the farmers' wing of the CPP, was founded in 1953 and later renamed the United Ghana Farmers' Cooperative Council (UGFCC). Kofi Dɔnkɔ was member number 165-A of the UGFCC branch in Takyiman.²⁷ Cocoa was the main source on which the colonial export economy depended, but it also was the source of the revenues through which the CPP attempted to overcome this dependence.²⁸ Cooperatives farms and self-help practices in several Takyiman villages were part of a wave of agricultural cooperatives that, after political independence, were responsible for marketing approximately 40 percent of the total cocoa produced. Nkrumah's government feared that the cooperative movement was becoming an economic as well as a political force in rural areas and ordered the movement disbanded, members' assets confiscated, their economic functions transferred to the Cocoa Marketing Board, and the Department of Cooperatives dissolved.

In late 1950s the UGFC urged the expulsion of foreign firms from the domestic cocoa trade, but it came into conflict with private traders (many of whom belonged to cooperatives) over control of the cocoa trade. In the early 1960s more than half of Ghana's cocoa was produced in the Asante-Bono region, where cocoa farms were worked principally by indigenes and where "chiefs" seldom sold land outright to "strangers" or "temporary visitors" but "rented" land on a system that was dependent on farmers' actual achievement in clearing and planting.²⁹ In 1961 the UGFC became the sole buyer of Ghana's cocoa and maintained this commercial monopoly until Nkrumah was ousted from power in 1966.³⁰ The CPP greatly depended on the cocoa fiscal surplus to expand the public sector and to redistribute it for national development; the UGFC's monopoly removed local middlemen-farmers and farmer cooperatives from the local cocoa trade, but created new bureaucratic intermediaries (i.e., those running large commercial farms) who managed to use the UGFC for their own interests.

While there were certainly political and economic weaknesses in the use of the UGFC as an instrument of CPP strategy, the CPP's basic economic failure was its monocultural economic structure. These cooperatives also failed because they lacked resources, management capacity, and adequate technical support; successive governments would adopt the *nnoboa* system for farming.³¹ The undermining and near collapse of agricultural cooperatives as well as the institution of chieftaincy during the Nkrumah regime have a shared but contradictory history. On the one hand, Nkrumah proclaimed building the new nation on indigenous values, but, on the other hand, he sought to destroy indigenous institutions underwritten by those values. He led an anticolonialist movement for political independence but ended up using rather than replacing colonial instruments of the state (e.g., the Cocoa Marketing Board) and the central government in draconian ways. A year after political independence, for instance, the CPP swiftly passed the Preventive Detention Act (1958) that legalized the detention of CPP opponents without trial; this included the detention of J. B. Danquah, a former Nkrumah ally and one of Ghana's leading scholars and jurists. As readers will recall, Danquah fought in the courts not only for recalcitrant and high-profile "chiefs" such as Ofori Atta I but also for Takyimanhene Akumfi Ameyaw III, who made the greatest strides in the protracted Asante-Bono dispute that morphed into a nationalist movement for Bono unification. Indeed, the hopes that accompanied the elevation of Nkrumah to pan-African greatness and president of Ghana were thematically followed by corruption, political centralization, party politics, and dissatisfaction within the armed forces. A series of military personnel would seize power over the next few decades, beginning with the 1966 coup that removed Nkrumah from office.

When Nkrumah and his supporters ushered in political independence from colonial rule and named the new nation "Ghana" in 1957, Kofi Dɔnkɔ and other healers in Takyiman formed an association comprising akɔmfoɔ/abosomfoɔ and named it Kɔmpan Adɛ Pa. The name takes its origin from the phrase *akɔm panin yɛ adee pa* ("ancient akɔm is a good thing"), which was consciously structured as a self-affirming call ("ancient akɔm") and response ("is a good thing").³² Associated with this phrase was a cloth analogy: the process of culture, embodied by akɔm or indigenous spirituality, is akin to an ancient cloth that is worn, washed, and passed on to succeeding generations without losing its significance. Although it is unclear why the association was formed then, where the association was established and by who may have much to do with the social and cultural transformations underway in the 1950s, as the colony transitioned to an independent nation. In the inauguration of a national identity that subordinated cultural specificity as Bono, Asante, Gã, Hausa, or Dagomba—in favor of "Ghanaian"—the fabric of indigenous cultures lacked the protection of the state, and the most central arenas of human life—spirituality/religion, education, health, and language—were vulnerable to predation by missionary institutions empowered by the state. Whether in the hands of European missions or converted Africans in their "independent" churches, the Christian ideology was the blood that flowed through the circulatory system of the nation, feeding the major organs of churches, health facilities, and schools. And like a virus, that ideology reproduced and diffused itself using indigenous institutions as hosts.

Soon schools rather than elders educated the young, bibles and hymnbooks were translated into indigenous languages, lexicons and dictionaries were created by missions in all the major local languages, clinics and hospitals preached the gospel to patients, and churches brought these strands together as the *only* place to worship "God" and *his* son in the phenotypical image of a European/white male. Was this the "beloved country" Kwame Nkrumah said was "free forever" during his independence speech on 6 March 1957? Although Nkrumah proclaimed that the people of Ghana were "no more a colonial but a free and independent people," he did indicate that Ghana's independence was impossible without the "support of God," and at the end of his speech he requested that his "fellow Ghanaians" ask for "God's blessing." One of the underexplored ironies of the nationalist and independence moment in twentieth-century Africa, and in Ghana no less, is how anticolonialist and political leaders were thoroughly schooled in mission settings and why they allowed, even promoted, the colonial missionary ideologies and assaults on indigenous cultural forms and ideas while they claimed to value things "traditional." While here is not the place for such an exploration, the very name and timing of the healers' association in Takyiman suggests a localized response to those assaults, the protection missions received from the central government, and local officeholders who saw the missions as opportunities to enhance their standing as "modern."

❇

THE ONE OR TWO mission church-schools in Takyiman failed to win over but a few individuals to their ideological camp. In the early 1950s this woeful record would change with the establishment of the Holy Family Hospital, which emerged from the collaboration between the Takyimanhene and the Society of Catholic Medical Missionaries (SCMM). Where schools and churches failed, the only hospital in Takyiman would enjoy greater staying power and function as the principal conduit for Christian ideology and proselytization through the guise of medical service. Naturally, the hospital also functioned as an ideological counterpoint and therapeutic competitor to the healers of Kɔmpan Adɛ Pa, who had previously monopolized the dispensation of curative treatments to the community. Between 1952 and 1953, the chairperson of the Takyiman Local Council (TLC) and the Holy Family Dispensary in the town of Berekum, west of Takyiman, outlined plans for a maternity clinic and dispensary at Takyiman. A proposed contract between the "Chief and Elders of the State of Techiman" and the SCMM detailed the allotment of ten to twenty acres: the deed would be in the name of the SCMM, and the dispensary or "Holy Family Health Center" in Takyiman would follow the structural plans of the Berekum dispensary.[33]

The parties agreed that the Holy Family Medical Mission would assume full responsibility for building and maintaining the proposed facility in exchange for "outright and unconditional grant of money and title to land." The TLC agreed unanimously to finance the building with £4,000 and twenty acres of land. No additional grants, however, would be made to the mission from the TLC because the mission expected financial support for the project to come from patient fees, though the government would fund the twenty-seven mission hospitals in the country shortly after independence.[34] The Sister Superior of the mission Anna Dangel stated, "there is no intention of developing the project into a Hospital but that they hoped that it would feed their Hospital at Berekum," and if justified, they might run an ambulance service between Berekum and Takyiman.[35] During the planning stage for what would be the Holy Family Hospital (HFH), the Roman Catholic Hospital in the small town of Hwidiem was the only hospital serving the entire Ahafo region, and it had plans to extend services elsewhere in August 1961. This expansion of services would have been too late and too far a distance for Takyiman's townspeople, where a local hospital was needed. The Takyimanhene and his elders did everything in their powers to persuade missions rather than the government to build such a health facility.

In 1954 the Medical Mission Sisters erected Takyiman's first European health care facility, the HFH. The hospital was managed by a team but governed by the Catholic Diocese of Sunyani through the Diocesan Health Committee, which functioned as the board of directors.[36] The Medical

Mission Sisters were not the only mission invited to establish a hospital; they just happened to be the only ones who accepted the invitation. In fact, at the end of 1954, Techimanhene Akumfi Ameyaw III invited the Seventh-Day Adventist Mission of the Gold Coast, based in Kumase, to build a hospital in Takyiman and offered land to that effect. The mission's president, Howard J. Welsh, informed the Takyimanhene that they did not have the money or staff for another hospital but would keep his letter of invitation on file for future consideration.[37] Soon after it became clear to all parties that the HFH would be the principal hospital in town, frustrations with the hospital's capacity or its inability to meet preconceived expectations erupted. In May 1956 the Takyiman leadership requested a "special Doctor" who could "treat cases of [a] serious nature, such as operations" since "the female so called Doctors in the said Clinic [i.e., the HFH] are unable to treat any sickness of any length seriousity [sic] but always refer cases which are not at all serious to Berekum." If such a medical doctor did not arrive, they demanded the "[Holy Family] Maternity Clinic changed to a Government Clinic in order to get [a] qualified Doctor in the Clinic."[38]

Although it remains unclear whether this demand was ever met, the HFH weathered the turbulence and in 1960 stood as the uncontested biomedical facility in the town, serving, at least in theory, some 8,700 to 8,755 townspeople arranged among 511 households. The early records for the HFH are scant or missing, but if it functioned like its contemporary mission hospital in the Asante town of Agogo, then sources for the latter open a window into the former. The Agogo hospital, like the HFH, remained under church ownership, held church services on hospital grounds, and began every operation with a prayer. Since the 1950s, doctors had increasingly been fully committed to the task of evangelization, engaging in or facilitating daily services for patients, bible readings to outpatients before consultation hours, devotions, the Lord's Supper, celebrations of Christmas, joint bible study, and Christian staff associations at a "Christian" hospital.[39] The Agogo hospital's idea of a community—and this idea was a generally shared missionary characteristic across Ghana—was a mission "hospital community," not a "village community," wherein the hospital's engagement with villagers commonly focused on schooling and morality and the production of a "modernized Christian elite" drawn exclusively from the church community. In 1961 the building of the largest church in Takyiman, the cathedral of St. Paul, was completed, giving the Catholics two reinforcing pillars in a town becoming less anomalous and being pulled more into the Christianizing and legal orbit of the republic.

Tempting as it is to believe the rise in the numbers of Catholic churches and hospitals in places like Takyiman had something to do with Nkrumah's affinity to Catholic missions—he attended and later taught in such schools—his government's hand in Takyiman affairs was much more explicit in the creation of the Brong-Ahafo region and the Brong-Ahafo Regional House of Chiefs. The first republican constitution of Ghana in 1960 drove the need for new or updated "customary laws," which became matters of law rather than of fact to be evidenced by witnesses. This new conception of customary laws meant that accurate and up-to-date ones had to be aggregated and filtered through Houses of Chiefs or Traditional Councils, whose opinion on a customary law in question may be furnished to the courts.[40] On 13 February 1961 Takyiman officeholders submitted their "customary laws" to the clerk of the Brong-Ahafo Regional House of Chiefs in Sunyani. Some parts of the document reveal the self-representation of Takyiman through its leaders and confirm some of the enduring trends in cultural understanding and social configuration. In either case, spiritual culture permeated all such laws and a sampling of them—associated with festivals, funerals, and taboos—should suffice.

Throughout Bono lands, especially Takyiman, the Tanɔ River remained deeply sacred, and transgressions necessitated purification rituals in "accordance with custom."[41] Taa Mensa Kwabena still ritually consumed newly harvested yams first, after which officeholders and townspeople may eat them. This occasion was celebrated through the annual Fofie "yam" festival in which a ritual meal of mashed yam (ɛtɔ) was prepared for deceased male and female stool occupants.[42] The other major state festival, Apoɔ, was enlarged to a twelve-day celebration marked in its beginning by the Takyimanhene traveling to the sacred ancestral grove of the polity.[43] The Apoɔ festivities were open to everyone, and during the celebration the laws of the land were relaxed without retaliation. During these state celebrations, no funerals, wailings, or drumming were permitted. In noncelebratory times, a range of taboos regulated social life. For instance, farming on Friday and Sunday were tabooed. But the most numerous and most serious taboos were channeled through spiritual forces that were a barometer of society's health and stability. Thus no one entered a "shrine house" wearing funerary cloth (*kuntunkuni*), desecrated a sacred grove or stream, buried a woman who died in childbirth before removing the child, cursed the townspeople or the state using a "Fetish," nor prophesied falsely on matters concerning the polity or of public interest. Women during their menstrual cycle did not enter a "shrine house" or proscribed sacred grove.[44] Furthermore, healers were required to attend state festivals and attend to individuals who sought consultation without prejudice or animosity. And in the all-important matter of funerals, "strong drinks" (other than beer or palm vine) were strictly prohibited for commoner funerals, and fasting for funerary purposes was restricted to three or fewer days.[45] Violators of any the above were duly fined, and the collected fees were used to purify the affected area, ritual object, or ceremonial process.

The "customary laws" detailed above were fashioned in the form of a declaration by the Takyiman Traditional Council, chaired by Takyimanhene Ameyaw Kwakye II, on the advice of the Brong-Ahafo Regional House of Chiefs but in accordance with section 58 of the 1961 Chieftaincy Act. Prominent healers like Kofi Dɔnkɔ were often consulted on matters of spiritual culture and indigenous notions of law, order, and the taboo regimen used to safeguard society. The declaration was then sent to the Regional Commissioner's office in Sunyani on 3 January 1962 and again on 7 November 1963. In the declaration, the Takyiman Traditional Council "decided to abolish funeral celebrations in its area of jurisdiction," but tempered this reasoning by acknowledging the "traditional significance" of funerals and proposed several guidelines to "mitigate high and unnecessary expenses." Those guidelines suggested offering soft drinks, *pito* (indigenous beer brewed from fermented millet), and palm wine at funerals and proposed that donations "conform with the old tradition of the State"; that is, the offspring of the deceased person should bear the cost of the coffin and the celebration of any funeral must be made within a week of the person's passing.[46]

The topic of funerals and of "customary laws" in general remained—and remains—part of ongoing efforts to "modernize" or, said differently, to bring those laws in line with the colonial and postcolonial legal and political frameworks adopted by succeeding governments. The awkward and often misguided interplay between foreign ideas of law and order and an indigenous episteme play out in comical ways (depending on the reader's sense of humor) that underscore the absurdity of a "free" nation governing itself by laws designed for its colonial captivity. A typical example should make the point clearer. On 5 May 1973, the Brong-Ahafo Regional House of Chiefs decided to study and recommend those customary laws "considered out of date and [that] need to be modernized" for approval and transmission to the government. They requested the regional administrative officer's advice concerning which areas of such laws "should be modernized or abolished altogether." A handwritten note on the bottom of an 8 October 1973 letter from the regional administrative office read, "Surely, the House should be in a better position to know what customary laws need modernization. After all they are the custodians."⁴⁷

❃

BY THE EARLY 1960s the principal custodian of the nation, Kwame Nkrumah, had survived two attempted assassinations (one by his own bodyguard), and perhaps these internal threats and the prevailing antisocialist mood in the capitalist centers of the world prompted the national referendum that made Ghana a one-party state in 1964. Joining hundreds of diasporic Africans in Ghana, Malcolm X visited the country in 1964, leaving "impressed by Ghana" and by "Nkrumah's desire for industrialization."⁴⁸ During these years, Kofi Dɔnkɔ worked jointly with Nana Ama Feintim, who was the ɔkɔmfoɔ, or female custodian, for Asubɔnten Kwabena. By then, Nana Feintim's younger sister Ama Fofie served as her assistant when the ɔkɔmfoɔ was in trance, carrying her *hyire* (powdered white clay) during akɔm ritual dancing.⁴⁹ Nkrumah's modernization agenda focused on the nation's vital transportation and electricity needs, which in the process restored Takyiman to its historic position as a nexus between southern and northern Ghana and further opened the town to greater Ghana and the world. Beyond the building of the Takyiman Secondary School on the site of an ancient market, in 1965 the government began to construct through Takyiman a highway between Kumase and Tamale and to build bridges over the Black and White Volta Rivers, making Takyiman the fastest and most popular route that linked northern and southern Ghana.

Although much work remained on the newly paved but incomplete roads between Kumase and Takyiman, the roads through Takyiman were one of the principal routes to northern Ghana, which, in contrast to contemporary modes of transport, relied on ferryboat on the Black Volta at Yeji. After the Akosombo Dam (a.k.a. the Akosombo Hydroelectric Project) was completed in the late 1960s, the Volta River at Yeji became a five-mile-wide lake, but ferry transportation became inefficient.⁵⁰ These modernizing developments under Nkrumah's regime are undeniable, even by his most ardent critics. But during 1964 and 1965, Nkrumah pursued his socialist and pan-African agenda with vigor, alienating (further) the concerns of Ghana's citizenry and partnering with anticapitalist forces in Asia, Russia, and other parts of yet-to-be-decolonized Africa. In February 1966, while in China en route to Hanoi, Nkrumah was overthrown in absentia through a military coup. Coup leaders then established the National Liberation Council (NLC), led by General Joseph Ankrah (figure 5.4). A year later

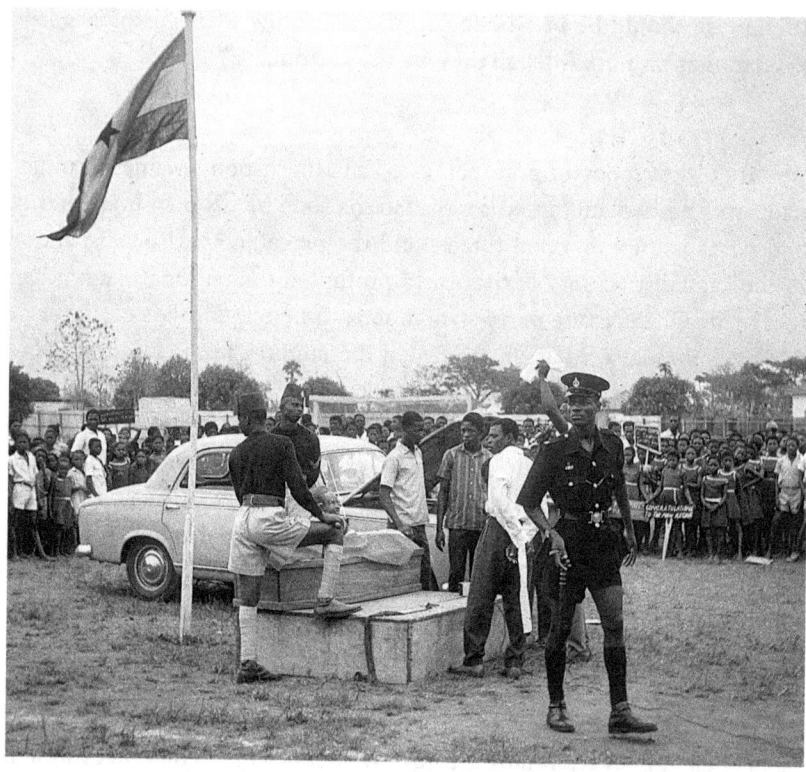

FIGURE 5.4. NLC rally. Mr. Acquah, speaker. From the Dennis Michael Warren Slide Collection, Special Collections Department, University of Iowa Libraries. Used courtesy of Greg Prickman, Head of Special Collections.

General Kotoka, one of the leaders of the military- and police-led NLC, was killed in an attempted coup, ushering in a pattern of military coups over the next two decades.

Against the sudden and politically violent transitions in national leadership, Kofi Dɔnkɔ welcomed a son named after him—Kofi Sakyi Sapɔn—and Takyiman welcomed a new Islamic religious organization from former British colonies and newly independent India and Pakistan. Muslims in Takyiman and under the ancient Bono kingdom were known commodities with established relations with Bono leaders, but they lived in self-isolated communities known locally as zongos (der. Hausa: *zango*).[51] During the beginning of Akumfi Ameyaw III's reign, a Muslim leader from the Hausa Zongo in Wankyi, Mallam Baba Enuwa, heard about the Takyimanhene's recent misfortune while in the Northern Territories and offered his reli-

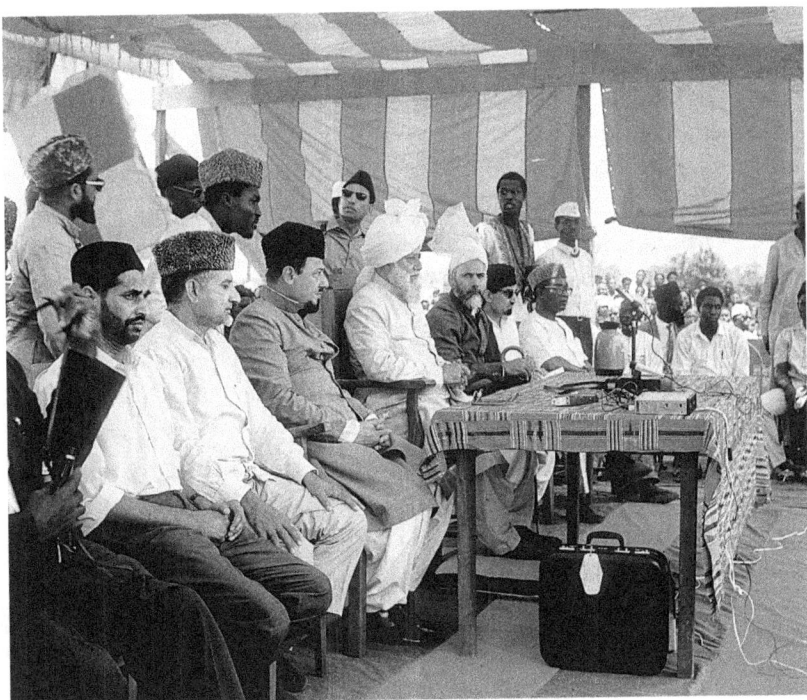

FIGURE 5.5. Ahmadiyya meeting, 1970. From the Dennis Michael Warren Slide Collection, Special Collections Department, University of Iowa Libraries. Used courtesy of Greg Prickman, Head of Special Collections.

gious assistance on the basis of cordial relations between Muslims and leaders in Takyiman. Baba Enuwa wrote, "my daily prayer is that may Allah (God) deliver you from the hands of your enemies and give you long life and prosperity. Further that Allah may cause your division to be an important division."[52] Before the mallam embarked on his trip to Mecca, he paid a visit to the Takyimanhene.

During the transition between Akumfi Ameyaw III and his successor, Kwakye Ameyaw II, Maulvi Abdul Wahab Bin Adam became the first African Ahmadiyya missionary trained in Pakistan, returning to Ghana in 1960 and becoming the first regional missionary for the Brong-Ahafo region. The formal opening of an Ahmadiyya mosque in Takyiman occurred on 1 October 1960 (figure 5.5).[53] Originally from the Asante region and schooled at the Ahmadiyya Secondary School in Kumase, Adam settled in Takyiman in 1964 and served as regional head of the Ahmadiyya mission until 1969. The Ahmadiyya movement was founded by Hazrat Mirza

Independences   157

Ghulam Ahmad (ca. 1835–1908) of Qadian, a Punjabi town in India, who claimed to be a spiritual reformer. The Ahmadiyya mission was established in 1921 at Saltpond, where they opened a school in 1926–27.[54] Four decades later, the mission claimed 304 branches with 170,000 members, 174 mosques, 40 primary and middle schools and 4 secondary schools, and a monthly English newspaper (the only Muslim paper in Ghana), the *Guidance*.[55] Orthodox Muslims in India and Pakistan rejected the legitimacy of the Ahmadiyya movement, forcing its members to establish its headquarters in England and embarking on a vigorous missionary project through the building of mosques in Asia, Africa, Europe, and elsewhere. Their presence in Ghana has been less than welcome. Sectarian, ritual, doctrinal, and "ethnic" tensions pervaded Muslim communities in Ghana with almost endemic factional strife, litigation, and disputes that often led to unrest and riots. Orthodox Muslims from northern and southern Ghana reject the largely Fante Ahmadiyya movement, which consciously imitated Christian missionary methods, building over 150 mosques and schools since 1957, although many students and teachers do not belong to the movement and the bulk of Fante Ahmadiyya remain illiterate. The large number of Ahmadiyya mission schools and widespread illiteracy among adherents undermine the popular view of Islam and literacy.

The choice of Takyiman for the Ahmadiyya mission may owe something to the historic relations between Muslims and its townspeople, but this only partly explains why Kofi Dɔnkɔ was so widely respected by Muslim women and men in Takyiman and why they were among his returning pool of patients seeking his therapeutic expertise and counsel. In Kofi Dɔnkɔ's diary entry for 10 October 1966, he or his scribe noted the "settlement of household cases," but also that "Tua Appau, Sisilasehene [leader of the Sisila people], he offered the land on Bamiri road called Nyinakofiase to the fetish Asubɔnten."[56] The Sisila were found in the predominantly Muslim region of northwest Ghana. Each Takyiman-based zongo community had their community-appointed leader, whose title was a combination of the cultural group's name and the Akan term *ɔhene* (e.g., Sisilahene), thus incorporating that group into an Akan sociopolitical order (figure 5.6). The Sisilahene "Tua Appau" more than likely resided in one of the Takyiman zongo communities populated by his people, and the land was offered as an in-kind gift of thanks to Kofi Dɔnkɔ on behalf of Asubɔnten Kwabena. This payment of land was no small gesture. In many ways the act shows the working relationship and mutual respect between adherents of an Islamic theology that supposedly abhorred "fetishism" and an *ɔbosomfoɔ* who,

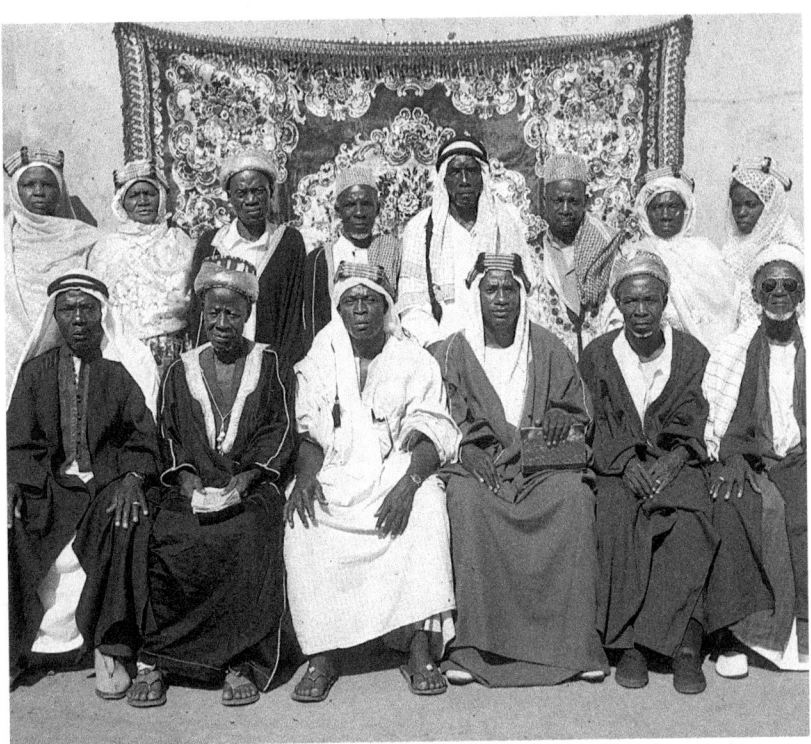

FIGURE 5.6. Zongohene Fie, Takyiman, 16 September 1970. From the Dennis Michael Warren Slide Collection, Special Collections Department, University of Iowa Libraries. Used courtesy of Greg Prickman, Head of Special Collections.

through his "shrine," served all members of his community, regardless of religious affiliation.

Once again, we might recall that Kofi Dɔnkɔ traveled to northern Ghana on numerous occasions, befriending and learning from Islamic healers but also attracting a significant number of clients who traveled to Takyiman for its markets, zongo communities filled with Muslim residents, and Kofi Dɔnkɔ's healing services. The description of the land given by the Sisilahene to Kofi Dɔnkɔ matches a large tract of land surveyed in 1974 and described as "the property of Obosomfo Kofi Donkor."[57] The land measured 135 acres. The size of the land in comparison to that of contiguous farms gives us some measure of Kofi Dɔnkɔ's and Asubɔnten Kwabena's value to their community, especially among those who held a set of beliefs different from Kofi Dɔnkɔ's. As described in his October 1966 entry, Kofi Dɔnkɔ's "shrub farm" (figure 5.7) was located off the Bamiri feeder road to Takyiman

Independences 159

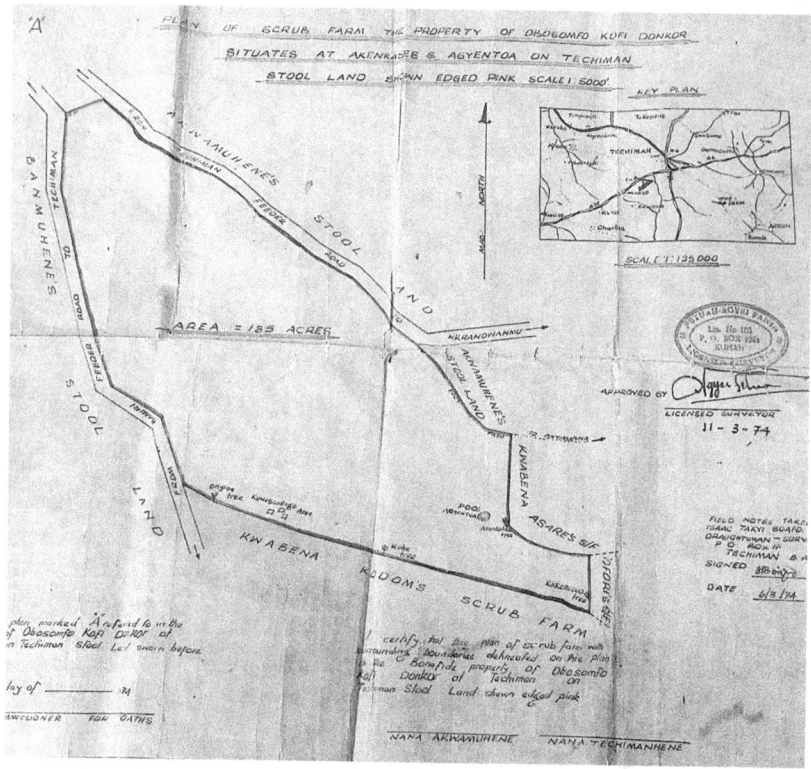

FIGURE 5.7. Survey of Kofi Dɔnkɔ's shrub farm, ca. 1975. Nana Kofi Dɔnkɔ Collection. Used with permission.

and nestled between stool lands belonging to the Akwamuhene and the Banmuhene, west and north of the surveyed farm. To the south and east of the 135-acre farm lay the much smaller "shrub farms" of Kwabena Kodom, Kwabena Asare, and an individual recorded as Ofori. Within the boundary of Kofi Dɔnkɔ's farm were the "Agyentoa" lake, "kokonisuo tree [*Spathodea campanulata*]," "kube [coconut] tree," and an "onyina tree," for which the land was named—Nyinakofiase ("under Kofi's *onyina* tree"). The onyina, or silk cotton tree (*Ceiba pentandra*), is both sacred and a treasure trove of medicinal applications. The site and name of the farm could not have been more fitting for a healer, especially one who lived at a time when the cultural ethos he represented began to receive less protection from the state and where state officials became more consumed with their own interests than those of the polity.

IN SEPTEMBER 1966 THE Takyiman polity celebrated its annual Fofie "yam" festival. The Takyiman Traditional Council issued this statement to the Ghana News Agency: the "Yam Festival is the celebration of the anniversary of the day when yam was first tasted and declared food by the 1st chief of Techiman at Bonomanso after it had been discovered by an elephant hunter [Takyi Firi] centuries ago immediately [after] they settled at Bonomanso." They explained that the festival was significant for three reasons. First, the citizens renewed their allegiance to the Takyimanhene. Second, the Takyimanhene paid tribute by offering sacrificial sheep and cooked yams (εtɔ) to the ancestors, prayed for the prosperity and health of the townspeople, and purified the blackened stools of past state leaders at the sacred grove. Third, the Takyimanhene thanked the townspeople in his palanquin and displayed indigenous cultural forms, and presented meat, yams, and other foods to strangers as tokens of love.[58] Taa Mensa Kwabena played no small role in the Fofie festival, and the absence of any mention of it and its ɔbosomfoɔ Kofi Mosi or Asubɔnten Kwabena, and of Kofi Dɔnkɔ, has an explanation. The prepared write-up given to the Ghana News Agency about the festival came from a council that was embroiled in conflicts with Takyimanhene Kwakye Ameyaw II, and from council members, including the Takyimanhene, who strove to fall in line with the "modernizing" trend of the nation (figure 5.8). They also began to abandon the historic spiritual-political contract between spiritualists (keepers of the community's culture and values) and officeholders (custodians of the community's land and servitors of its inhabitants).

New "chieftaincy" laws empowered local officeholders to deal with local matters (e.g., marriages, land disputes) and to implement changes to those laws, but few if any were concerned with protecting their indigenous cultures and institutions from the predaciousness of fanatical clergymen and Christianized politicians, which came under the guise of a constitutional "freedom of religion." Under the surge of Pentecostalism that swept through Ghana in the late 1960s and early 1970s, and the cowering of indigenous "chiefs" to its presence, Christian schooling and orthodoxy began to take control over processes of socialization in the hands of kin as well as of health and healing in the hands of healers who served their communities. In 1967 Owusu Brempong witnessed the last large and formal *bragorɔ* puberty rites in Takyiman.[59] The "customary rites" for marriage would die a slower death. As an example of the eroding socialization powers of kin and community, not to mention a strategy some claimed worked against teenage pregnancies, the disappearance of bragorɔ was emblematic. On

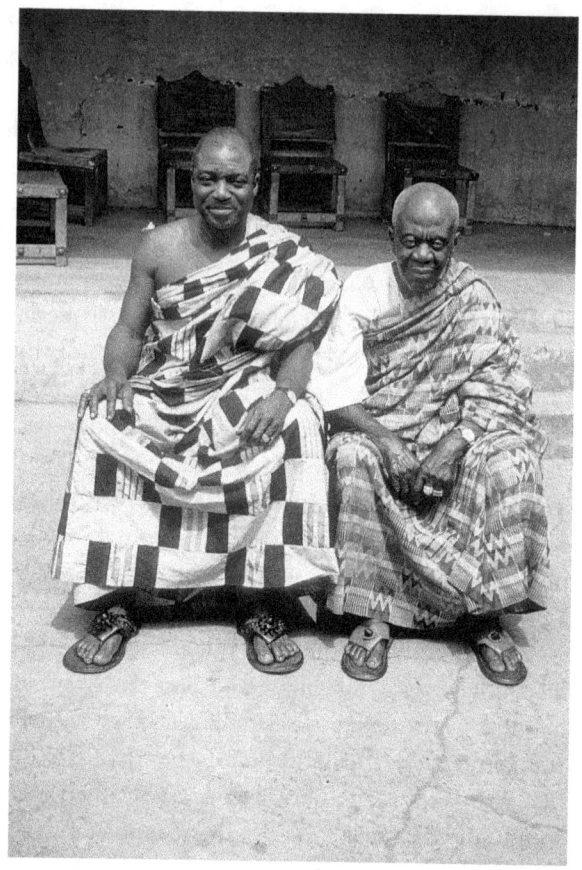

FIGURE 5.8. Takyimanhene Kwakye Ameyaw II and his father, 23 January 1971. From the Dennis Michael Warren Slide Collection, Special Collections Department, University of Iowa Libraries. Used courtesy of Greg Prickman, Head of Special Collections.

16 July 1968, the fifty-five- or fifty-six-year old Kofi Dɔnkɔ recorded, "my wife Afua Munfie delivered a female child on Thursday . . . the child's name is Yaa Badu (father's name Kofi Donkor)."[60] At the end of the year, Kofi Dɔnkɔ "performed the customary rites" for "Kwaku Agyeman [who] married Akua Abrese" as "the head of the family."[61] It is doubtful that Yaa Badu would participate in a formal bragorɔ when she became of age, although the marriage rites performed for Kwaku and Akua would remain common among Yaa Badu's generation but less so for her children.[62]

The tensions between members of the Takyiman Traditional Council, on one hand, and between the political head (Kwakye Ameyaw II) and spiritual head (ɔbosomfoɔ Kofi Mosi) of the polity, on the other hand, reached their tipping point toward the end of the 1960s and into the early 1970s. In a March 1970 petition to Kofi Busia, head of state, on behalf of the elders and people of Takyiman, the petitioners noted that the "rising tension," grievances, and unrest of the people have created a situation that could become violent without government intervention. A majority of the people, the petitioners claimed, were "aggrieved by the stealing, corruption and misappropriation of public funds by the Techimanhene and a small group of followers who for fear of their lives, have to acquease [sic] in whatever thing the Techimanhene would do or say."[63] Adontenhene Kwame Opoku had drawn the regional administrative officer's attention to this matter in 1968, but the Takyimanhene, it was charged, unilaterally "declared that the Adontenhene was destooled on 29th September, 1969 without the knowledge or concurrence of the Adonten stool makers."[64] These "stool makers" had sent a petition to the Takyiman Traditional Council and the Brong-Ahafo Regional House of Chiefs, but received no response since the accused Takyimanhene was chair of both political bodies.

Destoolment charges were then brought against the Takyimanhene and filed with the Brong-Ahafo Regional House of Chiefs by the "principal kingmakers of the Techiman stool," citing the number of people beaten by followers of the Takyimanhene. Other charges included misappropriated monies collected on every load of cocoa during the 1963–64 cocoa season to be used for the Takyiman-Wankyi boundary dispute. Council members contended that no such dispute existed and the Takyimanhene refused to account for such monies received.[65] Last, council members conceded, with the closing of the Chieftaincy Secretariat, it remained uncertain to whom complaints in "chieftaincy affairs" should be made.[66] Noteworthy are the signatures to the petition to Kofi Busia, a native of Wankyi, for they included those of ɔbosomfoɔ Kofi Mosi and Nana Kwabena Mensa, ɔkyeame and subsequent ɔbosomfoɔ for Taa Mensa Kwabena. Kofi Mosi's strong opposition to the Takyimanhene sealed his fate. In a twist of fortune, however, the same members of the Traditional Council who, like Kofi Mosi, called for the destoolment of the Takyimanhene now joined the Takyimanhene in removing Kofi Mosi from his office as head of all healers in Takyiman.

By December 1970 several "Police Wireless Message[s]" concerning ɔbosomfoɔ Kofi Mosi tell us that the Takyimanhene and his elders planned to march to the Taa Mensa Kwabena bosomfie on December 26 and remove the ɔbosomfoɔ, "as he has been sacked from that office," and recover the ɔbosom's "[head] pad." This plan was likely to "bring about a serious breach of peace," the police reasoned; at the meeting where the decision was made, "the young men of the town [were to] be organized to [march] to that house," and the police needed reinforcement to patrol the town.[67]

The Wankyi district police and reinforcement from Sunyani came and both quickly resumed control of the situation. Kofi Mosi then handed over the sacred head pad (kahyire) to Tanɔboasehene Kwabena Dwomo, who was also the custodian for Taa Kora, for safekeeping on December 26. The next day, Nana Kwakye Ameyaw II ordered Kofi Mosi to "quit the fetish house."[68] The larger and more important story here is not one of public disturbance and securing the peace, but rather the very communal covenant of political and spiritual authority that held Takyiman society together. The highest authority in the township was still Taa Mensa Kwabena and its human representative, ɔbosomfoɔ Kofi Mosi, who were above the Takyimanhene. Kofi Mosi was also head of all healers in the polity, including Kofi Dɔnkɔ and healers representing some 234 "shrines" (175 were Tanɔ abosom).[69]

Perhaps emboldened by the new "chieftaincy" laws and the new government of Kofi Busia, the Takyimanhene rejected the order of things in Takyiman and sought to destool Kofi Mosi in retaliation for successful destoolment charges brought against him by Mosi and his principal accuser, the Adontenhene. The Takyimanhene arbitrarily destooled the Adontenhene against the protest of the Adonten family just before the impending Apoɔ festival, and this posed a problem for the Takyimanhene because the festival could not begin until Kofi Mosi and the Adontenhene performed specific ceremonies. Most importantly, ɔbosomfoɔ Kofi Mosi had to secure permission from Taa Mensa Kwabena to begin the festival. Mosi protested by refusing to do his part, and Kofi Dɔnkɔ and other important abosomfoɔ and akɔmfoɔ joined him in protest by taking refuge in the Taa Mensa Kwabena bosomfie dressed in funerary cloth and singing funeral dirges. Their collective protest, in dress and song, underscored the somber occasion. Appeals from the Takyimanhene failed to break the joint protest, although Kofi Mosi did vacate the premises on his own terms. The behind-the-scenes legal fees and discord exhibited were a substantial price for the polity to pay, but the rupture between political and spiritual authority came at a much greater cost.[70]

In terms of rampant discontent and political maneuvering, the debacle in Takyiman mirrored the politics in Ghana and the equally widespread dissatisfaction that plagued Kofi Busia's three-year tenure as prime minister. In 1969, Kofi Busia and his Progress Party rode an anti-Nkrumah wave and ushered in the second republic through elections held under a military government. Whatever appetite citizens of Ghana had for Busia quickly faded during the country's steep economic decline. Like his former rival Kwame Nkrumah, Busia was removed from office through a bloodless coup in January 1972 while he was away from the country. The coup was led by Colonel Ignatius Acheampong, who ruled under the guise of the National Redemption Council. The political and economic ills of the country confronted all. In some ways the Ghana Psychic and Traditional Healing Association established under the Companies Code (Act 179) on 25 August 1969 approached the country's illness seeking the same outcome as the various coup leaders. All coup orchestrators claimed dissatisfaction with the quality of civilian and military leaders alike, who they deemed to be frauds. Each regime focused on preventing or quickly removing such individuals from office. As Ghana changed its national leaders, the association changed its name to the Ghana Psychic and Traditional Healers Association on 15 February 1973, but the change opened the association to the fraud and opportunism members sought to avoid.

For healers like Kofi Dɔnkɔ, fraudulent individuals threatened all credible healers as dispensers of health care and repositories of cultural knowledge. In Takyiman and throughout the country, "opportunists secured stamps and documents of the defunct Healing Association, and set themselves up as the legitimate organization. Local officials and previously unlicensed healers easily overlooked the minor difference in this Association name when presented with the bogus official documents.... [Some opportunists were] apprehended in Techiman, Brong-Ahafo, for obtaining money from healers in the small villages. Mr. James Donkor [who worked with healers, anthropologist Michael Warren, and the HFH] exposed this fraud."[71] The country was in crisis. Although Kofi Dɔnkɔ could not rescue the nation or a public body increasingly enthralled by Christianity and capitalism, his body of healing knowledge gave life to the career of an anthropologist who would share Kofi Dɔnkɔ's intellect and remarkable skill with the world beyond Ghana. More than any anthropologist, Dennis Warren would circulate, as well as profit from, Kofi Dɔnkɔ's accrued knowledge and reputation, placing in sharp relief an independent Ghana positioned to control its human and material resources, yet still exposed to the exploits of capitalists, neocolonialists, and the coming-of-age of African studies.

CHAPTER 6. **ANTHROPOLOGIES OF MEDICINE AND AFRICA**
"When the Whiteman First Came"

The healer trains his eye—so he can read signs. His training is of the ears—so he can listen to sounds and understand them. His preparation is also of the nostrils—life and death have their smells. It is of the tongue, and the body's ability to feel.
—AYI KWEI ARMAH, *The Healers*

After graduating from Stanford University in 1964 with a degree in biology, Dennis Warren entered the Peace Corps as a science teacher stationed at the Takyiman Secondary School. He spent two years teaching science, and one of his students was Owusu Brempong, who would become his "research assistant." While in Takyiman, Warren tells us, "I became highly interested in indigenous Brong concepts and systems of science. To further this interest I decided to complement my training in biology and chemistry and did three years [of] coursework in anthropology, linguistics (including Twi) and African Studies at Indiana University and returned to Techiman in July 1969 for a second stay."[1] By July 1969 he had married Mary Salawuh, who was born in Cape Coast but whose family was originally from former British colony and newly independent Nigeria (figure 6.1). Such interracial marriages were rare in the 1960s, and especially for white male anthropologists who were duly warned against "going native." Nevertheless, Warren returned to Takyiman, where Mary lived, to conduct his doctoral research in anthropology on Bono disease, medicine, and religion between July 1969

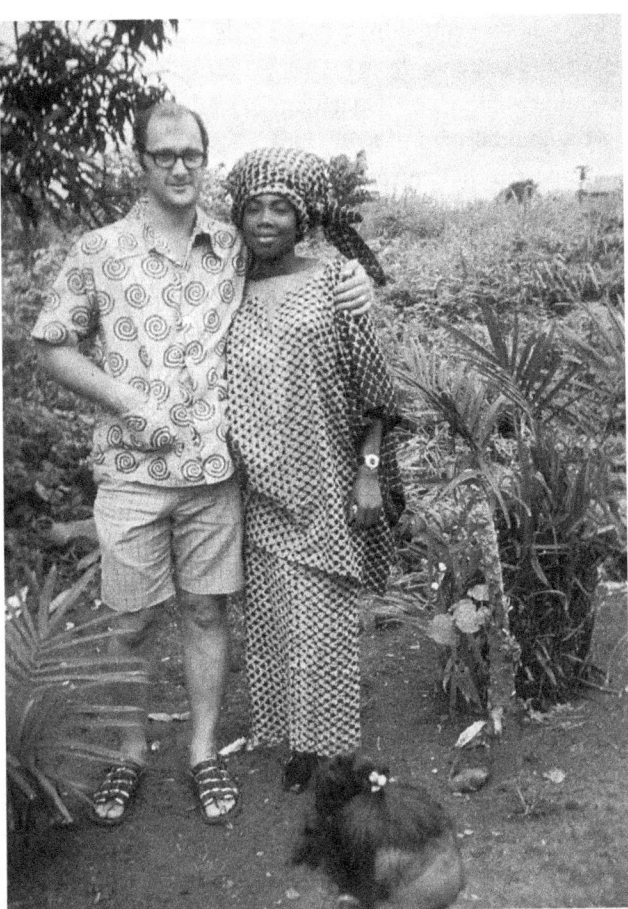

FIGURE 6.1. Mary and Dennis Warren, Takyiman, August 1973. From the Dennis Michael Warren Slide Collection, Special Collections Department, University of Iowa Libraries. Used courtesy of Greg Prickman, Head of Special Collections.

and June 1971.² Warren completed his dissertation in September 1973 and concluded, contrary to anthropologist Margaret Field, that the majority of Bono disease lexemes were conceptual and were defined in terms of natural causation rather than religion or "witchcraft." The baseline data for Warren's study derived from some 1,500 disease names arranged into a twelve-level taxonomic system expressed "by one venerated Bono priest-healer" Kofi Dɔnkɔ. The data gathered from Kofi Dɔnkɔ was compared with that from other informants within the same community as a check on the reliability of initial and primary informants, "the most important being Nana Kofi Donkor."

Because of its disease classification scheme, Warren's dissertation became one of the most cited in the field of medical anthropology, but Kofi

Dɔnkɔ's knowledge and intellectual history are little known or credited beyond his township and patients. In many ways Warren's dissertation, a database for subsequent writings on Ghana and his admirable academic career, was largely the mental map of Kofi Dɔnkɔ. As Warren himself explained, "it became apparent that one priest, Nana Kofi Donkor, possessed a knowledge of herbs and healing which surpassed that of the other professional healers in the area." The "Bono disease classification," a construct that became the hallmark of Warren's scholarly career, was *only* made possible by what Warren called Kofi Dɔnkɔ's "assistance" as a "major informant."[3] But Kofi Dɔnkɔ was more than an assistant or informant, for, as Warren conceded, "the largest sample of data was collected from Kofi Donkor, who provided highly detailed information on 204 different diseases," which came to "represent in skeletal form the Techiman-Bono disease classification as expressed by Nana Kofi Donkor ... [and the] thirteen levels in the disease classificatory system ... follow the intuition of the priest-herbalist Kofi Donkor."[4] Kofi Dɔnkɔ did not simply *inform* Warren's dissertation and subsequent work, which influenced the course of medical anthropology; Warren's foundational research on Bono medicine and disease was a codified fraction of the intellectual history of Kofi Dɔnkɔ. Rather than cast Kofi Dɔnkɔ as a victim, this chapter considers the relations between Dɔnkɔ and Warren as an allegory to the intertwined coming-of-ages of independent African nations such as Ghana and the academic study of Africa, set against global power relations and forces of exploitation. Within this setting, the chapter examines the politics of health and healing, more precisely attempts to integrate foreign and indigenous approaches or to propagate antiforeign institutions based on localized values, amid a series of military coups and economic crises.

❋

KOFI DƆNKƆ SHARED AN all-too-common predicament of Africans documented as informants, assistants, and interpreters: the banal exploitation of indigenous knowledge in the academic coming-of-age of African studies in European and North American universities. Such intermediaries in the circuit of knowledge production and the inequity of it all reveal the very real power relations between academia and the place of African ideas and peoples in it, and between Africa writ large and the outside world dominated by the five permanent members of the UN Security Council. Indeed, the academic study of Africa in non-African universities was a by-product of the relations of domination and exploitation, where its white/European male "founding fathers" shared much in common: access to capital (e.g., foundation monies); belonging to similar social, ideological, and cultural circles; and having taught at elite academic institutions in North America or Western Europe.[5] It is doubtful that Kofi Dɔnkɔ was fully aware of the intricacies in the asymmetric power relations between Ghana/Africa and the world, but experience and intuition made these relations so clear to him that he, at least initially, viewed Warren with deep suspicion and rebuffed Warren's first attempt to use him as an informant.

Kofi Dɔnkɔ's articulation of Bono therapeutics only came from the combined suasion of Owusu Brempong, now Warren's "research assistant," and his father D. K. Owusu, the "interpreter" for Eva Meyerowitz, when Warren's research was in deep jeopardy. Owusu Brempong recalls,

> When Mike Warren declared his intension to work on traditional medicine with me, there was a need to study with a specialist and I could not think of anybody but Nana Kofi Donkor, my own grandfather. One morning Mike and I decided to visit Nana Kofi Donkor to ask him to give us his help for the proposed enterprise. Sadly, upon arrival Nana Kofi Donkor was not prepared to work with us. He stated categorically that he was not prepared to work with any Whiteman because White men are cheats. Indeed, it was a very embarrassing situation, which I tried to elude Mike from it; I did not want him to know the conversation between my grandfather and me. I told Mike that he was busy and that we could come back later. That evening I went to my father Mr. D. K. Owusu and told him about what had happened at my grandfather's house. Upon hearing the news, my father laughed and said to me, 'I am not surprise[d] that was the character of your grandfather who he inherited.' He continued, 'You see, when the Whiteman first came to Takyiman, it was your grandfather and his colleagues who stopped him from staying here. My father *Agya* [Kwadwo] Owusu and his friends (the other priests), went to the bush and collected plenty of wasps in a gourd. At night when the Whiteman was asleep, my father and the other *abosomfoo* went to the Whiteman's abode to release the wasps into his room to stink him. Agya Owusu and the other priests felt that the Whiteman was tricky and was going to destroy our culture and traditions; therefore, they did not want him in Takyiman. The Whiteman then moved from Takyiman to Wenchi.' My father laughed despairingly, after his narration.[6]

At this point, Owusu Brempong is "apprehensive after hearing [his father's story]." He asked his father for advice and D. K. Owusu, in turn, told him to accompany him the next morning to Kofi Dɔnkɔ's house. Owusu continued:

> The next morning around 8:30 am I was at my grandfather's house with my father. After the initial customary greetings, D. K. Owusu went straight into the matter of concern. During his appeal, he alluded to his work with Eva Meyerowitz, which helped in the foundation of the Brong Ahafo Region and Takyiman's freedom from the Ashanti. After Papa's appeal, Nana Kofi Donkor turned to me and asked. "Do you say that he is a good Whiteman who will not cheat me?" I replied "Nana, he is a good man; he taught me at Techiman Secondary School therefore I have known him for a long time."

Owusu tells us that after the meeting,

> Nana Kofi Donkor agreed to meet Mike and I the following Friday and Papa and I thanked him by shaking his hand. The following Friday we readied ourselves with two bottles of schnapps and by 9:00 am, Mike and I were at Nana Kofi Donkor's house. This time he received us with opened arms. It was indeed a red-letter day for me and I felt very proud for the success of the first meeting. That day Nana Kofi Donkor was very generous. He slaughtered two tortoises for us and the stew and *kenke* [fermented cornmeal dough] accompanied the schnapps for the day. This was our first meeting.[7]

Over the course of three or four years, Warren referred to Owusu Brempong as his "research assistant," but Owusu insists he did 80 percent of the workload and some 95 percent of the interviews, transcriptions, and translations involved (figure 6.2). Warren reportedly took all the notebooks in which Owusu wrote the transcriptions and translations, including hand-drawn maps.[8] Warren had learned some of the Akan/Twi language, but he was, admittedly, never able to conduct an interview on his own.[9] When we think of the sheer labors involved in surveying some four thousand townspeople, interviewing hundreds of healers and officeholders, and transcribing and translating those interviews, Owusu's claim of doing the lion's share of the work for Warren's dissertation—and later career—is not without merit. In 1973, while Warren was nearing completion of his doctoral studies and had begun teaching at Iowa State University, the twenty-five-year-old Owusu Brempong was pursing his master's degree at the same

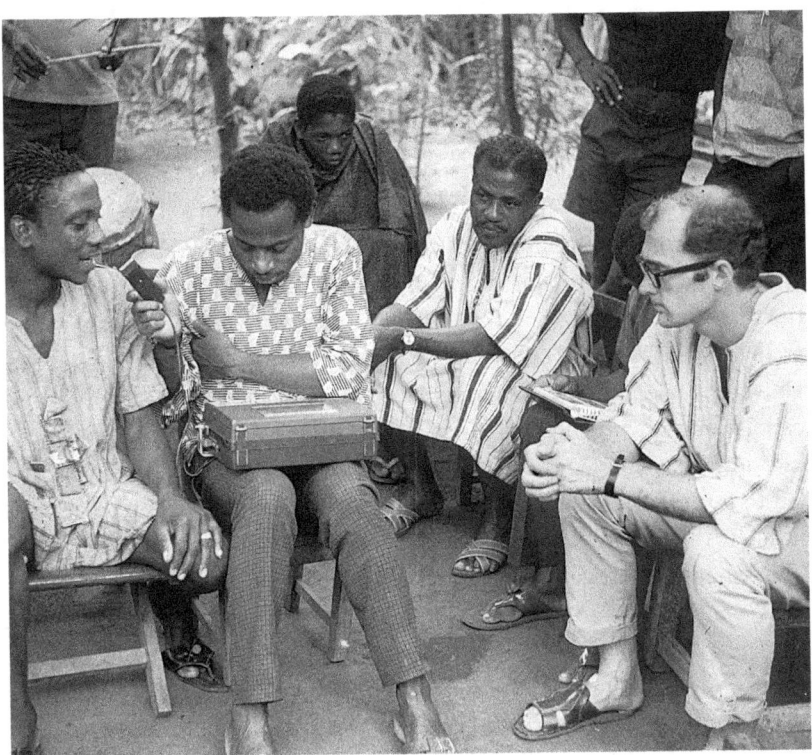

FIGURE 6.2. Nana Kwame Manu interviewed by Owusu Brempong (center) and Dennis Warren (right), 19 August 1970. From the Dennis Michael Warren Slide Collection, Special Collections Department, University of Iowa Libraries. Used courtesy of Greg Prickman, Head of Special Collections.

university with the help of Warren's recommendation, though the latter offered no financial assistance.[10] Owusu would go on to complete his doctorate at Indiana University and become a faculty at the Institute of African Studies, University of Ghana. Besides anecdotes about Warren providing some shingles for Kofi Dɔnkɔ's house, Kofi Dɔnkɔ also received no concrete benefits from his intellectual property. Meanwhile, Warren would go on to receive his doctorate as a result of his single-authored dissertation, publish numerous articles and present papers from the dissertation research, and eventually earn academic promotion, tenure, and distinction.

Unfortunately, and strangely, we only get glimpses of Kofi Dɔnkɔ's intellectual prowess during Warren and Brempong's research and through the published results. On the one hand, Warren wrote, "Kofi Donkor, an elderly priest-herbalist, was selected as the primary informant and in-depth interviews were conducted over several months until all of the lexemes were covered and a model for the traditional disease classification system was worked out."[11] But, on the other hand, the original audio interviews conducted between March and June 1970 were, "due to logistics problems," all "erased after translations were made since the tapes were needed to collect shrine histories."[12] It all seems more than coincidence that Owusu had to give Warren all the notebooks from *their* research, Warren *erased* the audio tapes with his "major informant" whose "classification system was ... the traditional model," and that Indiana University (where the tapes were archived) and Warren's collections at the University of Iowa and Iowa State University had none of the notebooks.[13] With headings in Warren's publications announcing the "Techiman-Bono Disease Classification System ... (according to Kofi Donkor's classification of 392 specific diseases)," we are left to imagine the contours of that "system" in Kofi Dɔnkɔ's intellect and healing, though we know that classification system became influential.[14] This schema inextricably shaped the Ghana research of Robert W. Wyllie (1983) and Helga Fink (1990), among others.[15] By default, Warren's work would have given us the only window into the ways Kofi Dɔnkɔ translated those understandings into social and therapeutic practice, if it were not for two recently discovered record books which Kofi Dɔnkɔ kept (figure 6.3). More on the content and implications of these record books in the next chapter. For now, we will settle on the insights Warren and Brempong's joint research provides.

In 1970, among interviewees and over four thousand townspeople surveyed, Kofi Dɔnkɔ was the highest-ranked healer in terms of "priests and shrines most frequently visited" (one-fourth more respondents than the state *ɔbosom* Taa Mensa Kwabena) and "herbalist most visited."[16] Tuesday and Friday were Kofi Dɔnkɔ's "shrine days." On the four occasions Warren and Brempong visited Kofi Dɔnkɔ, they saw fifty-two patients (twenty-nine males, twenty-three females): most were less than twenty years old; all came from within a thirty-mile radius of the township; and they were Christians, Muslims, and adherents to indigenous spirituality. On these documented occasions, Kofi Dɔnkɔ treated stomach ailments, convulsions, childhood diseases, and types of boils and edema using a range of diagnostic techniques. He palpated the patient's body and placed his lips, hands ("feel the joints, head, stomach, fontanel lightly touched"), or nose ("to detect disease odors through medicines on the healer's nose") to the patient's skin. He would use his "possessed state to diagnose"; he would note the patient's ears and eyes becoming pale and diagnosed impending

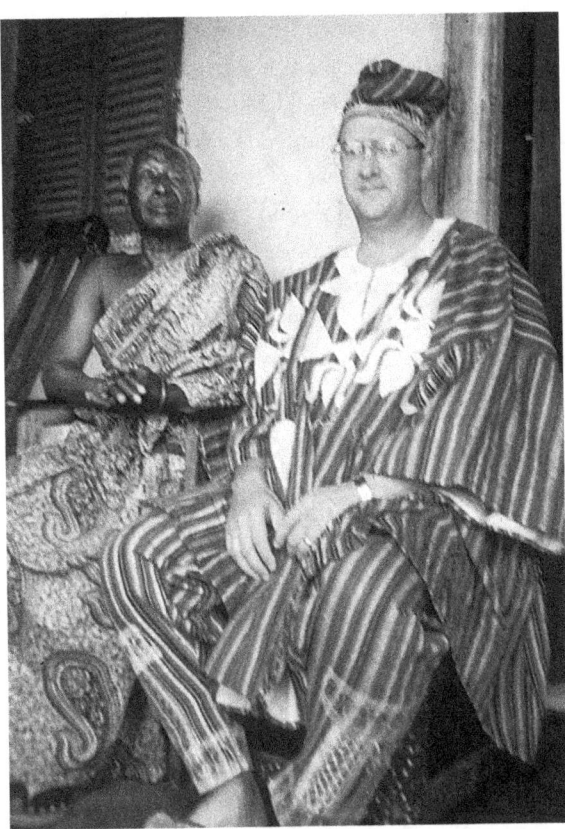

FIGURE 6.3. Dennis Warren seated with Nana Kofi Dɔnkɔ. From the Dennis Michael Warren Slide Collection, Special Collections Department, University of Iowa Libraries. Used courtesy of Greg Prickman, Head of Special Collections.

convulsions; he touched the engorged breasts, observed milk from them, and diagnosed small organisms on the breast; and diagnosed as a disease centered on the brain if a patient could not understand simple questions.[17] That twenty of the fifty-two patients Warren and Brempong observed were less than one year old underscores two persistent themes in Kofi Dɔnkɔ's approach to healing: he had a deep concern and affection for children and their well-being, and he often did not charge a fee for their treatment. In fact, Owusu Brempong, who was a child patient of Kofi Dɔnkɔ and saw him in action over decades, recalled how he was "loved by the women from Nigeria (Lagosians) because he healed and cared for their babies/children at no charge."[18]

❀

UNFORTUNATELY, MANY YORÙBÁ traders and individuals from Nigeria, including mothers to whom Kofi Dɔnkɔ provided therapeutic care, were forced to leave Ghana at the end of 1969 and into 1970 because of Kofi Busia's Aliens Compliance Order of November 1969. In 1970 Takyiman had a population of 12,068 individuals with 777 non-Ghanaians, many of whom were from Nigeria. The Busia government blamed the country's economic woes, labor and land crises, and increased crime (especially armed robberies) on "alien residents," and this spawned public hysteria against foreign nationals. An implicit but deeply significant undercurrent in this moment of economic turbulence, political ineptness, and social anxiety was the nascent wave of Pentecostalism that began to ravage the land and the psychic landscape of the populace. We have already seen how "foreign" religious movements held such a grip on the citizenry during the cocoa boom in the first half of the twentieth century. This was act two or three. In late September 1970, "a religious movement swept across Ghana in a matter of weeks, beginning in Accra with a rumor that the devil was actively catching people at night, and the one way to avoid capture was to write 'God is King' (top) and 'Good' and 'God' (bottom) of a cross on one's bedroom door. Within days, this sign appeared on virtually every doorway in the [Takyiman] township."[19] The Takyiman Secondary School's Scripture Union also became very popular as the teacher in charge claimed to have frequent visions of the "Holy Ghost."

The Takyiman population was now confronted with fourteen churches and five main mosques, two of which are Ahmadiyyan. Both Christians and Muslims sought to further their goals through schools, and thus most of the primary and middle schools were linked to churches or the Ahmadiyyan Muslim movement (figure 6.4). In the Asante heartland, its peoples welcomed the new Asantehene, Opoku Ware II (r. 1970–1999), who became a Christian. Because of the ritual obligations of his office, Opoku Ware II continued the reverence for the Golden Stool (*sika kofi dwa*) and propitiation of the ruling clan ancestors and the *abosom* of the reconstituted Asante nation. Like Kofi Dɔnkɔ, Opoku Ware II managed to distance himself from party politics, although he created a new stool, *nkosoɔhene* ("progress leader"), dispersed throughout his nation and awarded to foreigners to secure "development" funds for Asante's "progress."[20] Takyiman's efforts to stem the country's economic malaise sought not foreign investment but to tap regional trade. The township built a three-day market that attracted over ten thousand people a week and became a main source of income for the polity (figure 6.5).[21] Both Kofi Kyereme and Kofi Dɔnkɔ played active roles in creating the Takyiman market. One of Kofi Dɔnkɔ's trainees, Nana Kwasi Owusu, recalled, "I came to meet Nana Akumfi Ameyaw, the then

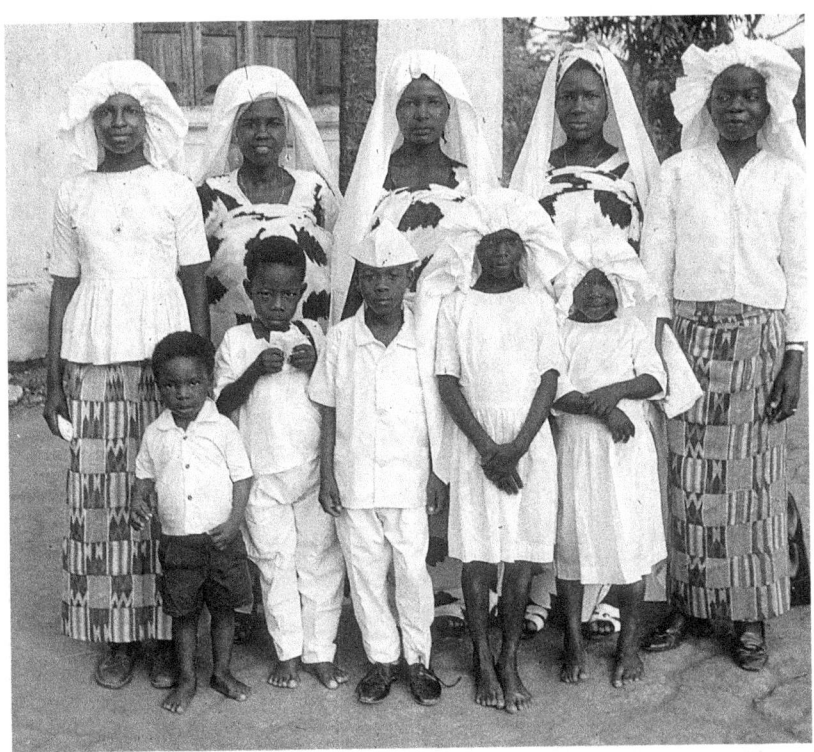

FIGURE 6.4. Ahmadiyya Mission in a group photograph, Takyiman, 1970. From the Dennis Michael Warren Slide Collection, Special Collections Department, University of Iowa Libraries. Used courtesy of Greg Prickman, Head of Special Collections.

Takyimanhene, who used to visit Nana Kofi Donkor. I used to listen to their conversations in the night concerning the building of Takyiman Market."[22] Another trainee from the Asante region, Yaa Kɔmfo, shared, "Nana Kofi Donkor told me the Takyiman Market was initiated using *akokɔhwedeɛ* [partridge or a kind of game bird with brown plumage] and other rituals performed. After that, the *akokɔhwedeɛ* was left to fly away and wherever it lands will be the extent to which the market will extend. I was not surprised when the last time I visited Takyiman the market has spread very widely like that.... This means that the prophecy was true."[23]

For the remainder of the 1970s, health and healing concerns permeated the lives of the Takyiman townspeople and in some ways, the citizenry of Ghana. Although the Ahmadiyyan Muslim mission opened their own hospital in April 1971, the Holy Family Hospital (HFH) remained the premier

Anthropologies of Medicine and Africa   175

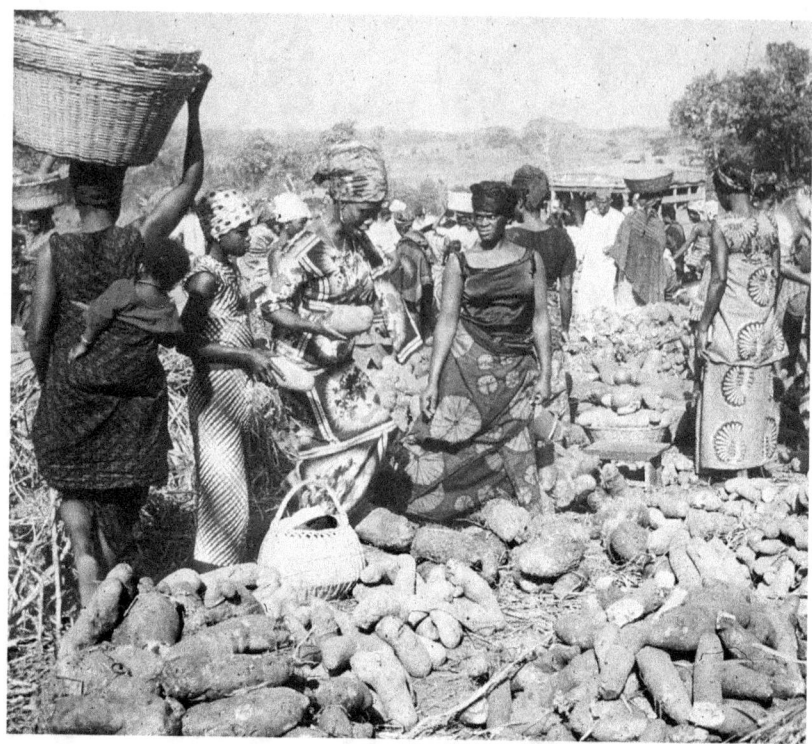

FIGURE 6.5. Selling yams, Takyiman market, 1970. From the Dennis Michael Warren Slide Collection, Special Collections Department, University of Iowa Libraries. Used courtesy of Greg Prickman, Head of Special Collections.

health facility in the township, and its annual reports provide unprecedented insights into the health and disease battles waged by biomedical staff and indigenous healers alike. An outbreak of an undisclosed epidemic disease was detected by the HFH in 1973, and many people, including the registrar for the Takyiman Traditional Council, were victimized by the unnamed disease; though it was unnamed, hospital staff did declare that it was neither cholera nor typhoid. Part of the problem of identification was that the hospital did not have the equipment to isolate the germ causing the disease. Sample tests were eventually sent to either Kumase or Accra for further study. In the interim, doctors and staff stressed the need for better sanitation in the polity and petitioned the Takyiman Traditional Council to that effect.[24] The infrastructural concerns about sanitation were not new, but new health facilities, such as the Forikrom Health Center built between Forikrom and Fiaso, could not ameliorate the problem. For

Takyiman's township population of some thirteen thousand, there were only there public restrooms (1:1,500 ratio) and thirteen public standpipes (1:1,000 ratio).²⁵ New Taakofiano, adjoining the township, was built as a "model village," yet it had no sanitary facilities and could not obtain water from Takyiman pipes because the pressure was too low. Consequently, many of the townspeople regularly traveled to contaminated streams to secure water because of inadequate water supply in the township, leading to 520 documented cases of river blindness (onchocerciasis) treated at the hospital.²⁶

For the healers' part in addressing old and new diseases, Kofi Dɔnkɔ remained committed to the vocation by healing and training new healers to do the same (figure 6.6). In 1975 or 1976, Kofi Dɔnkɔ trained seventeen-year-old Kofi Owusu of Pomakrom. When Kofi Owusu was five years old, he visited his grandmother, Nana Akosua Mframa, and he went into trance and danced like her. Owusu was then chosen to inherit her principal ɔbosom, Mframa ("wind"). When Kofi Owusu turned seventeen, his grandmother passed and

> so he was taken in as an apprentice by Nana Kofi Donkor.... While Kofi followed the strict rules of the apprenticeship, his brother Yaw helped Kofi learn how to read and write whenever he had the chance. Kofi Owusu spent three years as apprentice with Nana Kofi Donkor, and then he took over his grandmother's compound.... Kofi Owusu keeps all of the sacred holidays recorded in an exercise book given to him by his brother Yaw. He practices the important rituals as a priest healer, but he hasn't begun seeing patients on a large scale yet because he wants to earn enough money through farming to improve the compound.²⁷

Decades later, Nana Kofi Owusu remembered fondly, "I learned so many medicines from Nana Kofi Donkor."²⁸ The youthful Kofi Owusu joined a healing community led in many ways by Kofi Dɔnkɔ, paving for him and other young healers an integral and steady path in a changing, "modernizing" town and country.

Electricity arrived in 1976 in the Takyiman district, with an aggregate population of sixty thousand. The HFH located in the township was connected, and soon Takyiman became the headquarters for extending the electricity grid from the Akosombo Dam to northern Ghana.²⁹ The excitement created by the availability of electricity to the hospital, however, could not mask the particular stresses placed on its medical resources: the hospital had only one

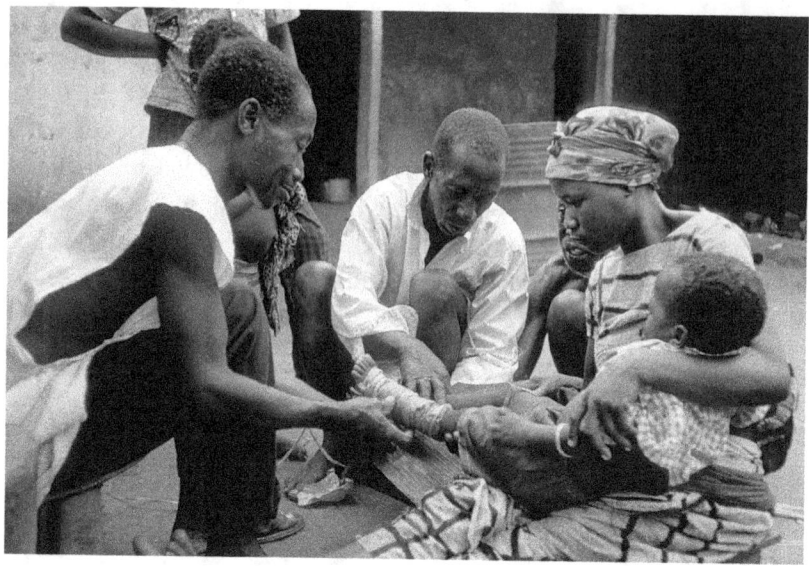

FIGURE 6.6. Kofi Dɔnkɔ treating a child with rickets who can't walk well, 1970. From the Dennis Michael Warren Slide Collection, Special Collections Department, University of Iowa Libraries. Used courtesy of Greg Prickman, Head of Special Collections.

medical officer (who was occasionally relieved by doctors on location), salaries were the biggest expense (at 55 percent of operating costs), and patient fees were the main source of income. The Takyimanhene chaired the thirteen-member HFH advisory board and sat on the governing board, but was powerless in the face of these structural challenges.[30] The townspeople were equally helpless against the scourge of malaria (*huraeɛ*), which continued to be holoendemic as evidenced by 18,455 cases recorded in the outpatient department in 1974, 17,290 in 1975, and 20,888 in 1976.[31] As Kofi Dɔnkɔ and the hospital came to find out, most of these malarial cases were with children under age five. Hospital staff observed a decline in hepatitis, but measles and onchocerciasis still were prevalent—the latter courtesy of the optimal breeding grounds for the *Simulium* (a genus of black flies) near the Tanɔ and Volta rivers. Although the government supplied all vaccines and some drugs for communicable diseases, their costs were prohibitive and they were less than effective against the chief maladies, as the "disease patterns in the area show[ed] little change."[32]

Cognizant of the stakes, local officeholders and biomedical personnel supported several heath projects in the Takyiman district to address the known afflictions. In the village of Baafi, a nutrition project that started in 1972 with the involvement of HFH staff in primary health care began to grow into a "community development project," with local people assuming much of the responsibility.[33] This effort was matched by a World Health Organization (WHO) project at Kintampo aimed at helping villages become more responsible for their own health through lectures and activities for traditional birth attendants (TBAS). The WHO World Health Assembly meeting in Geneva in May 1976 created a "Working Group on Traditional Medicine." Dr. Robert Bannerman, a well-known Ghanaian physician who would work closely with the Primary Health Training for Indigenous Healers (PRHETIH) program, served as the working group's secretary and facilitated communications between WHO and the Ghana Ministry of Health.[34] The Ministry reluctantly established relations with indigenous medicinal practitioners through its utilization of TBAS, its recognition of the Ghana Psychic and Traditional Healers Association (GPTHA), and its collaboration with the Centre for Scientific Research into Plant Medicine in Akropong under the direction Dr. Oku Ampofo. In the Asante town of Agogo, a rural health care program was introduced at the Agogo hospital, integrating TBAS into community-based services. Indeed, efforts to thwart malaria and ensure the well-being of mothers and their children were the prime foci of health care delivery in Takyiman and across the country.

In December 1977 the ownership and management of the HFH was transferred from the Medical Mission Sisters to the Roman Catholic Diocese of Sunyani, which was created in 1973 with jurisdiction for the entire Brong-Ahafo region.[35] Against the shift in management, shortages of medical officers remained the major staffing dilemma, while new additions to the cast of major diseases included typhoid fever (94 cases in 1976 to 481 in 1977), gastroenteritis (1,485 cases in 1976 to 4,213 in 1977), and other diseases facilitated by poor sanitary conditions and inadequate or unsafe water supply. Because the supply of safe and adequate water was a major problem in Takyiman, work was underway on the Tanɔso water project that began in late 1977 with the creation of the new Takyiman district and the inauguration of a new water project for it.[36] While officials at the HFH were "beginning to see the need [for] a 'Primary Health Care' department at the hospital with a person for full time coordination and training, TB [tuberculosis] follow-up and primary health services in the villages," Baafi villagers were helping to run its clinic and provide food for cooking demonstrations.[37] The newly established chest clinic for TB noted that screenings were unsuccessful because patients reported that their families quarreled with or shunned them.³⁸ Overall, hospital officials were slow to recognize that the health challenges in the district were relatively the same year to year and for the same reason: poor environmental sanitation. These officials argued that if nothing is done, "we shall always have the same disease pattern in the community."³⁹ But their view was partial and shortsighted.

Sanitation was part of the challenge, but the forest-savanna ecology in which Takyiman was situated had undergone rapid destabilization and deforestation due to the cocoa industry and mechanized farming approaches that turned a malaria "bush fire" into a nationwide inferno. No wonder "malaria still reign[ed] as the number one diagnosis on almost every OPD [outpatient department] card," and stubbornly remained holoendemic in most of the country with a notoriously high incidence rate.⁴⁰ By 1978 hospital officials finally conceded, "the disease patterns seem to reduplicate themselves every year," and local and national progress in the delivery of health care seemed to be on the horizon.⁴¹ Locally, the newly formed Takyiman District Council immediately supported the collective call for safe drinking water and a hygienic environment, and nationally the Ministry of Health gave greater policy attention to health care in villages; in the village of Baafi, communal labor built a second primary school, while mothers planted a large demonstration garden and men a cassava farm.⁴² Empowered by these developments, the HFH began to explore a program where the hospital's three doctors and staff worked with professional herbalists, while five TBAs trained at the HFH had their graduation ceremony during an international conference at Kintampo in July 1978. As things began to improve for the HFH and the community it served, the hospital was receiving fewer vaccines and drugs for communicable diseases from the government, which was, again, in turmoil.⁴³

❋

IN JULY 1978 ANOTHER bloodless coup forced Colonel Acheampong to resign and put General William Akuffo in charge of the country. His promises of civilian rule failed to materialize and the theme of widespread discontent set in. Almost a year later, in May 1979, Flight Lieutenant Jerry Rawlings attempted what turned out to be an unsuccessful coup. Rawlings was swiftly arrested but then freed by soldiers who supported his plot. On June 4, a Rawlings-led coup inaugurated yet another military government claiming that its purpose was to ensure free elections, end governmental corruption, and reverse the country's economic woes. After executing Acheampong, Akuffo, and other military leaders, Rawlings's Armed Forces

Revolutionary Council allowed national elections on June 18, and in September handed power over to the new president Dr. Hilla Limann and his People's National Party.[44] Limann would hold on to a short-lived presidency, unable to excavate Ghana from its economic stagnation through very unpopular economic reforms. Under these shifting political and economic conditions, the townspeople of Takyiman and Kofi Dɔnkɔ no less survived on what they knew best: farming and cooperative economics through kin and clients. Although unable to heal the wounded economy of Ghana, Kofi Dɔnkɔ's repute as an exceptionally skilled healer had reached Europe, where a German man, for instance, requested his help to forestall the man's impending economic troubles.

In two undated letters (ca. late 1970s to early 1980s), one Aribert Keil of (West) Berlin in East Germany wrote to Kofi Dɔnkɔ for assistance with a divorce that was to ruin him, specifically, the loss of his house in socialist East Germany and money in the bank. In return he initially promised Kofi Dɔnkɔ a car. The second letter, however, contained more urgency: "Now Nana [Kofi Dɔnkɔ], I am having bigger problems which all day becoming bigger and bigger now my wife is working underground in order to collect all my properties from me through one lawyer in Germany, whilst I have work [sic] for twenty years (20), and all my bank accounts will go to her." Urgency was perhaps an understatement. Aribert exclaimed with deep anxiety, "I am fed up, please help me or I promise you 1,000 DM [Deutsche marks] and a car if you can able to KILL this woman or you let her ran [sic] away from my house. I want this within one month after you receive this letter. For this moment what should I do? Please Nana if you're able to do this, write me quickly."[45] No other letters from Aribert were uncovered among Kofi Dɔnkɔ's documents, and it is likely the healer simply ignored Mr. Keil or indicated (through a scribe) that he was prohibited from taking human life in accordance with the ethical code of his profession. Alternatively, the thousands of Ghanaian migrants in East or West Germany since the 1970s probably provided Kofi Dɔnkɔ with the referral and perhaps the means to reject Mr. Keil's multiple requests. The point of this story about Mr. Keil highlights not only the diffusion of Kofi Dɔnkɔ's prowess beyond Ghana but also the reception of "African" therapeutics in an East Germany, where millions were leaving the Roman Catholic and Protestant churches. Ultimately, however, Kofi Dɔnkɔ was more concerned with regenerating or saving human lives than with terminating them. It was during this time that he accepted the offer to join a new health project for healers and their healing communities.

During the June 1979 election period, the PRHETIH program was inaugurated in Takyiman with a handful of herbalists who registered for the program under field coordinator and Peace Corps volunteer G. Steven Bova. Bova later became a well-known pathologist and cancer researcher. What attracted individuals like G. Steven Bova or Dr. Bannerman to the PRHETIH program was the research into indigenous medicine by Warren and Brempong, which featured Kofi Dɔnkɔ's vast knowledge and which facilitated the first of several integrative health projects in Africa. In the 1970s Ghana was one of the first African nations to host health initiatives such as the Damfa project in Greater Accra, the Brong-Ahafo Rural Integrated Development Project in the Kintampo district, varied United Nations Children's Fund–sponsored training projects, and the PRHETIH project that operated between 1979 and 1983 in Takyiman. On the basis of the PRHETIH experience, numerous projects of a similar nature were initiated in the Bono localities of Berekum and Dormaa, as well as the film initially entitled *Bono Medicines* (1982) and later renamed *Healers of Ghana* (1993). Kofi Dɔnkɔ and his son Kofi Effa were featured in *Bono Medicines* and both participated in the PRHETIH project in 1979 (figure 6.7).[46] During the inaugural ceremony for the PRHETIH program on 7 June 1979, "Nana Kofi Donkor stated that 'all of us are involved in improving the health of Techiman inhabitants; just as the right hand washes the left, and the left hand the right, our mutual collaboration in this project can only benefit our people.'"[47] This spirited message soon fell on deaf ears.

Besides challenges with transportation to regular follow-ups with healers—HFH staff hoped the purchase of a Yamaha motorbike would resolve this matter—the most fundamental problem that concerned HFH staff who worked with the PRHETIH project was the trainees. "Trainees (healers) reception and retention of lessons," wrote HFH project members, "is also slow and calls for a lot of restraint and patience. In fact the training (teaching) session is visited with all the problems connected with [an] adult literacy programme."[48] Many healers who signed up for the PRHETIH program soon discovered the project's one-way transfer of knowledge and skill rather than a mutual exchange between biomedical workers and healers, as Kofi Dɔnkɔ envisioned, for "improving the health of Techiman inhabitants." Though healers were problematized, healers and doctors in Takyiman were clear about the benefits and limitations of the therapeutic tools in their respective toolkits. Apparently, this reality was an inconvenient truth for the biomedical establishment to swallow. And so, hospital and national health officials, convinced of their superior approach

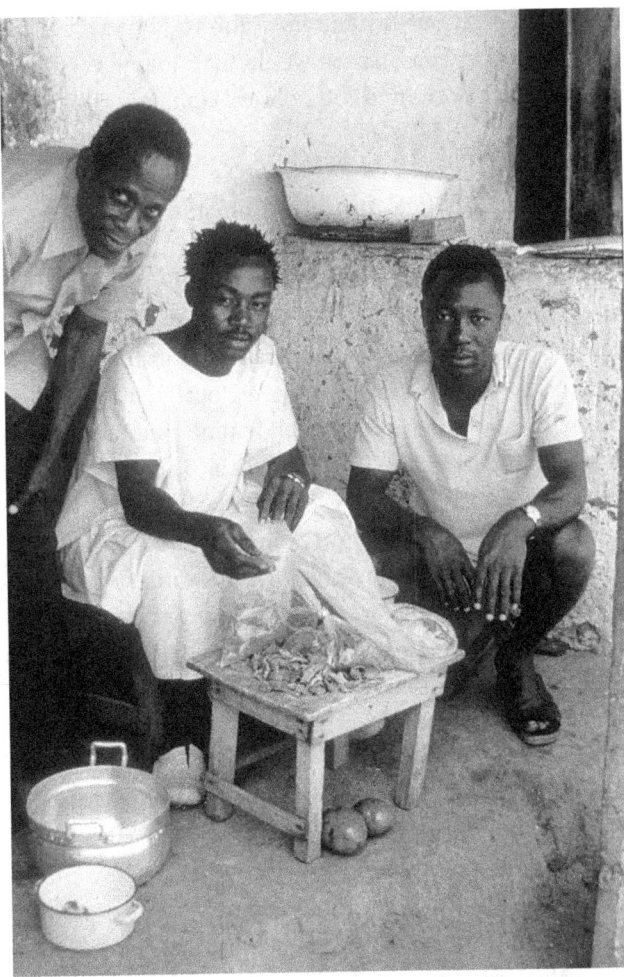

FIGURE 6.7. Nana Kofi Effa (middle), n.d. From the Dennis Michael Warren Slide Collection, Special Collections Department, University of Iowa Libraries. Used courtesy of Greg Prickman, Head of Special Collections.

to health, took the high ground and dug into the position that healers required training in basic biomedical care. The "Ministry of Health personnel who [worked with the PRHETIH program] were not very considerate of traditional healers," recalled Sr. Elaine Khols of the HFH and the Medical Mission Sisters, though she "was impressed by the sincerity of the healers we worked with and their concern for healers who were not properly doing their work."[49] As Ghana adopted a national policy of primary health care and district hospitals like the one in Agogo were formally integrated into the national health care system, such hospitals, like the Ministry of Health, generally rejected "traditional medicine." Instead, they focused on health and missionary education while government grants-in-aid went

Anthropologies of Medicine and Africa 183

to hospitals rather than indigenous healing institutions. Healers and the people's healthcare system they represented would have to find their own ways to survive in the current economic and political climate.

❉

GHANA'S ECONOMIC AND political troubles from the 1970s had encroached upon the 1980s, and the ubiquitous cancer of corruption—or at least the charge of pervasive corruption—infected each regime. Ghana squandered its dominant position as a global producer of cocoa, as production declined precipitously and as the country's support for president Limann quickly faded. The awkward tango between local politics and the forces of the global marketplace meant that each regime paid more attention to the prospects of removal by military coup than to engendering the prosperity of the country. As Jerry Rawlings's recurring calls to terminate corruption generated broad popular support, Limann's inept administration as well as corruption within the government and wider society cannibalized his ruling party, opening the doors for yet another Rawlings-led coup in December 1981. The December 31 "revolution" followed a series of military efforts to take power from Limann, but where those attempts failed, the December 31 attempt reigned in the near anarchy and social distress facing the country.

Through the "revolution," Rawlings established the Provisional National Defense Council (PNDC), through which the country was managed, with Rawlings as chairperson. The PNDC seized power, suspended the constitution, dissolved parliament and the governing councils, banned political parties, and detained indefinitely and without trial those deemed threats to national security—eerily reminiscent of the Nkrumah regime. In place of these governing structures the PNDC installed military committees to pave the way for a promised democracy, while engendering greater public involvement in the fight against the national malady of corruption. Although authoritarianism was no stranger to Rawlings and his PNDC, they were able to halt the country's steep economic slide and stabilize its temperamental politics through a mixture of socialist and liberal policies. The broad benefit to average citizens under PNDC rule is still being debated. Nana Kwasi Appiah, a former student of Kofi Dɔnkɔ who trained during the PNDC period, noted, "I remember it was [the] PNDC era where there was a redenomination exercise, so it became very difficult for me, even travelling from my hometown (Saase) to Takyiman for my *akɔm* training for the first time. Kerosene was also in short supply and people had to queue to buy kerosene for their lamps since electricity was only in the urban centers of Ghana, leaving most of the rural areas dependent on kerosene."⁵⁰ Rawlings's push to create the conditions for anticorruption and "democracy" was no cure for the ills of the country, while healers who attended to the country's majority rural population had to engineer their own way out of the thick fog of competing forces.

While Rawlings staged his December 31 coup using the prop of corruption and the rhetoric of revolutionary change, a quiet but no less important revolution was taking place among opposing forces in the enjoined arenas of health, culture, and ideology. The revolution of ideas and practice took place between representatives of indigenous culture and spirituality drawn from the ranks of prominent healers and of biomedical workers of African and European origin who accepted the ideology of white/European superiority in all things that mattered. Most of Ghana's and Takyiman's population lived in a world touched by politics in only abstract ways. The biomedical workers at mission hospitals, such as the HFH in Takyiman, were situated in a web of individuals and local institutions that mattered in the lives of indigenes, strangers, and visitors. By the summer of 1981, Kofi Dɔnkɔ and other healers involved in the PRHETIH program had renamed the project "Abibiduro ne Aborofoduro Nkabom Kuo" (African Medicine and Western Medicine Integrated Group), marking a significant shift in their understanding of what was a stake and in asserting their right to be "equal" partners rather than empty receptacles of biomedical knowledge.⁵¹

An April 1981 report prepared by Mary Ann Tregoning of the HFH, anthropologist Dennis Warren, Peace Corps volunteers and PRHETIH field coordinators G. Steven Bova (1979–80) and Mark Kleiwer (1980–81) also suggests that healers were not passive receptacles. Rather, healers approached the one-way flow of "Western" medical knowledge with tact and from their own self-understandings. The PRHETIH sessions that focused on medicinal herbs "were most enthusiastically received" (figure 6.8), whereas healers disregarded "those sessions that consisted primarily of advice or description" and about "family planning," which received "such a low rating" that the authors of the report surmised this was "probably because contraception was antithetical to the beliefs and practices of this highly natalistic society. In fact, one priest-healer, Nana Kofi Donkor, revealed that his giving advice regarding contraception was an anathema to his shrine."⁵² While organizers of the PRHETIH project envisioned a health revolution wherein healers could be used in national health delivery systems within

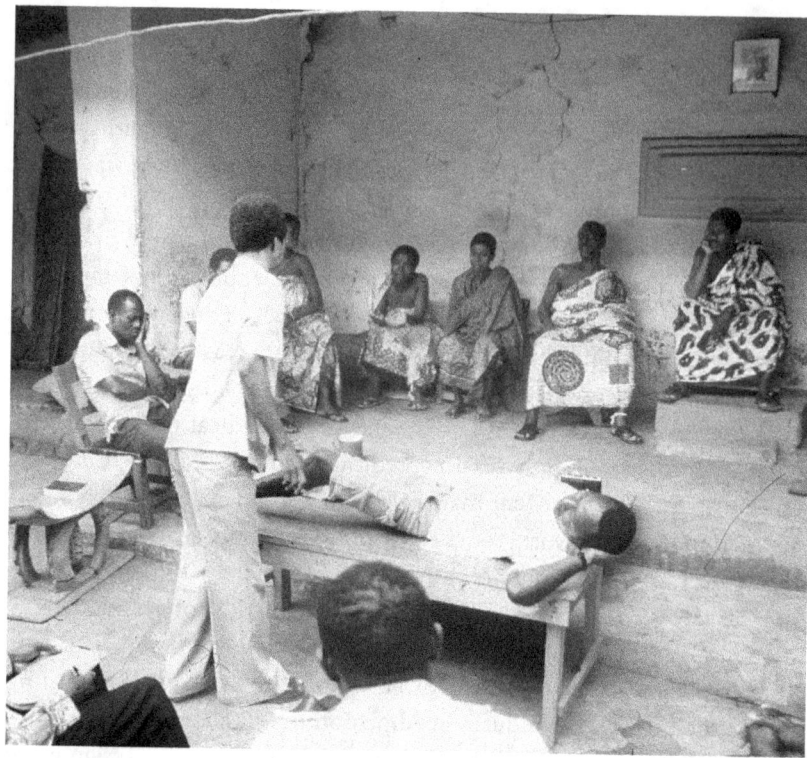

FIGURE 6.8. Session 11, First Aid, PRHETIH program. From the Dennis Michael Warren Slide Collection, Special Collections Department, University of Iowa Libraries. Used courtesy of Greg Prickman, Head of Special Collections.

and outside of Ghana, the healers' rebellion against their prescribed role and the pejorative view held by the Ghana Ministry of Health toward them placed project organizers and their backers in a precarious position.

With an estimated healer-to-general-township population ratio of 1:300,

> most of the traditional healers interviewed [for the PRHETIH project] practice their skills upon demand. They typically return from a morning of farming to find a friend or neighbor waiting with a patient. The most prominent healer in Techiman Township, Nana Kofi Donkor, is an exception to this, however. He has set aside Friday (the principal Techiman weekly market day), and Tuesday as his special healing days. On a typical Friday, one finds seated lines of 10–20 patients waiting to consult the healer, each patient with a wooden chip with a number painted on it, modeled after a similar practice at the

Techiman Holy Family Hospital. Nana Donkor does see patients upon demand on other days of the week if he is not at farm or in the forest collecting herbs.[53]

Kofi Dɔnkɔ led the revolution not only in how healers practiced their evolving craft but also in the ways in which healers and biomedical practitioners worked toward the health of the community in which both served, albeit from different epistemologies.

When GPTHA regional secretary and PRHETIH field officer James Donkor helped prepare a report on the PRHETIH project, which optimistically acknowledged that "the project continued steadily this year," this optimism was based on some promising results.[54] The final two groups of healers from Takyiman had completed the PRHETIH coursework, while healers from the localities of Krobo and Tuobodom were interviewed for two additional cohorts.[55] Guided by Kofi Dɔnkɔ and his exemplary practice, healers who completed the PRHETIH program also had a decisively immediate impact on health outcomes for the Takyiman community. The PRHETIH project was managed by the HFH, which, broadly speaking, served some 83,000 patients in the Takyiman area in 1981, with patients coming from a forty-mile radius. This wide net encompassed three other mission hospitals in the Brong-Ahafo region stationed some 18 miles away (Ahmadiyya, Wenchi Methodist, and Nkoranzaman hospitals), four health centers (Nkoranza, Tanoso, Nkyeraa, and Kintampo), and the government hospital in Sunyani about 39.5 miles away. The HFH received an average of 300–350 patients a day, but the 44 healers who received primary health training were an integral part of the 26 percent decrease in the outpatient department and of the more than 80 percent drop in the number of diagnoses of malaria, gastroenteritis, respiratory tract infection, and skin diseases by that department in 1981.[56] Most of the maladies, according to HFH reporting, "could [and did] receive first line treatment in the villages and/or be prevented by decent water supply and sanitation facilities," though malaria remained the most intractable health problem for all.[57]

As Mark Kleiwer departed for the United States to attend medical school, Jeff M. Stein arrived in Ghana to replace Kleiwer as PRHETIH field coordinator for the 1981–82 term; he had watched Kleiwer and others participate in the making of the *Bono Medicines* film featuring primary health care workers and "the traditional healers in the [Takyiman] area."[58] In the summer of 1981, the Scott Dodds Productions company, based in Lone Rock, Iowa, shot footage for the 16mm documentary film titled *Bono*

Medicines (later retitled and released in the 1990s under Films for the Humanities & Sciences as *Healers of Ghana*). The company also produced a study guide for use in college classrooms in order to dispel stereotypes about "traditional medicine" in "developing nations." In the guide, the narrative script and English translations of interviews reveal just how central Kofi Dɔnkɔ's ideas were to the making and aim of the production and of the PRHETIH project. Because such a project was revolutionary in health care delivery in the "postcolonial" world, it was apropos that the first PRHETIH training sessions were held at Kofi Dɔnkɔ's compound, providing the setting and the plot for the film. In the beginning of the film, Kofi Dɔnkɔ's close friend and colleague *ɔbosomfoɔ* Kofi Owusu of Krobo poured libation. Nana Owusu spoke, "[Onyankopɔn], accept this drink. The filmmakers are here with us. See that their equipment functions properly. We pray their efforts will result in *a truthful representation*, and that they will have a safe journey home. Let no evil befall us. And let the Techiman area prosper through this film."[59]

Not long into the film, Kofi Dɔnkɔ is featured, examining a small child. He comments, in English translation, "I can cure many kinds of diseases, including cold, fever, retroversion of the uterus, and others. If I had to describe all the diseases I [have] healed, it would take a large volume. My spirit reveals to me in dreams which medicines to give to my patients. The spirit tells me whether to use the roots, the bark, or the leaves of a tree. The spirit may direct me to pound the stem of a specific tree into medicine for a particular patient. So it always works, if it is the will of [Onyankopɔn]."[60] At Kofi Dɔnkɔ's compound, film narrator Harold L. Cannon tells us, "Instructors from Holy Family Hospital and Ghana's Ministry of Health begin the first of fourteen weekly training sessions to educate the healers in the basics of western primary health care. . . . Kofi Donkor's first training group, comprised of his apprentice herbalists, learned how to instruct parents to prepare protein-rich, nutritious foods for their children."[61] On this initial cadre of healer-participants, *ɔbosomfoɔhene* Kwabena Mensa poured the following libation: "[Onyankopɔn], here is drink. Mother earth, here is drink. Today, herbalists, priests and priestesses, and doctors have all united. And we are meeting to consider our medicines so that we may administer them better. Take this drink, and let us prosper from our endeavors here. Let success attend the work of all herbalists and health workers. It is our tradition from the ancient times, and we will not discard it."[62]

There is no doubt that healers envisioned their partnership with biomedical workers from no position of deficit, and more importantly, medical staff and doctors also recognized, in some respects, their shortcomings as well as therapeutic areas where healers were decisively more effective than they. Dr. Willem Boere conceded, "The more total approach of the indigenous healer to illness is probably best reflected in the treatment of psychiatric diseases and psychosomatic diseases.... Usually, when these illnesses occur, I advise the patient also, besides drug treatment, to consult a traditional healer." Sr. Mary Ann Tregoning of HFH joined the chorus, reminding viewers of the film that "for quite a while now we've referred patients to them that have psychiatric illnesses.... [We] have known for a long time that [healers] are [also] very skillful in fractures. In fact they often get quicker and better results than we get with the traditional casting and splinting in the hospital."[63] Fittingly, at the end of the film, Kofi Dɔnkɔ remarked, "Previously, the doctors did not understand what we were doing. But now they work with us. The doctors find that there may be sickness of a spiritual nature that they cannot cure, and they will send that patient to us for treatment."[64] Dr. Boere concurred: "I think it is better in the long run to cooperate with the healers than to fight them."[65]

By February 1982, seventy indigenous healers had been trained in basic biomedical care through the PRHETIH program, and another forty would be trained between 1982 and 1984. These new classes of healers were slated to help ease the flow of outpatient attendance to the HFH, which accounted for an average of 420 outpatients per day in 1982. Sometime that year, HFH husband and wife physicians Willem and Magda Boere, however, returned to Holland to practice medicine, while Roland A. Foulkes, an African American field coordinator, joined the PRHETIH project and worked with the healers-in-training between 1982 and 1984. After his Peace Corps tenure, Foulkes returned to college and would become a sociocultural anthropologist. Sisters Mary Ann Tregoning and Elaine Kohls were HFH administrators who both championed the PRHETIH project. Tregoning was the hospital matron and nursing supervisor who was "perhaps the most outspoken advocate of the PRHETIH project," whereas Kohls was an administrator for over eleven years and was among the first to propose the PRHETIH project (figure 6.9). Kohls, however, would leave the HFH and Takyiman to study in the United States in 1983.

Elaine Kohls recalled, "Yes, I was at HFH Techiman from 1970 to 1983 and we had developed a training program for the traditional healers, mainly on first aid on how to treat diarrhea, fever, etc. and who to refer to the hospital. We trained about 80 all together in groups of 6 to 10 depending on the specialties.... I knew Kofi Donkor but at this point remember very

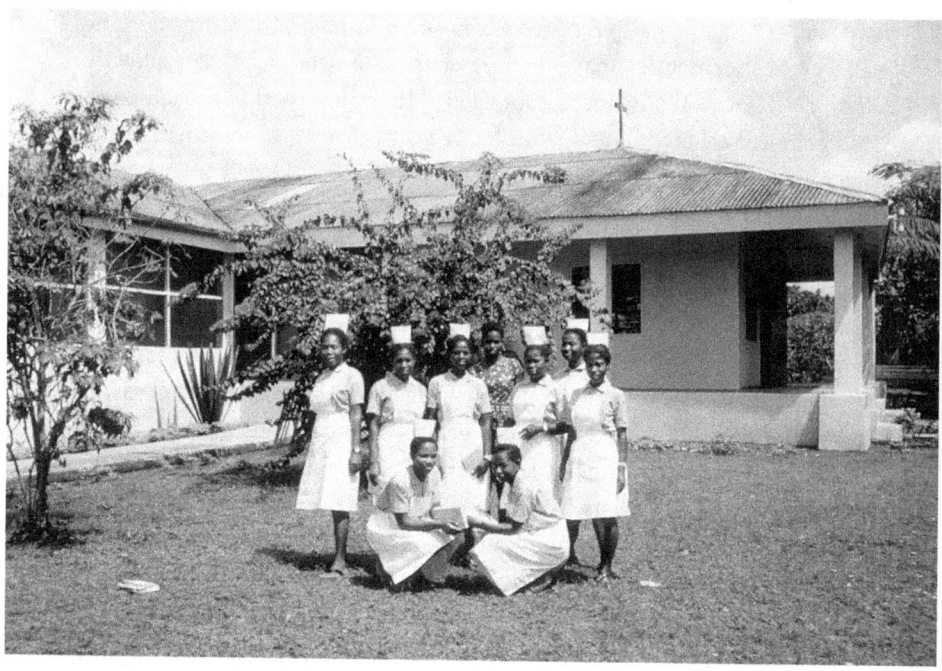

FIGURE 6.9. Takyiman Holy Family Hospital nurses, 1970. From the Dennis Michael Warren Slide Collection, Special Collections Department, University of Iowa Libraries. Used courtesy of Greg Prickman, Head of Special Collections.

little—too many years ago!"[66] For the citizens and strangers residing in Takyiman, the personage of Kofi Dɔnkɔ was as difficult to forget as the protracted socioeconomic crisis of 1983. Between 1982 and 1983, several unsuccessful coups and opposition groups (using Togo as a base of operations) concretized a low point in Ghana's relations with its West African neighbors, leading to a forceful repatriation of more than a million Ghanaian nationals from Nigeria in a period of unprecedented drought and forest fires. Kofi Dɔnkɔ's former student Yaa Kɔmfo remembered the "1983 economic crisis [as a time] where a lot of farmlands in Ghana got burnt by bushfires that actually brought about hunger and drought."[67] Hers was no understatement. Under these conditions, Rawlings's PNDC regime introduced the first phrase of an Economy Recovery Program sponsored by the World Bank and International Monetary Fund (IMF), restructuring Ghana's economic priorities to meet World Bank and IMF conditionalities. Those conditions formed the bedrock of the infamous and devastating structural adjustment program that induced an economic conservatism in

Rawlings's Ghana. The net result was a devalued currency, the elimination of subsidies, and other measures of economic austerity.

❋

ALTHOUGH THE SOCIOECONOMIC crisis of 1983 only confirmed for Rawlings the correctness of the December 31 revolution/coup, it also affirmed the persistent ways in which Ghana's populace responded to one crisis or another and principally through indigenous, grassroots initiatives. Just as health care was framed by the PRHETIH project as an (asymmetrical) partnership between indigenous therapeutics and biomedicine, so too were members of Rawlings's PNDC framing the historic moment as one between indigenous and foreign forms of remedy. One such member was Kwabena Damuah, who was an original member of the seven individuals who formed the PNDC and remained so until his resignation in late 1982. After his resignation, Damuah founded an organization called Afrikania Mission that grew out of the 1981 Rawlings-led coup, poor socioeconomic conditions, and the rise of Christian sects amid suspicion of all things foreign, especially "missionary" Christianity and foreign religions.

Damuah's Afrikania organization would morph into a movement, attracting a lot of attention precisely because of its cultural position of African/Black pride and identity, its siding with the "revolution," and its self-branding as a "reformation" of what some label African Traditional Religion.[68] According to Damuah, "Afrikania mission ... is committed to the study, defense, preservation and promotion of African values.... [The movement] is called Afrikania because it is rooted in the African experience ... It is the restructuring of the African Traditional Religion."[69] To realize this aim, as articulated by one Akosua Kwakowa while in trance, "Afrikania mission must bring about unity among all shrine priests, priestesses, and herbalists."[70] Established on 22 December 1982, the movement had several incarnations (e.g., Afrikanianism, Godianism, Sankofa/Amen-Ra), during which a number of branches opened throughout Ghana to spread its core ideology. Some of these branches were established in the Brong-Ahafo regional capital of Sunyani and in the major town of Takyiman.

Kofi Dɔnkɔ was a member of the "Techiman district branch" of the Afrikania Mission. Although Kofi Dɔnkɔ poured libation at some branch meetings, he went to only a few of them. About one hundred members in Takyiman belonged to the branch, but Kofi Dɔnkɔ's distance from the branch and its activities may be explained by the group's decision to meet only on Sundays and by Afrikania organizers preaching from the

Christian bible and speaking from the position of Christian rather than indigenous beliefs. In the "Bye-Laws for the welfare of the members of Afrikania Mission—Techiman district branch," Kofi Dɔnkɔ was listed as chair of the Welfare Committee (i.e., "a benevolent society within the Afrikania Mission"), while Kwabena Mensa was district chairperson. Other members and their posts included ɔkɔmfoɔ Kwadwo Bɛkoe (treasurer), Kofi Ampɔnsa (member), Kofi Adu Gyamfi (financial secretary), J. B. Ojukwu (vice-chairman of committee), and Kofi Kyereme.[71]

Kofi Adu Gyamfi was chosen by Damuah to be an Afrikania "priest" and organizer for the Brong-Ahafo region. The branch functioned as a committee within the Afrikania organization, and the Takyiman version was a "welfare [and financial] committee" that "covers anybody who will become a member of Afrikania Religion."[72] The benefits provided through this committee included "(a) naming of a child; (b) marriage; (c) relief of sickness; (d) advice and assistance where necessary in connection with their work; (e) burial and funeral expenses; (f) free will donation to a member who may lose his/her relative; [and] (g) settlement of all disputes and other matters." Members were obliged to contribute two thousand cedis and pay fifty cedis as monthly dues.[73] Although the organization issued a stiff warning that "any member who fails to attend Afrikanian Traditional Religious Meetings and activities for three consecutive weeks will be fined six hundred cedis (¢600.00)," this had to be enforced.

Kofi Dɔnkɔ's stature, much less his documented place in the branch's hierarchy, makes his healthy distance from Afrikania seem without penalty and justified. Afrikania preached a message of propagating indigenous ideas and spiritual practice, and these ideas certainly resonated with Kofi Dɔnkɔ. But if that was the case, what explains Kofi Dɔnkɔ's infrequent participation in Afrikania meetings and activities? Damuah's biography suggests why prominent healers such as Kofi Dɔnkɔ were initially supportive but remained deeply suspicious of and kept some distance from the Afrikania Mission. Kofi Dɔnkɔ would have spotted Damuah and his cast as proverbial wolves in sheep clothing: Afrikania's rhetorical claim to indigenous spiritual culture boiled down to a "performance" as spiritualists, but without the requisite rites, rituals, and learning demanded by a healer's rigorous training. In many ways Afrikania was the organizational form or embodiment of Damuah's conflicted Christian past, which remained his frame of reference for thinking through and talking about indigenous spirituality. By 22 December 1982, almost a year after the Rawlings-led coup, Damuah resigned from his twenty-five-year post as a Roman Catholic priest.

Born in April 1930 at Asankrangwa in the Western Region, Vincent Kwabena Damuah was ordained in the year of Ghana's political independence at age twenty-seven, but he showed little concern for politics until he joined the PNDC—for which he was suspended by the Catholic Church. Between his suspension and leap into electoral politics, Damuah underwent a crisis of faith, and influenced by the "revolutionary" moment and its antiforeign sentiments, became a fervent advocate of "traditional religion" in Ghana. Hoping to start his own religiously induced revolution, Damuah assumed the name "Osofo Okomfo Kwabena Damuah" in December 1982. The honorifics preceding Damuah's name confirmed Kofi Dɔnkɔ's suspicions. The term ɔsɔfoɔ has the contemporary gloss of church pastor, but its meaning and use predate Christianity in the Gold Coast and Ghana. We have already seen how, in the Akuapem area where the Basel Mission settled in the nineteenth century, the concept of ɔsɔfoɔ was analogous to the ɔbosomfoɔ in Takyiman. The term ɔkɔmfoɔ also has stubbornly indigenous roots and uses. The crisis that prompted Damuah's reawakening as well as the ideological ambiguity that plagued him and his organization remained unresolved, but was explicitly coded in the "pastor-healer" title (ɔsɔfoɔ-ɔkɔmfoɔ) he chose for himself.

Damuah and his Afrikania Mission rejected Christian claims as the only way to salvation and demanded reparations from colonialists and missionaries, but he did not abandon Christianity nor his socialization and training under its views and values.[74] Damuah claimed he resigned from his Catholic post to "reactivate the African Traditional Religion to take its leading role among the religions of the world," but why should he and not "real" practitioners such as Kofi Dɔnkɔ take this vanguard role?[75] In fact, like Kwame Nkrumah, who became politicized and steeped in the pan-Africanism grown outside of Africa, Damuah spent twelve years in the United States, where he obtained his doctorate at Howard University and taught for a few years. When he returned to Ghana in the late 1970s, he also came back to the Catholic Church, ordaining some nine priests by 1983. In 1989 Damuah detailed a "miracle" at the shrine house of ɔbosom Kwaku Aberante. There, we are told, a seventeen-year-old ɔkɔmfoɔ named Akosua Kwakowa gave "virgin birth" to a baby boy through and according to this ɔbosom's prophesy. The town celebrated, though "the people who attended the delivery [of the baby] were all said to be Christians."[76] For Damuah, this seismic "miracle" demonstrated to Afrikania adherents and to disbelievers that "traditional religion" was on par with Christianity.[77]

In the Afrikania handbook, Damuah explained that "we should be ourselves and create our own forms of worship from our own perspective," but his frequent references to Christian ideology to justify the worth of "our own forms of worship" undermined rather than extolled the virtues of African spirituality on its own terms.[78] Damuah died in 1992, and much of the ideological ambiguity that plagued Damuah flowed into his successors, beginning with his immediate heirs, Komfo Kofi Ameve and Osofo Komfo Atsu Kove. Using Christian theology as a model, Ameve declared the creation of "written scriptures of African Traditional Religion" and envisioned the training of Afrikania priests through a seminary. Kove claimed the dual honorific as Damuah did and praised the founder "for the role he played in the cause of the emancipation of African spirituality," though Damuah and Afrikania had tenuous contacts with indigenous healers and with an "African spirituality" outside of a Christian guise.[79] Both Ameve and Kove, however, categorically lacked the qualifications and lived experiences in the very "traditional religion" they claimed to propagate. Against the rise in neo-Pentecostalism and charismatic churches, leadership struggles within Afrikania materialized after Damuah's death. Schisms and legal conflicts ran their course throughout the organization, including its nationwide branches and the millions claimed as members.[80] Although these conflicts and succession disputes plagued the colony-turned-nation, there was no sign that Ghana was immune from coups or the uncertainty and unrest that would require remedy in the Rawlings years.

CHAPTER 7. **UNCERTAIN MOMENTS AND MEMORY**
"Our Ancestral Spirits, Come and Have Drink"

The healing work that cures a whole people is the highest work, far higher than the cure of single individuals.
—AYI KWEI ARMAH, *The Healers*

While Afrikania founder Kwabena Damuah was building a theological army for the fight over Ghana's soul and collective psyche, Jerry Rawlings's Provisional National Defense Council (PNDC) government was in a fight for its own survival and the revolution it sought to legitimate. The PNDC struggled with organized labor over wages and privatization, students from the country's three universities under the National Union of Ghana Students who were influenced by Christian revivalism and antisocialist sentiments directed at Rawlings, and a coup attempt to remove the PNDC from office. International Monetary Fund (IMF) conditionalities affecting workers and students were announced in April 1983, and university students violently clashed with a workers' counterdemonstration and PNDC supporters in Accra. Students protested, sometimes escalating to violence, against the PNDC regime and its "anti-worker and anti-student policies imposed by the IMF and World Bank," and called for an end to these policies.[1] Unable to generate mass support for their cause, student agitation was suppressed by government closures of the universities and government use of those institutions to train rank-and-file cadres of the revolution.² In June, Sergeant Abdul Malik and other military exiles based in Togo led a coup in the capital of Accra, but PNDC government soldiers captured the "rebels" and executed Malik and company by firing squad.³ All soldiers were ordered to return to their barracks under curfew, and military and police forces were deployed to suppress dissidents. Hundreds were detained for suspected involvement or offering moral support for the coup attempts, and *Free Press* newspaper staff were arrested for their strident criticism of the PNDC government.

While the PNDC devalued Ghana's cedi currency in dramatic fashion and searched for a coherent economic policy, cities and towns across the country had to figure out how to live in a time of great flux. But living in uncertainty was a recurrent theme in the lives of Ghana's citizens and strangers. Flanked by national politics and unrest, this chapter argues, an aging Kofi Dɔnkɔ showed no sign of yielding to either volatility or mental decline. Takyiman and Kofi Dɔnkɔ were mutual gateways for migrants fleeing conflict and seeking therapy, while he elevated and expanded his healing practice independent of—though in some partnership with—Takyiman's foremost hospital. If Kofi Dɔnkɔ held in place community bonds and partnerships with local and foreign actors, so too did his passing in 1995 occasion a reverse in the partnership between the Holy Family Hospital (HFH) and healers and a resurfacing of tensions in his family, community, and nation. It is therefore at the scale of towns and their villages that we might approximate the meanings of national politics and economic policies, the ebb and flow of people's lives in local contexts, and the memory of those who served them well over a lifetime.

❀

TAKYIMAN REMAINED A crossroads between the northern and southern halves of Ghana, and in towns of its relative size and stature, agriculture continued to be the most important economic activity and source of subsistence. However, the high cost of living and food prices, the great drought, the forced return of over 1 million Ghanaians from Nigeria, and stagnant wages led to elevated incidence of malnutrition, especially among children. The Takyiman district population numbered around 103,000, but the HFH served a population twice this number, and as we might expect, a significant share included children. The Takyiman township of 25,000 inhabitants lived among the second-largest food market in Ghana and a large but fluctuating immigrant population from northern Ghana, facilitated by respectable roads and its weekly market. One North American visitor to the township in the summer of 1981 described the market this way:

> Beginning every Wednesday evening, a stream of cars, trucks, and buses streams into Techiman from all directions, as merchants prepare their shanty market stands. But it's not until Friday that things get into full swing. Row upon row of miniature storefronts cater to some 100,000 shoppers each week. You can buy, it seems, anything: dried fish, car parts, plastic shoes, smoked snails on a stick, colorful funeral cloths, western clothes (the vendors joke they are from deceased Europeans), knives, antibiotics, herbs and animal parts for [therapeutic] preparations ... the list is endless. You can even get a haircut or have a watch repaired. Haggling is pervasive. Shopkeepers try to drown one another out, vying for attention in a dozen languages. Prayers are echoed as Muslims kneel on prayermats, their portable mosques. The place bustles with vitality and excitement.[4]

The added stress caused by drought and forest fires on food producers and suppliers in Takyiman, and the economic austerity enacted by the government, forced the township and the nation to manage crisis and economic conservatism the best they could. Kofi Dɔnkɔ and family members farmed cocoa and root crops; his son Kofi Sakyi Sapɔn received some of his father's land for cocoa and subsistence farming during the widespread forest fires of 1983. Residents in the neighboring village of Oforikrom also produced cocoa but terminated this practice in 1983 after fires destroyed most of the cocoa plantations.[5] Kofi Dɔnkɔ hired three Mossi persons originating from northern Ghana to work on his four acres of land and cocoa farm; he also had several workers from Bonduku.[6] Through cooperative farming and hiring migrant laborers who shared in the farming output, individuals and families like that of Kofi Dɔnkɔ effectively handled the consequences of forest fires, drought, and late and inadequate rainfall during the rainy season.

The year 1983 was a tough one for most of Ghana, and the HFH, like other institutions serving large swaths of the population, suffered from the challenges confronting those under their care. The five mission hospitals, ten government health centers, and eleven community clinics within a fifty-mile radius of Takyiman had to grapple with a constant shortage of essential medical supplies and drugs, which the mission hospital regularly received through the Christian Health Association of Ghana. These low supplies for an extremely large number of patients were further compounded by deteriorating electricity supply for half the year, scarcity of vehicles and spare parts, shortages of diesel and motor oil, and a broken water pump, which, taken together, severely affected sick people in remote locations. Indeed, as HFH officials accurately reported, 1983 was "a difficult year for the hospital... in the face of many problems."[7] With water, food, and electricity shortages all year—electricity was rationed to one evening a week—there was a 300 percent increase in the number of children admitted with malnutrition and anemia.

Statistics from HFH served as a barometer of the community's health patterns: the hospital reported a 25 percent drop in the number of measles admissions (a disease affecting only children), reflecting decreased morbidity, but a double-digit rise in the number of deaths from pneumonia, hepatitis, and anemia—equating to a 3.9 to 4.6 percent increase in mortality. Children experienced serious problems of cross-infection, especially with patients who remained hospitalized for long-term care and in spite of relatives who provided basic care, food, and companionship by sleeping on the hospital's floors and benches. The hospital also witnessed high incidence of maternal mortality among pregnant women with jaundice, caused most likely by hepatitis. Among the women admitted with this condition, 30 percent died, deeply affecting unborn children and pregnant women.[8] The village nutrition clinics in Krobo, Boankron, and Baafi promoted hygiene and health among this same population of women, but from the perspective of the clinics, "unfortunately many mothers in Ghana still put more faith in medicines than in good food."[9] Besides the usual culprit of malaria, the major health conditions and common causes of death in 1983 were measles, pneumonia, and gastroenteritis caused by the chronic deficiency of clean water supplies.

The HFH trained more traditional birth attendants (TBAs), and the work with indigenous healers continued with training sessions and leprosy clinic lectures.[10] Healers like Kofi Dɔnkɔ were equally involved, even in their old age, in populating the community with newly trained healers and in treating the social and physical ailments of patients, as Kofi Dɔnkɔ did through his "Donkor Herbalist Clinic" (figure 7.1). Kofi Dɔnkɔ was one of the principal trainers of Nana Kwasi Badu of Takyiman, then, as he had been, a thirteen-year-old trainee. In 1994 the thirty-four-year-old Badu recalled, "I was trained by another priest-healer named Nana Kofi Donkor. The training lasted about seven years and now I have been working as a healer myself, for fourteen years."[11] Populating a country of just over 12 million people with indigenous healers meant the rural inhabitants that constituted 70 percent of Ghana's population had a first line of care

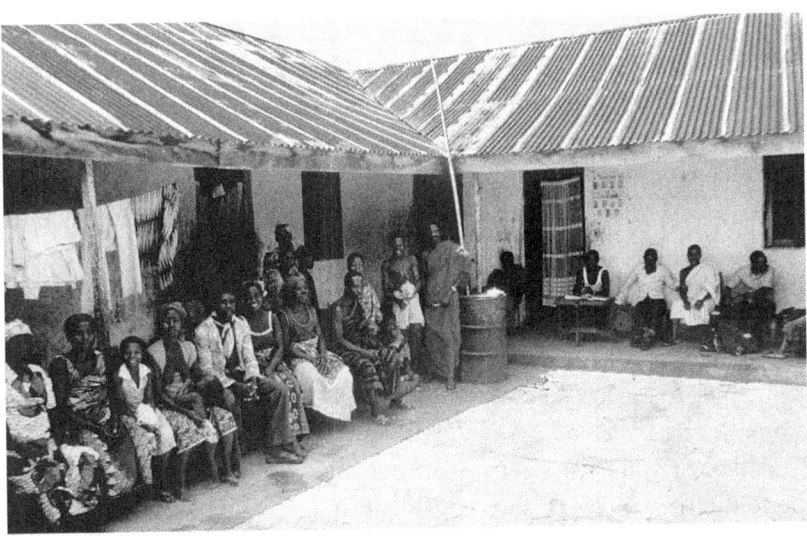

FIGURE 7.1. People waiting in line at Kofi Dɔnkɔ's compound for treatment. From the Dennis Michael Warren Slide Collection, Special Collections Department, University of Iowa Libraries. Used courtesy of Greg Prickman, Head of Special Collections.

to deal with the cumulative psychological trauma, social burden, spiritual yearning, and physical toll of 1983 and early 1984. Besides, of the estimated 1,665 registered medical physicians (including dentists), only 801 practiced their craft. The 3,685 professional nurses and 6,827 auxiliary nurses were insignificant when weighed against the composite needs of a growing and anxiety-ridden populace, especially outside of the urban centers where those medical practitioners were primarily stationed.

By 1984 and 1985, Ghana had one of the highest birthrates in the world (at fifty per one thousand individuals) and, with an improving economy, one of the highest rates of population growth in Africa, though under the dreaded structural adjustment regime. In light of economic "progress" made under its guidelines, the IMF issued additional loans to the Rawlings administration, which replaced its National Defense Committee and Workers' Defense Committee with Committees for the Defense of the Revolution.[12] The rhetoric of revolution underscored the persistence of real or imagined coup attempts, in addition to the detention of political prisoners, but it also translated into strong ties with socialist governments in Cuba and Libya and strained diplomatic relations with the United States. At home, Kofi Dɔnkɔ and other farmers across rural Ghana constituted two-thirds of the population and counted among the strongest backers of Rawlings's populist politics, but the Rawlings regime reduced its assistance to farmers following structural adjustment prescriptions. Farmers and other rural folks responded by turning to traditions of self-help organizations and cooperatives, remaining committed to the revolutionary ideals espoused by Rawlings. The HFH, in fact, formed a "Committee for the Defense of the Revolution in response to the call of government for the people at the grassroots to become more personally involved with the purpose of the revolution. Meetings are enthusiastically led and attended by [HFH] staff members."[13] The hospital's decision to actively side with the ruling government, however noble, owed something to the "sizable subvention grants" for salaries the HFH received from the PNDC regime.

Although Kofi Dɔnkɔ received no such subvention from the government, he continued to serve the two largest constituents of government support: workers and the rural population. In early 1985, for instance, he saw male patients like Kwabena Busumwa from Subenso (Subinso) and female patients like Akua Abrafi from Takyiman. In a dispatch dated 28 May 1985, Kofi Dɔnkɔ dictated a letter that indicated an officer named Eva Abrankroh of the Post and Telecommunication Corporation in Kumase was "found fit for duty." In particular, he stated, "I am happy to report that the Officer Miss. Eva Abrankroh of your Corporation has now recovered completely from her illness and is therefore fit for full duties with effect from Wednesday 29th May, 1985."[14] In broader terms, Kofi Dɔnkɔ's attention to the community and corporal needs of Ghanaians went beyond his old age and immediate surroundings to embrace citizens, strangers, migrants, local and state enterprises, and foreign researchers seeking this therapeutic knowledge and care (figure 7.2). His location in Takyiman became ideal, for he could obtain the best medicines from the forest and savanna, intellectually sharpen his ideas among a range of patients and therapeutic practitioners from both halves of the country, and make the case among healers to participate in some of the first health projects between indigenous and biomedical specialists in Africa.

The Takyiman town and district boasted populations of 25,000 and 103,752, respectively, as the unparalleled "gateway between the north and the south" of Ghana.[15] The increasing flow of would-be settlers and transients made land and therefore housing in Takyiman a premium and highly contested resource. The morass of land litigations that began in the nineteenth century continued unabated, and even selfless and politically disinterested individuals like Kofi Dɔnkɔ could not escape the trappings of

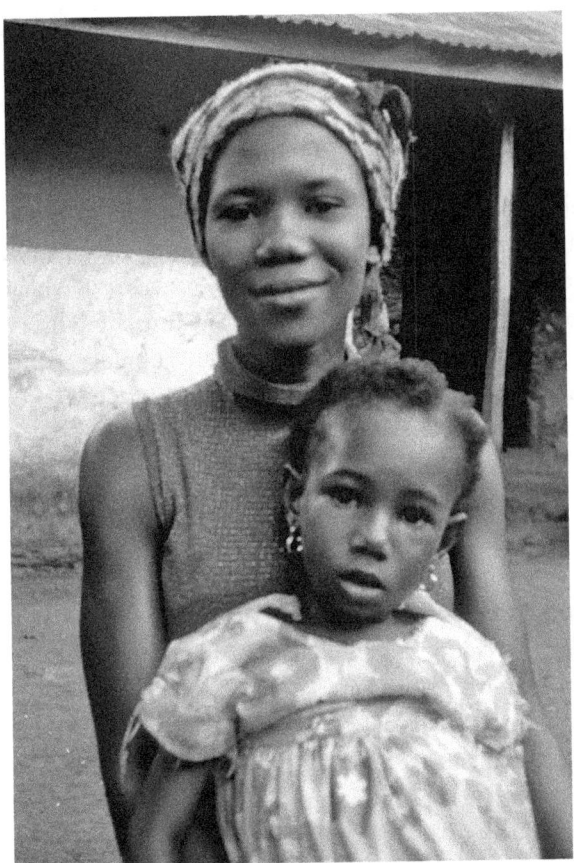

FIGURE 7.2. Mother with sick child at Kofi Dɔnkɔ's compound, 1970. From the Dennis Michael Warren Slide Collection, Special Collections Department, University of Iowa Libraries. Used courtesy of Greg Prickman, Head of Special Collections.

legal disputes related to land. In 1985, Bamirihene Nana Kwabena Mframa claimed that land originally granted to Kofi Dɔnkɔ and his family when they emigrated to Takyiman was in fact part of Bamiri stool land. Nana Mframa insisted the land should return to his stool, ignoring one simple fact: Akwamuhene Nana Owusu Gyare had given Kofi Dɔnkɔ and his family some 350 acres of land to settle shortly after their migration from Old Nyafoman.

The land in question contained, at the time, four building plots and was located on the outskirts of Old Takyiman. This location was chosen precisely because Asubɔnten Kwabena tabooed the dogs and goats found in larger numbers inside the township. Eventually, the matter was brought before the land litigation part of the Sunyani High Court—the highest court in the Brong-Ahafo region. The case was called three times before the court. In each instance, Nana Mframa failed to appear; for Kofi Dɔnkɔ's part, his three witnesses led to a final settlement of the case with the court ruling in his favor. This case was not the only land litigation in which Kofi Dɔnkɔ participated, but the others were minor disputes requiring no court intervention and were settled amicably. Kofi Dɔnkɔ's family members explained that a central factor in the resolution to these disputes was the "forgiving person [Kofi Dɔnkɔ was, since he] usually forgave his offenders."[16] The veracity of this statement is not important; rather, these cases point to the ongoing fight for land in a town and country with shifting populations and housing needs. It seems clear that the ultimately frivolous cases in which Kofi Dɔnkɔ was party convinced Rawlings's PNDC to institute compulsory land registrations to reduce the high incidence of land litigation.

The bustling market town of Takyiman remained a magnet for food producers, merchants, consumers, and seasonal migrants, making housing a prized and scarce commodity and making sanitation and the maintenance of human health enduring challenges for healers and hospital staff alike. HFH officials lamented the "chronic deficiency of clean water and general sanitation" that contributed to a range of diseases.[17] With only sixty-seven beds and a dearth of housing in town, many patients found accommodation with friends and relatives, which permitted many ill patients to be treated as outpatients and allowed for early discharges.[18] For those the HFH could accommodate, a small pastoral care team was established along with weekly meetings and prayer with patients to build a sense of Christian community.[19] Each Wednesday, the St. Paul's Parish prayer group met with staff and prayed with and for patients.[20] If accommodations were a serious problem—and they were—having only a single doctor on staff at the HFH from mid-February to August 1985 was a more fundamental problem for which the hospital had no solution. Left untreated, therefore, were the major yet consistent medical concerns: Tuberculosis was a big problem, the disease patterns for admission were the same as in the previous years, and the four leading diseases were malaria, gastroenteritis, skin disease, and chest infections. Malaria and gastroenteritis accounted for 65 percent of all general outpatient attendance—some 65,346 outpatients in 1985.[21] Naturally, the hospital recorded and the townspeople experienced high rates of death among adults (as meningitis, tuberculosis, and hepatitis accounted for 49 percent of adult inpatient deaths) and children who suffered and died from pneumonia, anemia, malnutrition, hepatitis, and convulsions.[22] What is revealing here is that most of these health conditions and diseases among children were treated especially by Kofi Dɔnkɔ, and because of acutely low attendance at village clinics established by the hospital, we may suspect that many mothers took their child(ren) to one or more indigenous healers.[23]

For reasons not fully clear, the available records strongly suggest that the relationship between the HFH and healers was strained with the collapse or termination of the Primary Health Training for Indigenous Healers (PRHETIH) program, which, HFH officials argued, "folded up in 1985 due to some socio-economic problems."[24] In addition, James Donkor, the HFH staff member who was the link between the hospital and healers in the PRHETIH program, died as a patient at HFH in 1985.[25] In that year, HFH officials wrote, "Thanks to the initiative of thirteen members of the Psychic and Traditional Healers Association of Techiman, it will now be possible to re-establish our former good relationships with these indigenous healers from the area."[26] Sister Therese Tindirugamu of the Medical Mission Sisters of Uganda joined nurse-midwives at HFH in early 1985 after six months of Akan/Twi language studies.[27] Tindirugamu recalled, "I myself worked as young sister and nurse at Techiman Holy Family Hospital, for only three years, from January 1985 [to the] end of December 1987. During that time, I am aware that some of our sisters—the Medical Mission Sisters at the hospital[—]worked in collaboration with many traditional healers around Techiman at the time."[28] "At the time I was in Techiman," Tindirugamu continued, "the Matron of the Hospital was Ms [now Nana] Elizabeth Dwamena and her mother was the Queen Mother of Techiman at the time."[29] The "Queen Mother," of course, was Nana Akua Abrafi, who held the Takyiman ɔmanhemmaa position when Dennis Warren began his dissertation research and when Warren and HFH officials helped to initiate the PRHETIH project.

Although HFH officials promised but did not complete an assessment of the defunct PRHETIH project, they wrote in 1986 that "we hope that we will be able to revive the good working relationships we once had with the traditional healers and herbalists of Techiman Traditional Area. On the last day of November 1985, 13 healers came to the hospital for discussions about the past and our hopes for the future. We poured libation as a sign of reconciliation, and we agreed to come together in the near future."[30] Throughout 1986, HFH officials actively pursued "continued negotiations with the healers of PRHETIH to review the relationship with HFH and to conduct a post-training survey."[31] HFH and PRHETIH officials knew it was in their collective interest to cooperate with rather than alienate healers, but this simple idea never seemed to have achieved any staying power. The consequences of an ineffective and one-sided partnership were obvious to all. Primary health-care activities filtered through nutrition clinics at the village level began in 1972, but the constant low rate of use by villagers, especially the target population of women, made them unsuccessful. Six new clinics and thirteen drug dispensaries opened in the Takyiman district in the mid-1980s, but with 105 villages in a district consisting of 111,097 individuals, these outlets for health care and medication paled in comparison to the number and remoteness of the target populations.

As the second-largest town in the region possessing the second-largest weekly food market in Ghana, Takyiman's location made it a notorious nest for fluctuating or mobile people, which only made worse the major health complaints of malaria, diarrhea, gastroenteritis, and skin disease.[32] The hospital's delivery of curative services, HFH officials argued, was hindered by poor drinking water, sanitation, and refuse disposal. Although the prevalence of measles fell significantly, this was due less to the hospital than to the intensive antimalaria campaign throughout the country.[33] In effect, the hospital needed to join forces with healers more than healers needed to collaborate with the hospital. The HFH instead remained besieged by social and health conditions it could not adequately address alone, and listed among its priorities for 1987 was to "visit and supervise the trained healers."[34] Regardless of the ambiguous relations between the hospital and healers, Kofi Dɔnkɔ's commitment to his craft, his patients, and his community did not waver in his old age. During the annual Kwabena festival for Asubɔnten Kwabena on 30 September 1986, Kofi Dɔnkɔ carried the ɔbosom in his village of Kɔmfokrom ("healer's town") and into the Takyiman township. There the townspeople celebrated Kofi Dɔnkɔ's life work and one of their most important *abosom*, and affirmed community bonds and service to community—all of which Kofi Dɔnkɔ embodied.

❁

IN 1981 A NORTH American visitor to Kofi Dɔnkɔ's compound was struck by its apparent "state of perpetual pandemonium." At sixty-eight or sixty-nine years of age, Kofi Dɔnkɔ and his healing practice showed little sign of slowing down. The visitor continued:

> One can arrive any given morning to the sound of wild drumming, and the sight of a half-dozen young priests and priestesses covered in white powder, gyrating wildly across the compound. Occasionally one falls unconscious, eyes rolled back, only to be helped back up to continue dancing. Amidst this clamor, older priests demonstrate how to grind roots, bark, and leaves into medicines, and how to sacrifice and butcher goats, providing food for priests and deities

alike. For Kofi Donkor is a teacher, initiating young trainees into the priesthood... [and] when we arrived at [Kofi Dɔnkɔ's compound, the...] initiates were undergoing intensive possession experience and training.³⁵

As this training session for the morning ended, "a more reserved crowd quietly filtered in and took orderly seats on a bench along one wall. They were outpatients, come to Kofi Donkor's weekly clinic to employ his healing knowledge. Each held a small piece of wood with a number brightly painted on it, an idea Donkor picked up at a modern hospital."³⁶ Kofi Dɔnkɔ's ability to adapt an effective technique or procedure without undermining the cultural and intellectual platform on which his healing practice stood was precisely why he was so effective and why the hospital—and biomedical practitioners in general—was constrained in holistically treating patients. Patients were not simply diseased organisms. They had histories, aspirations, differed dreams, ancestral linkages, and a range of material and psycho-emotional experiences that, in one lived moment or another, weighed heavy on the individual and community. Viewed from this perspective, Kofi Dɔnkɔ argued convincingly, "'it is always better for a patient to consult a traditional healer. We are more conversant than western doctors, and it is our rapport with patients that leads to our success.'"³⁷

Healers like Kofi Dɔnkɔ delivered some 70 percent of the health care in the Takyiman district, and of the over 45,000 villages that accounted for three-fourths of Ghana's total population, we can suspect the picture in Takyiman reflected that within the country writ large. Doctors at the HFH, such as physicians Willem and Magda Boere, had no doubt of the healers' capacity and what role they should play in Takyiman and in the national health-care system. Willem conceded that "the healers have the potential to help us with our overwhelming caseload.... I already refer patients with psychiatric diseases to Kofi Donkor's place." Willem continued, in a remarkable statement that should not be taken lightly: "It is difficult to find convincing evidence that *our* medicine [i.e., biomedicine] is more effective than theirs. Take snakebite, for example. Seventy percent of the snakebites in this area are nontoxic. So if a patient with snakebite consults a traditional healer, he will always care seventy percent. But we with our antivenom, on the other hand, can cure seventy-five percent. But that is just not convincing statistically."³⁸

Overall, Willem was right. The number of patients that flowed daily through Kofi Dɔnkɔ's compound supports Willem's case. One day in summer of 1981,

[a] woman carrying a small child and holding the token marked with a bright number 'one' took a seat opposite [Kofi] Donkor. Serene and grandfatherly, he immediately put the mother and child at ease. His popularity was obvious. Nearly 40 patients had come that day, some from more than 30 kilometers away.... After receiving medicine, each patient had his or her condition and treatment recorded in a large record book, and a small payment was elicited. This payment was purely a token gesture, to foster a bond of obligation between patient and healer.... It is only after a cure has been effective that proper compensation can be offered.[39]

More statistically convincing are two surviving record books Kofi Dɔnkɔ kept during the 1980s, providing an unprecedented "big data" view of a "modern" healing praxis and the communities served.

In a 1980 interview Kofi Dɔnkɔ asserted, "My work is like that of a medical doctor and so anybody can come to me."[40] This English translation or the statement itself, however, deserves further attention. Kofi Dɔnkɔ was ɔbenfoɔ—one with a high degree of knowledge and skill within a system of spiritual practice and cultural acumen. Counterparts are rare and cross-cultural comparisons are imprecise, but if we had to pin down the term ɔbenfoɔ to something familiar, that something would be a doctorate degree for healers, for ɔben is another term for medicine, properly called aduro (pl. nnuro). Although the ɔbenfoɔ knows the properties of and uses for all types of indigenous medicines, they employ aduro rather than aduto, medicine of neutral value but whose outcome is fashioned by the intent of the user. Some healers, or those individuals supplied by healers, aim the aduto with their ill intent and "throw" (i.e., leave or deliver through spiritual means) the aduto to cause destruction or malice on another person.

The target of successful aduto develops a sickness and becomes a diseased person. In some cases the recipients of aduto, who may retaliate with their own deployment of aduto, can transform an individual into an invalid or cause an epidemic in a community. Said diseased person or community may seek out the hospital and a medical doctor. But they soon realize neither hospital nor doctor can heal, though they might offer some relief. Patients need ayare-sa, the holistic act of healing. Therefore, in 70 percent of the encounters between a range of illnesses and infected patients, the patients consult or seek therapeutic intervention from indigenous healers. In these encounters and in cases where doctors referred patients to him, Kofi Dɔnkɔ was the embodiment of ɔben (medicines of highest potency)

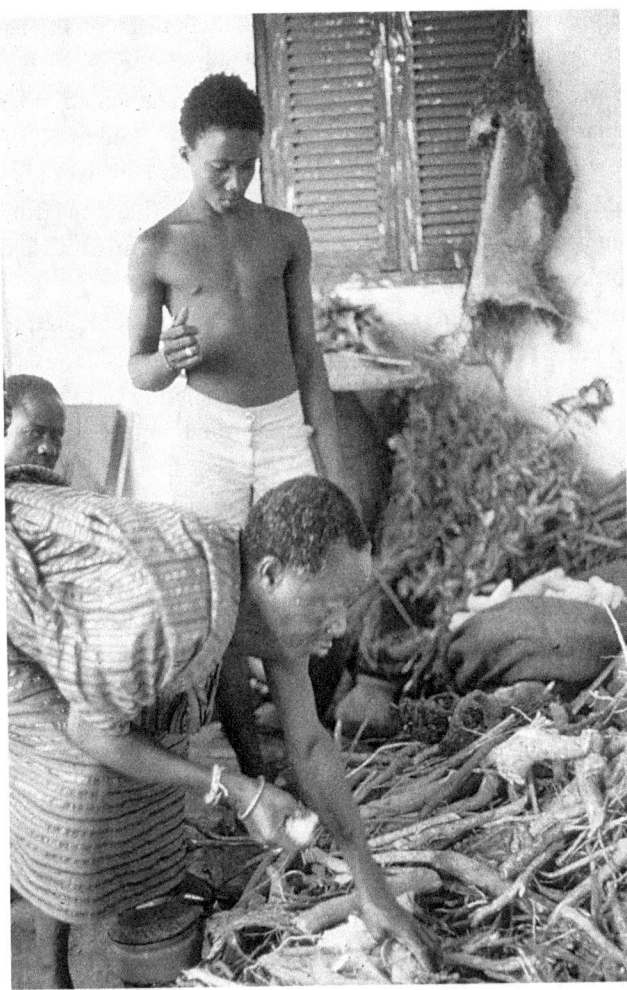

FIGURE 7.3. Kofi Dɔnkɔ. From the Dennis Michael Warren Slide Collection, Special Collections Department, University of Iowa Libraries. Used courtesy of Greg Prickman, Head of Special Collections.

and appropriately known as ɔbenfoɔ to all who remained "amazed at his endurance when it came to [healing] his patients. Nana [Dɔnkɔ] would sit in the same spot for hours, talking and diagnosing his patient."[41]

The efficacious delivery of *health* with *care* was the hallmark of Kofi Dɔnkɔ's healing practice (figure 7.3). Sadly, we have few statistics for the daily workings of his healing craft, but record books that he kept during the 1980s brings his practice into sharper relief. Those record books also allow us—within reason—to imagine his previous decades of practice. As noted previously, the "condition and treatment [of patients were] recorded in a large record book," but two such books and a collection of index cards together disclose some remarkable insights into at least 70 percent of the

Takyiman community and beyond. In fact, Kofi Dɔnkɔ's reach was transnational—as both a trainer of healers and a healing practitioner. Nonetheless, patient data were kept on loose, unorganized, and fragmented index cards and in two large notebooks with the heading, "Kofi Donkor Herbalist Clinic Nyafoma—Techiman B.A." For instance, on 20 February 1987, Kofi Dɔnkɔ treated Adwoa Fordjour (Fodwoɔ) and Ayuba Muhamed from Dɛɛma using small, two-by-two index cards with "outpatient card" and "bring this card on each visit" written on each respective side.

These cards, or at least what remains of them, were too fragmented to derive a reliable picture of the individuals and families he treated. The two surviving record books, however, are much more fascinating in their details and revealing in the profile generated for individual patients and the broader communities to which they belonged. While the first record book ("book 1") recorded 2,073 patients between 1982 and 1988, the second book ("book 2") contains records of some 5,670 patients who visited Kofi Dɔnkɔ between November 1982 and December 1986.[42] From this total of 7,743 patients we can determine a respective average of 1,291 and 1,936 patients per year. If we multiply the 1,936-yearly average by the sixty or so years of Kofi Dɔnkɔ's healing career, which seems more accurate, he would have diagnosed and treated over 116,000 patients, assuming he worked on non–shrine days as well. Although we are working with incomplete and literally tattered records and will never know what revelations complete records would have made possible, these imprecise numbers more than justify Kofi Dɔnkɔ's acclaim and legacy.

For the 2,073 patients recorded in book 1, there exists strong, statistically significant relations between patients and the variables of occupation, age, village, and region of origin. Where patients listed their occupation, a sample size of 585 revealed 65 percent of the patients were farmers, followed by traders (16 percent) and students (3.1 percent). Of the total number of patients recorded, 84.3 percent originated from the Brong-Ahafo region, with 15.1 percent from the Asante region, several individuals from northern Ghana and the Volta region, and one person named Afia Douhs from Togo. Although the average age among patients was eighteen years, Kofi Dɔnkɔ cared principally for children ages one to three years and adults ages twenty to thirty years. Individuals aged thirty made the most visits to his healing center, but many infants who had not yet turned one year old also received his therapeutic offerings. Of the 108 patients who made the most frequent visits, the majority came to Kofi Dɔnkɔ's compound for healing services in 1984, followed by 1987, 1986, and 1983.

Readers may recall that Ghana had one of the highest birth rates in the world during 1984–85, and this might explain the ages of those who paid the healer a visit, as well as the volume of visits. Although most of Kofi Dɔnkɔ's patients hailed from the Brong-Ahafo region, only 28 percent came from his adopted township of Takyiman. The remainder came from outside the township—some 12 percent from Akomadan, 4.8 percent from Aworowa, 4.6 percent from Nkenkasu, and 4.3 percent from Tanɔso—but within the Takyiman district and Brong-Ahafo region. If the geographic reach of Kofi Dɔnkɔ's practice was noteworthy, his wide appeal among patients who self-identified their religious orientation was equally remarkable. Of the 682 who disclosed their religious affiliation, 31.2 percent were Roman Catholic; 16.7 percent, Muslim; 14.4 percent, Methodist; 9.5 percent, Seventh-Day Adventist; 4.7 percent, Presbyterian; 4.5 percent, True Church members; and 4.1 percent, Pentecostal. Six individuals identified themselves as members of Musama (an "independent African church"), three as members of African Faith Church, and two as Halaluya.

We can presume the more than 1,200 individuals who did not identify religious affiliation were adherents of the spiritual culture that Kofi Dɔnkɔ embodied, precisely because that spirituality was not a separate institutional form and practice outside of the culture they lived. Kofi Dɔnkɔ identified and treated hundreds of illnesses, and the ones patients most often reported were illnesses centered on the stomach or abdomen, fever with jaundice, illness affecting the flesh or innards, illness associated with childbirth, malarial fever, and illness preventing pregnancy. Forty-eight individuals came "for medicine." The treatment protocol or method for delivering medicines for most of these illnesses involved a combination of drinking the medicinal preparation and receiving it through enema, bath, or *dudo*. Dudo is a type of medicine consisting of various herbs, barks, and roots kept in a black pot with water; the liquid is used for bathing as a preventive and cure, and the ingredients are specific for each ailment. Most monetary payments for treatment consisted of twenty to forty Ghanaian cedis (40 percent) and one hundred cedis (23 percent), though in-kind payments of chicken, eggs, and alcoholic drink were included in practice. One-fourth of the patients in book 1 identified themselves as married, with 10.4 percent indicating "under husband" (i.e., a woman who is married). The married couple who individually or jointly consulted Kofi Dɔnkɔ the most was Yaa Donkor and Kwaku Nyamekyɛ. Kwaku was a sixty-year-old farmer and Methodist from the Asante region—the village or township of Akomadan to be precise—who visited Kofi Dɔnkɔ six times "for medicine" and the other times for

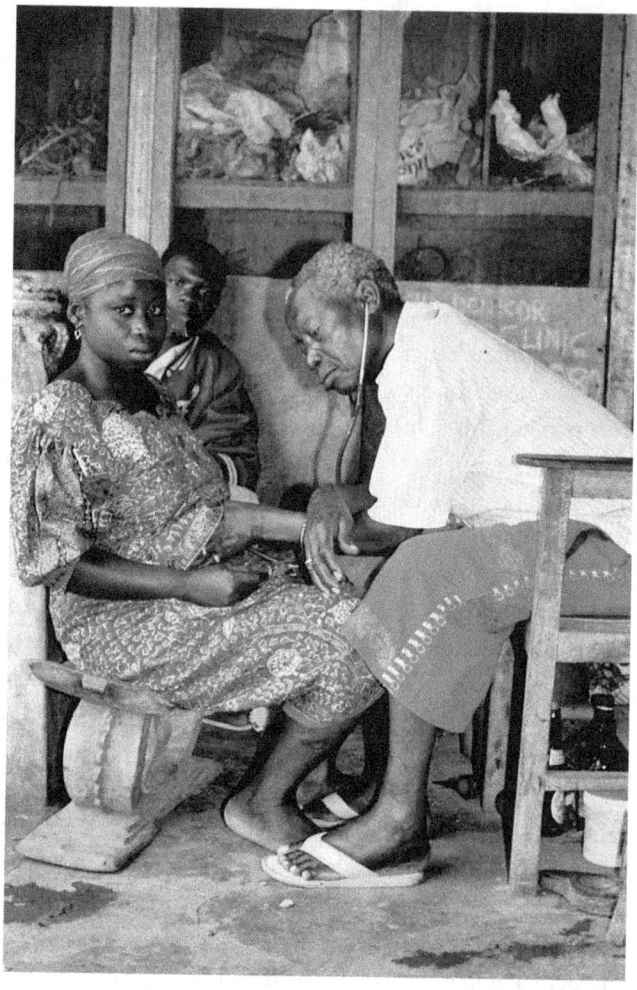

FIGURE 7.4. Kofi Dɔnkɔ with a patient, 1991. From Nana Kofi Dɔnkɔ Collection, in private hands, Takyiman, Ghana. Used courtesy of Kofi Sakyi Sapɔn.

afflictions resulting from "negatively charged" medicines. Apparently, the sickness derived from ill-intended medicines (aduto) were severe and protracted, causing Kwaku to make frequent visits to Kofi Dɔnkɔ's compound in search of protective and nullifying medicines.

In book 2, the number of patients more than doubles that recorded in book 1 but for a shorter period. Between November 1982 and December 1986, some 5,670 patients flowed into Kofi Dɔnkɔ's compound (figure 7.4). Just over one-fourth originated in the township or district of Takyiman, whereas the rest—mirroring the profile given in book 1—came from Akomadan (10.6 percent), Aworowa (6.4 percent), and Afrancho (3.9 percent). Both

Akomadan and Afrancho are in the northern part of the Asante region. The patients from these locales consisted of infants or toddlers (several months to three years old) and adults ages twenty to thirty-five, per the entries for the 3,209 individuals for whom age was listed. The average age was nineteen years old. Consistent with book 1, the most frequently treated illnesses were those associated with childbirth (11.2 percent), pregnancy (5.9 percent), malarial fever (5.7 percent), abdomen and innards (4.7 percent each), and fever with jaundice (4.2 percent). Although book 1 included treatments administrated through baths, enemas, and oral application, book 2 added vapor therapy, steam baths, and nasal drops to Kofi Dɔnkɔ's repertoire. Unique to book 2 is the robust data on payment (*aseda*, "giving thanks").

Of the 2,076 patients from whom payment data was recorded, approximately one-fourth (22.2 percent) gave thanks with 400 cedis, an alcoholic drink, and a chicken. Some 11 percent did the same except gave 200 cedis; 7.1 percent the same apart for 600 cedis; and a combined 8.4 percent who made the same offerings but with either 100 or 140 cedis. We should bear in mind that aseda was given only after the patient declared that their illness—social, physical, psychic, or otherwise—had been effectively treated. Patients were empowered, and payments were thus contingent upon empirical outcomes. Because women's illnesses topped the list of most frequently treated ones, it should not surprise us that women paid the most often, for either themselves or for their children. The top women in the latter category were Adwoa Manu, Grace Yeboah, Alima Kramo, Abiba Kramo, Adwoa Akoma, and Adwoa Amponsah. In this list we see the three major types of patients ordered by religious affiliation or spiritual adherence: *kramo* is the Akanized Malinke term for a Muslim, *Grace* was a Christian name received through baptism or upon entering school, and *manu* (second-born child) and *akoma* (heart) represented the indigenous spiritual culture. Most intriguingly, Adwoa Manu and Grace Yeboah were among the patients who made the most visits to Kofi Dɔnkɔ's healing facility. And why not? Kofi Dɔnkɔ identified and treated some seven hundred illnesses, as evidenced in books 1 and 2.

※

IN 1988, WHEN BOOK 1 ends, the Ghana Psychic and Traditional Healers Association issued a "Certificate of Competence and Authority" to "Oduyefo—Okomfo Kofi Donkor." The certifying document indicated that Kofi Dɔnkɔ was "a member of the above association and has been critically examined by the Board of Examiners of the National Executive and

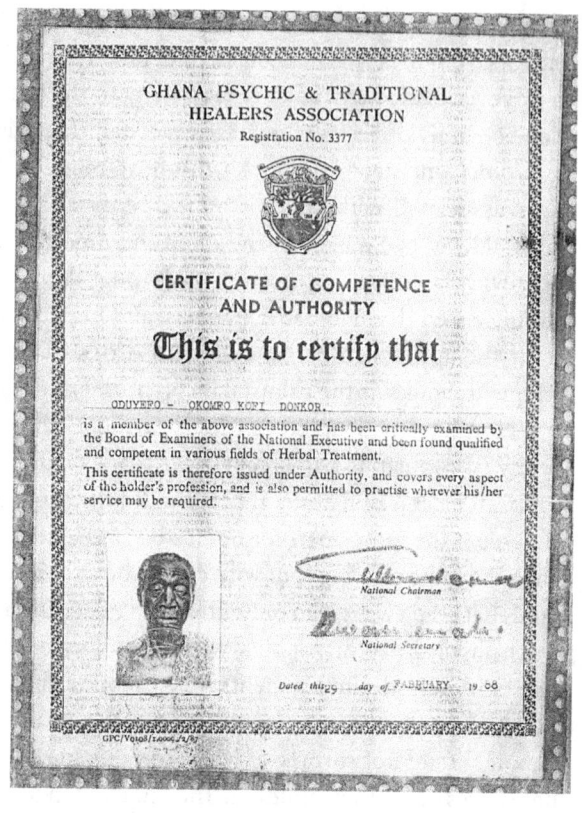

FIGURE 7.5. Kofi Dɔnkɔ's certificate from the Ghana Psychic and Traditional Healers Association. From Nana Kofi Dɔnkɔ Collection, in private hands, Takyiman, Ghana. Used courtesy of Kofi Sakyi Sapɔn.

has been found qualified and competent in various fields of Herbal Treatment."[43] The certificate was issued on 29 February 1988 with a picture of Kofi Dɔnkɔ and signatures from the national chairperson and secretary. Kofi Dɔnkɔ also had a membership card, and although empty, it contained the aims and objectives of the association (figure 7.5).[44] As a member of the Takyiman community and its subset of healers, Kofi Dɔnkɔ also played the ubiquitous role of attending funerals as family head (*abusuapanin*) and prominent healer. Attending to life as a healer also meant attending to matters of death and temporal transition, all filled with ritual obligations, observances, and participation in the mundane ebb and flow of community life.

On 20 June 1984, Kofi Dɔnkɔ attended, for instance, the funeral of *ɔbaapanin* Nana Amma Tabuaa, the fifty-four-year-old "Queenmother of [New] Kenten" who had recently passed.[45] This was typical, and funerals were usually held on Saturdays. Most funerals, regardless of the deceased's social standing, were announced on small two-by-two or three-by-three cards, indicating the chief mourners, kin, and invited personalities. Kofi Dɔnkɔ was frequently invited, and in one way or another, the majority of those mourned had been his patients or relatives of his patients. But like the index cards that recorded patient information, the back of these funerary announcements was also used to record important life information. A note on the back of the funeral announcement for Kwadwo Krah dated 5 January 1988, for instance, read, "we functioned from morning to evening and had an amount of five hundred and thirty cedis (530.00). With the above amount old man [an affectionate term for Kofi Dɔnkɔ] authorized me to give 300 [cedis] to his wife as feed allowance and also one hundred cedis (100.00) to buy pito. It has now left with 180 cedi."[46]

Kofi Dɔnkɔ the healer stood at the unending precipice of temporal life and death, and on the back of that funerary announcement card, he accounted for life's priorities. He and his family worked "from morning to evening," earned 530 cedis that day, gave most of his daily earnings to his wife Afia Monofie, bought *pito* (a beverage with low alcoholic content brewed from fermented millet) to share with family, and saved the rest. Although profound in his understanding of disease and medicine, Kofi Dɔnkɔ was deeply pragmatic, engaging in community affairs and in many of the mundane activities of other Ghanaians. On 2 September 1990, Kofi Dɔnkɔ and his elder sister ɔkɔmfoɔ Adwoa Akumsa and family participated in a "send off party" for Mr. J. K. Tuffour at the community center in Takyiman. Tuffour had recently retired from the police force after twenty-eight years of service.[47] One striking example of participation in mundane activates concerned the national weekly lotto that was established as the Department of National Lotteries in 1958.

The Department of National Lotteries would morph into the National Lotto Authority in 2006, after having its processes automated in 1979 with mechanized lotto coupons. Kofi Dɔnkɔ probably played the national weekly lotto since the 1960s, though only two lottery tickets dated 17 September 1988 were found among his papers. Lotto players choose five numbers from one to ninety, and winners would cash in their prized coupons at regional offices. Kofi Dɔnkɔ would have done so at the regional office in Sunyani. As one can imagine, the lotto was extremely popular during the political and economic turbulence of the 1960s to 1980s. The lotto's steady popularly continued into the early 1990s as economic decline in Ghana—before the Gulf oil crisis—raised petroleum prices by 2 percent, affecting transport and foodstuff prices. For a largely farming population, Ghana's common folks bore the brunt of the weight, and this burden grew, with inflation pegged at 37 percent. Farmers and families like that of Kofi Dɔnkɔ stubbornly pushed their lives through the jagged contours of Ghana's unstable political economy.

By 1990, claims of subversive activity and executions by firing squads were reoccurring themes, along with criticism of PNDC policies, while the second phase of the Economic Recovery Program and extradition treaties between Ghana and its eastern neighbors were implemented under Rawlings's vision for Ghana. Rawlings's National Commission for Democracy expanded Ghana's administrative districts from 65 to 110 and officially recognized the newly created Upper West Region. The commission also presided over national efforts to register voters for district assembly elections across the country, instituted a new minimum daily wage (set at 460 cedis in 1990), and sought to provide a roadmap for the political future of Ghana; clergy meeting in 1990 asked for a debate on this future. An opposition group called the Democratic Alliance of Ghana, based in London, echoed the clergy in protest and demanded multiparty constitutional rule. The Movement for Freedom and Justice in Accra joined the chorus. Rawlings's ruling administration did not ignore these calls for transition, but Rawlings wanted to be the architect of that transition. In this moment of flux more than half of the cocoa and coffee plantations were sold to private individuals and businesses in Ghana and abroad, signaling yet another reordering of economy policies along lines praised by the IMF and World Bank.

In Takyiman, the district too had been restructured, reducing the land mass by 25 percent and shrinking its population.[48] With only 39 percent of the majority rural populace of Ghana having access to safe water and 43 percent to health services, the HFH had little choice in reviving the PRHETIH program through the appointment of Samuel Oduro-Sarpong as program coordinator in October 1990. Oduro-Sarpong prepared for the 300 identified healers and the 124 ready for training.[49] Another important focus at the HFH was educating staff on HIV/AIDS, given the increase in HIV-positive cases from seven to twenty-three.[50] However, not even a nascent HIV/AIDS challenge could refocus the apparent misguided use of limited resources. The HFH used its government subvention for salaried workers who focused on daily prayer, their Christian community, and encouraging pastors "from different churches . . . to visit their parishioners," while only 9 percent of government expenditures went to health care but 26 percent to missionary-based schooling. Meanwhile, the prevalence of malaria and measles increased by 30 percent, resulting in many deaths.[51]

In 1991, the seventy-nine- or eighty-year-old Kofi Dɔnkɔ was paid a research visit by Margaret Yeakel-Twum, a student associated with Michael Warren. Yeakel-Twum's observations at Kofi Dɔnkɔ's compound provide an important snapshot of his healing practice and the patients he treated. Yeakel-Twum described Kofi Dɔnkɔ's "shrine room" as a "dark room with two small windows, each with a light grate covering the opening." Inside "there were nine [abosom represented by brass pans] that were housed in this shrine room."[52] In the compound area transformed into a clinic, she recorded,

> I would arrive at the clinic and find patients waiting to be seen. Some patients stayed at the clinic for extended treatments or if their homes were a long distance away. Many of the patients who sought out Kofi Donkor did so on references from friends or relatives, often traveling from far away areas. Those who waited did so very patiently and quietly, never seeming to be in a hurry to leave. There were days when those who were waiting were not doing so for treatment but to bring payment of some sort for previous services rendered. At this clinic, no one was turned away if they could not pay and payment was not expected until the treatment was effective. Women would proudly bring in babies to show Kofi Donkor, proving that his treatments for their infertility had worked again.... Infertility was one of the major complaints of women who came to the clinic, which was presented as always a women's problem.[53]

Yeakel-Twum observed Kofi Dɔnkɔ treating boils (*mpɔmpɔ*), malnutrition (*asenam*), snakebites (*ɔwɔka*), and many other conditions, but she regarded his "clinic" as surprisingly unique because the HFH continued to refer patients to him. "There were other herbalists in the area who had clinics in their compounds," she continued, "but Kofi Donkor's seemed [to] be the oldest and most established clinic in this area."[54] Kofi Dɔnkɔ's healing facility was well stocked with herbs gathered locally and from afar, arranged in a cabinet containing a wide range of dried bark, roots, and leaves. A fresh pile of medicines laid in the middle of the compound, and Yeakel-Twum "was always amazed [when] Nana Kofi Donkor would stand up from his chair, put his crutch under his arm, hobble over to this pile and proceed to point out to his son or another family member the pieces of plant material he needed to work with. Nana [Dɔnkɔ] had slipped and broken his hip about a year ago and was dependent on the crutch for mobility."[55] For her, "it truly was fascinating to watch this process, as I knew very well that Nana

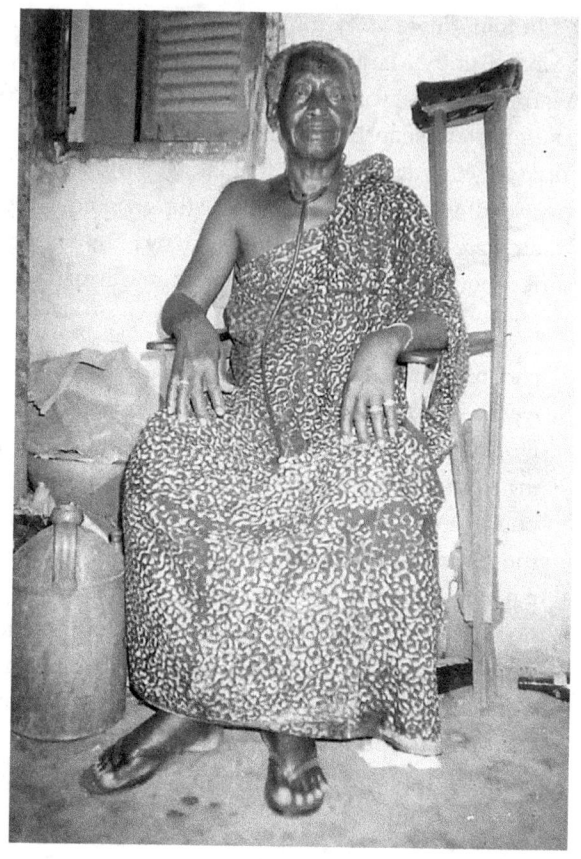

FIGURE 7.6. Kofi Dɔnkɔ with crutches and a gifted stethoscope. From Nana Kofi Dɔnkɔ Collection, in private hands, Takyiman, Ghana. Used courtesy of Kofi Sakyi Sapɔn.

knew exactly what plant the root, stem or bark originated from." In addition, while "Nana [Dɔnkɔ] used his extensive knowledge of herbs in his diagnosis, he also used a stethoscope that had been given to him as a gift from a visiting African-American. He would listen, in particular, to the breathing of the youngest patients who were brought in for treatment" (figure 7.6).[56]

Through his "herbal clinic" Kofi Dɔnkɔ also taught and certified healers trained under his leadership. On 22 December 1991 he had a letter written for his kin and recent healing graduate, Akua Asantewaa, authenticating her status as Asubɔnten Kwabena ɔkɔmfoɔ. In the letter, Kofi Dɔnkɔ dictated that "this is to certify that Nana Akua Asante[waa] Asubonteng Bono Priestess has been an apprenticeship at the above clinic for a period of four years. During her period of stay, she studied the following: Bono traditional culture, Bono medicine and traditional religion. [She] was trained/joined Primary Health Care Training for Indigenous Healers Programme in [sic]

24th June 1981 by Holy Family Hospital Techiman. Her conduct is good and respectful. I recommend her for traditional healing license and certificate." The letter was signed with Kofi Dɔnkɔ's thumbprint or index finger print inside the stamped seal of the "Nana Kofi Donkor Herbal Clinic."[57] Kofi Dɔnkɔ also trained Kwasi Appiah and Kwasi Owusu around the same time. Both hailed from the Asante region. Appiah's family migrated from Koforidua to farm cocoa in Asante. He trained for the ɔbosom Akumsa his great-grandparents had used to build their town, whereas Owusu trained for an ɔbosom his uncle had found in the forest and brought to their village of Boɔho (eight miles north of Kumase) in the 1970s. While Appiah returned to his hometown after graduation (and visited Takyiman intermittently), Owusu remained in Takyiman, bought a plot of land, built a house, initiated his own healing practice, and in the process named his first son after Kofi Dɔnkɔ—Kwame Sakyi.[58]

Alongside Kofi Dɔnkɔ's training and certification of healers, the reconstituted PRHETIH, under new field coordinator Oduro-Sarpong, represented a different certification process centered on the imperatives of biomedicine and the Christian orthodoxy gripping the nation.[59] The reincarnation of the PRHETIH program came with some new faces among its personnel and some changes from within. Oduro-Sarpong was the first Ghanaian and non–Peace Corps field coordinator, and joining him was HFH matron Elizabeth Dwamena, who was a manager of the PRHETIH program. After studying the Dormaa Healers' Project and attending courses in Kumase and at the Centre for Scientific Research into Plant Medicine in Akuapem, Oduro-Sarpong recruited 180 of 300 herbalists for the PRHETIH program. He also mapped out year-end goals: register all herbalists in the Takyiman district, train healers and graduate them from the program, construct an arboretum, and establish a "databank on all healers in the district," which would allow for follow-up visits and supervisions. Through Oduro-Sarpong, changes were made to the PRHETIH emblem on its certificates, from the "old one [that] portrays a doctor and a fetish priest" to one that would "portray a leaf crossed with a hypodermic Syringe."[60] His reasoning was rooted in the aforementioned imperatives: the "former emblem does not represent all the categories of the healers who are made up of Christians, Muslims, Fetish Priest(ess) and 'Ordinary' herbalists. The new symbol will signify the cooperation between all users of herbs (leaf) and all Western Medical practitioners (syringe)." The new changes to the revitalized PRHETIH program were publicized through press releases to the *People's Daily Graphic*, the state-owned daily newspaper.⁶¹ The Ghanaian state, under Rawlings's PNDC, also reveled in this mood of change.

❋

TAKING THE LEAD from the PNDC, a new constitution was crafted and put to a vote in May 1992. The ratified constitution paved the way for freeing political prisoners, abolishing indefinite detentions, a free press, and multiparty elections (set for November) and parliamentary elections (toward the end of December). The PNDC formed a new party, the National Democratic Congress (NDC), and offered Jerry Rawlings as its presidential candidate. Rawlings captured the presidency with almost 60 percent of votes from registered voters, while historian Albert Adu Boahen, representing the New Patriotic Party, was the closest contender with some 30 percent of the electorate. Former president Hilla Limann received less than 7 percent of the vote. Not surprisingly, the NDC won the lion's share of the parliamentary seats—189 of 200. Sworn in on 7 January 1993, President Rawlings ushered in the fourth republic, built on a constitution that drew upon United States and British models. In fact, in true neocolonial fashion, Ghana civil and criminal law remained rooted in British common and criminal law *after* constitution reforms.

Although the constitution provided immunity for PNDC action over the previous decade, the political and economic volatility during that period could not be so easily managed. That instability had, among other things, led to an irreversible surge in Christianization in Ghana and transformation in the people's outlook and values as expressed through popular culture. For instance, gospel music and cassette tapes became ever so popular, prompting local musicians and artists to migrate to the churches and for church music to be shorthand for popular music. Emigration to Europe—especially Germany and England—also cross-fertilized local music by having overseas Ghanaians, who were influenced by Caribbean-based reggae music or electronic instrumentation, produce a fusion of indigenous and foreign styles that became increasingly popular in Ghana. But Christianization not only cast a wide net over Ghanaians and their diasporic populations; it also led to a specific rise in Pentecostalism, whose pace of diffusion was both frenetic and fanatic. In fact, while Kofi Dɔnkɔ was hospitalized at the HFH over three consecutive months in 1995, Christian fanatics constantly sought to evangelize him while he was in and out of the hospital and gravely ill. We might imagine that in the early 1990s this scene—sometimes with even greater ferocity—would be replayed among the forty-nine general hospitals, hundreds of rural health clinics, and countless private health facilities across the fourth republic.

In 1994 the HFH was named a district hospital for Takyiman, qualifying it for more government funding and enabling it to offer greater care for the poor. However, the hospital had to celebrate its fortieth anniversary amidst the rebuilding of its maternity unit, which had been destroyed by a tornado the previous year. Unlike the care provided by the HFH, the government's care for the poor through its community health insurance plan was duly criticized for its inability to improve health care to the impoverished, but more so for its inability to address adequately the politics and "ethnic" clashes that erupted in northern Ghana. The subplot to these clashes was the cumulative effect of military and civilian rule, inflation, currency devaluation, failed structural adjustment schemes, and indebtedness. Following the 1992 presidential election, Ghana's inequalities and antagonisms ran beneath a veneer of democratic progress and an almost unquestioned acceptance of things foreign. In 1994, "ethnic" rivalries over political authority in the Northern Region exploded into violence and bloodshed, killing some five hundred people and forcing thousands of refugees to Togo. The Northern Region is the largest of Ghana's ten regions, populated by numerous yet distinct linguistic and political groups. The imposition of Akan statecraft and British colonial administration favoring one group over another created tensions and divisions between centralized and "chiefless" societies, represented by the Dagomba and Konkomba, boiling over into outright civil war.[62] In short, the minority Konkomba asserted their political independence by pushing for a paramount chief, but they circumvented the Dagomba ruler, Ya Na, who represented the largest group in the region.[63]

The violence that erupted, however, pointed less to the politics of chieftaincy per se than to the failure of independence politicians to balance sociopolitical development in the two halves of the country. The reinstalled Rawlings government of 1994 imposed an extended state of emergency and dispatched the national armed forces to the area. Negotiations began after several people were killed in the regional capital of Tamale, but these were marred by claims of plots to overthrow the government and by opposition parties withdrawing from the reconciliation process. By August, a peace agreement was reached and a cease-fire went into effect, allowing a negotiating team to focus on its task of facilitating stability. Ironically, the new president returned to old tactics of arresting individuals who allegedly conspired to overthrow the government and charged them with crimes against the state. Further arrests and killings in the region worked not to resolve the tensions but rather to increase suspicion and conflict among the participants involved and toward the new government. Kofi Dɔnkɔ had traveled often to northern Ghana, learned from its healers, and had many patients who traveled from that region for his therapeutic offerings. Kofi Dɔnkɔ's approach to the people of Ghana was simple: treat all, regardless of their political or religious standing and affiliation, with an affirmation of their humanity and with care. The Rawlings regime and consequently the people of Ghana would have benefited greatly from such a balanced and human approach.

The conflicts that erupted in northern Ghana had consequences for the rest of country. With newly paved roads between Tamale and Takyiman and between Takyiman and its regional capital of Sunyani, "people [were] mobile," as HFH officials observed.[64] The extended state of emergency, however, placed travel restrictions on all movement to and from northern Ghana. Once again, Takyiman was the crossroad between northern and southern Ghana, and so the restrictions emanating from the conflicts affected those who needed hospitalization or the indigenous therapeutics offered by Kofi Dɔnkɔ and company. Also affected were the flow of goods and services, and the thousands of food producers and the commerce they transacted at the Takyiman market. The Takyiman market was the largest three-day market and the township was the fastest growing commercial center in the country. Approximately 90 percent of its residents were farmers who planted cassava, yams, maize, and beans and engaged in small-scale trading, whereas 2 percent were full-time merchants and just over 5 percent were civil servants. The conflicts affected the arrival and departure of people, produce, and manufactured goods through the commercial hub that was Takyiman, as well as the number of inpatients and outpatients at the HFH, both of which decreased during the protracted conflicts.[65]

For Takyiman inhabitants, the six doctors at the HFH translated into one doctor per 20,133 individuals, while the nine mission hospitals (seven Catholic, two Protestant) in the Brong-Ahafo region served about 69 percent of the regional population.[66] Through HFH records we can see what features all mission hospitals shared but also what programs made the HFH different in its response to the present exigencies. In May 1971 the HFH developed a credit union called Abosomankotere ("chameleon") with 165 members, and reports in 1994 suggest the credit union "continues to thrive with 201 members."[67] The HFH responded to the 130 HIV/AIDS cases brought to the hospital with an educational campaign targeting every village in the district, including schools.[68] To help fight against malnutrition and anemia, the active

169 HFH-trained TBAS were deployed alongside the 201 PRHETIH healers located in ten communities, yet "no further training" was envisioned for these healers; efforts were geared toward the "supervision of trained traditional healers."[69] While leaders of diverse cultural groups grappled with the burial of indigent and abandoned group members, the HFH was challenged by a new life-and-death matter: abortion.[70] Of the sixty-eight cases of induced abortions, about half were done by inserting herbs deep into the vagina; 22 percent of those undergoing an abortion were married women who explained that they did so because the last baby was born too young, whereas 47 percent were unmarried women whose reasoning was no trade or a low level of schooling.[71] The unborn, the living, and the deceased remained entangled because they embodied community in both its transformations and its transitions.

For Kofi Dɔnkɔ and family, life and temporal death were not statistical matters but rather the filaments of the human experience. On 17 April, 7 May, and 12 June 1995, Kofi Dɔnkɔ was admitted to the HFH. While there, Christian fanatics tried their hardest to convert him, but their theological arguments failed. Kofi Dɔnkɔ, we are told, could not accept that he had "sinned" and that Jesus would cure his illness if he confessed these "sins." Gravely ill, he proclaimed that he had committed no acts of negativity toward anyone. During the three months he was in and out of the hospital, Catholic priests also sought to convert Kofi Dɔnkɔ through baptism. According to Kofi Dɔnkɔ's family, the healer "understood the pastor's language, but [Kofi Dɔnkɔ] gave [the clergyman] a good [proverbial] response and did not change his beliefs."[72] On 8 August 1995, Kofi Dɔnkɔ, around age eighty-four, made his transition to *asamandoɔ* at his compound in the "healer's town." In observance of that moment, family and community appropriately exclaimed *ɔkɔ akuraa* ("she/he has gone to the village"), *ɔkɔ baabi* ("she/he has gone someplace"), and *dupɔn kɛsee atutu* ("a great tree has been uprooted").

Relatives nearby described his transition in the following way. Kofi Dɔnkɔ expected to pass seven days before he did. As a child's belonging in the world requires waiting seven days inclusive before they are named—and therefore registered as a member of the community—so too healers reserve this right on their way to an ancestral community. On the seventh day, his wife Afia Monofie prepared for him pounded yams made into a dough (*fufu*) and a light soup (figure 7.7). While eating, Kofi Dɔnkɔ fell to the ground, shaking, in front of the eating table. He then went into his bedroom, followed by some family members who witnessed the healer fall

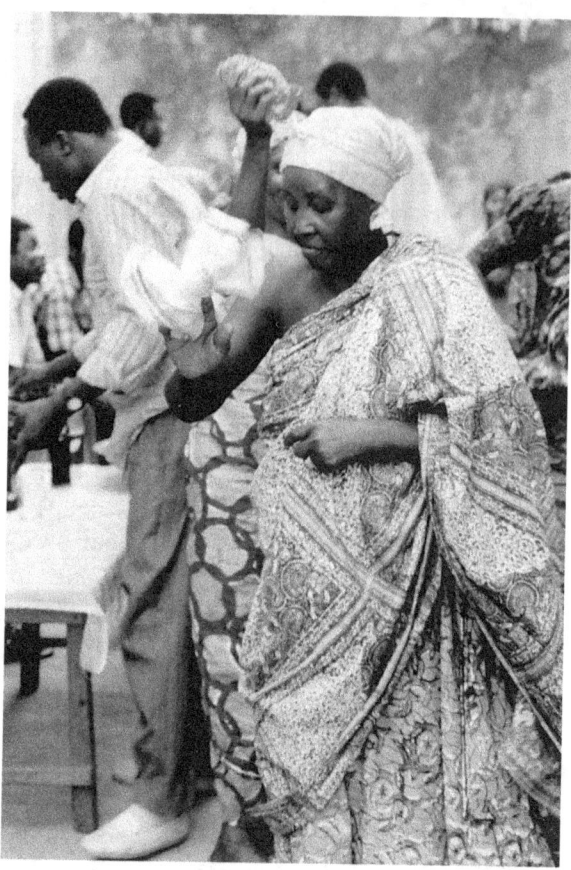

FIGURE 7.7. Afia Monofie, 1991. From Nana Kofi Dɔnkɔ Collection, in private hands, Takyiman, Ghana. Used courtesy of Kofi Sakyi Sapɔn.

again, but this time into a deep trance state. He requested those with him to remove the iron bracelet (*kaa*) on his hand and the iron ring (*kawa*) on his finger. Water and schnapps were brought to the room almost immediately. Water was poured on Kofi Dɔnkɔ's mouth before the animating life force—which had fought so hard to stay on earth around 1913—left his physical body. Kofi Dɔnkɔ's passing occurred when preparations were being made for the annual "yam" or harvest festival. For this reason, funerary plans were put on hold and his body was sent to the HFH mortuary for preservation—*nana kɔ aduro mu* ("Nana [Dɔnkɔ] went into medicine"). The body would remain there for several weeks while the community and his family sorted out their mutually overlapping affairs.

Yaw Mensa, a teacher and storekeeper in Accra, was called back to Takyiman by his uncle Kofi Dɔnkɔ and his mother Adwoa Akumsa to learn "home affairs." The forty-eight-year-old Yaw was assured he would inherit the ɔbosomfoɔ position held by Kofi Dɔnkɔ. Yaw recalled, "when my uncle was in the hospital, my uncle told me . . . he called one of his brothers Kofi Ankoma and the ɔkyeame Kofi Ɔboɔ and told the family he was old and that he needed feedback from them, since he wanted to pass everything onto me."[73] According to Yaw Mensa, the family had an opportunity to voice their support or opposition, but their nonresponse infuriated both Kofi Dɔnkɔ and Yaw's mother Adwoa Akumsa. Kofi Dɔnkɔ then transitioned during the impasse. Kofi Ɔboɔ, however, felt he should be the one to inherit Kofi Dɔnkɔ's position, for "Kofi Dɔnkɔ . . . knew if he passed away I would carry on the practice."[74] Conflicts over inheritance were nothing new to Ghana, to Takyiman, or to families like that of Kofi Dɔnkɔ. This contestation, however, signaled the end of an era of prominent healers who helped balance the countervailing forces of the township and society, and split the family into opposing sides.

Family members either supported or rejected Yaw as the next ɔbosomfoɔ, though Yaw's ɔbosomfoɔ training proceeded well under the collective guidance of Boɔtwerewa Kwaku ɔkɔmfoɔ Kofi Asimadu, Taa Kwasi ɔbosomfoɔ Kofi Kyereme, and Taa Mensa Kwabena ɔbosomfoɔ Kwabena Mensa. The ensuing familial conflict "nearly broke the whole family into parts," and explains why "it took a few months before appointing a successor" to Kofi Dɔnkɔ.[75] Be that as it may, in the moment of Kofi Dɔnkɔ's passing, family and community all agreed: the healer deserved a state funeral, the highest burial honor (figure 7.8). Kofi Dɔnkɔ's body remained on view for seven days before the burial, while thousands of individuals from near and far paid the first of several periodic respects to a person who embodied the best of them and what they could become. Everyone from market women to dignitaries to Christians and Muslims attended his funeral, which was a wholly indigenous affair with akɔmfoɔ wearing white clay on their faces and bodies and with drumming, dirges, and dancing that celebrated his temporal life. The brass pan that contained the "shrine" of Asubɔnten Kwabena, the ɔbosom that protected his early life and supported his longevity, was removed from its wooden stool and placed on a small bundle consisting of the *nyamya* plant. This ritual gesture held a week after the public funeral meant those in spirit, joining the mortals, were in a state of mourning—*abosom kɔ ayiyɛ* ("abosom attends the funeral").

❋

IN THE WAKE of Kofi Dɔnkɔ's temporal transition from kin in the flesh to relations in spirit, historic tensions resurfaced between Asante and Takyiman

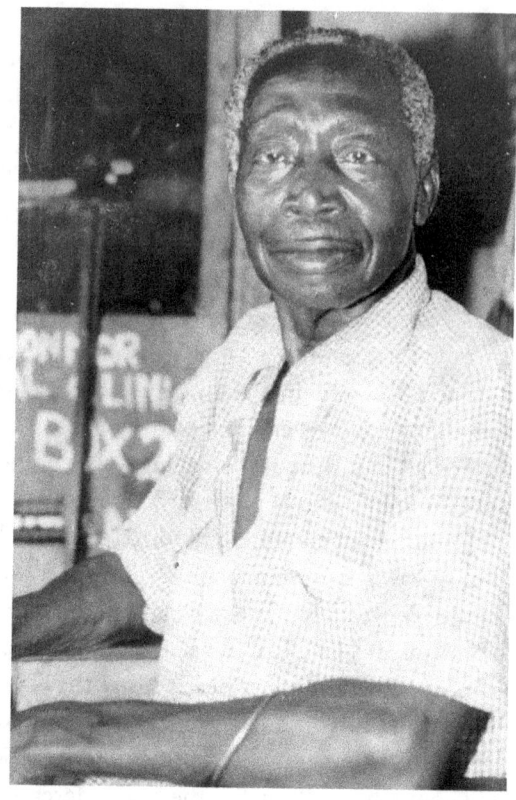

FIGURE 7.8. Photo taken of Nana Kofi Dɔnkɔ, 1994. It was placed on T-shirts worn during his funeral celebration in 1995. From Nana Kwaku Sakyi Collection, in private hands, Miami, Florida. Used courtesy of Nana Kwaku Sakyi, photographer.

and among prominent cultural groups in northern Ghana. An equally important rupture between the government and the civil service joined the moment of localized and national unrest. In February 1996, six or seven individuals were killed in the Takyiman district during riots, destruction to property, and fighting over which indigenous political actors had real "chieftain" authority. The conflicts erupt in and around four of the historically disputed villages that were on Takyiman lands but at one point had been under nominal Asante rule. The leader of the Asante people, Asantehene Opoku Ware II, elevated the status of subordinate "chiefs" in the Takyiman district to the same standing as the Takyimanhene, the district's indigenous leader.[76] Supporters and opponents of the Asantehene's move responded to his political gesture not by confronting the Asantehene but through violence against fellow Takyiman residents. Over a hundred people were killed. An imposed curfew followed by a joint committee consisting of leaders from the main parties were instated shortly thereafter. In the southern part of the country—in the Asante capital of Kumase and the nation's capital in Accra, to be precise—widespread but peaceful protest over the newly imposed valued-added tax (VAT) was met with a violent response that left several dead. Organized by the Alliance for Change, the *Kume Preko* ("kill me at once") protest demonstration of 100,000 people in Accra rejected the exorbitant living costs and the newly imposed VAT of 17.5 percent, which the Rawlings government introduced to generate income. The driving force, however, came from IMF and World Bank pressures embedded in their structural adjustment scheme.[77] The Kume Preko demonstration represented over a decade of IMF and World Bank–authored privatization, currency devaluation, public spending reductions, and political liberalization, on one hand, and deep poverty (especially in conflict-ridden northern Ghana) and debt to those multinational institutions, on the other hand.

The IMF and World Bank, in short, provided loans with interest and conditionalities that made countries like Ghana more indebted by assuming a debt they could not repay. Loans begot more loans and downgraded credit, and increased debt became a lever for managers of the IMF and World Bank to exert control over or coerce indebted countries. Although the VAT was suspended and the old sales tax reinstated following the public protest, the infection of IMF and World Bank prescriptions had already run its course and made the government powerless to keep its own promises. Teachers and nurses went on strike for salary increases and improved working conditions, but an agreement was reached between the teachers and the government only in December 1995. Shortages of nurses and doctors would require more protracted attention.

The five doctors in the entire Takyiman district stemmed from the limited number of trained physicians but also the blatant refusal of available and government-trained doctors to assume postings assigned by the Ministry of Health. Ironically, inflation had increased the cost of medical supplies and the number of doctors engaging in private practice. For the HFH, the shortage of nurses and doctors was no surprise, and the "chief elders and townspeople" knew this when they formally recognized the HFH during the annual *Apɔɔ* festival in April.[78] Equally unsurprising was the recognition of "no essential change in disease pattern in top ten conditions treated," though malaria accounted for 33.7 percent of consultations and the hospital had begun to produce Mosbar (an insect repellant) in August.[79] The year after Kofi Dɔnkɔ transitioned, there was surprisingly nothing about healers in HFH activities or with regard to goals and prospects for the following year. And there is nothing in the HFH records to explain this abrupt absence. Was Kofi Dɔnkɔ the connective tissue between the hospital and the community of healers? Or was the project to integrate two distinct worlds of culture and therapeutics something that belonged to an era, and that era went with the person who embodied it?

With that era also went several prominent healers within Kofi Dɔnkɔ's family and community, and all within the harvest "new year" season. Some background is important here. The forest fringe has long been a locus of Bono settlement and the tributaries of the Tanɔ River, home to historic and revered Tanɔ abosom. The forest fringe was also home to the indigenous oil palm, especially along the rivers that perforated the landscape. Both yam and oil palm are critical indigenous food crops whose cultivation archaeologically places the Bono—and the broader Akan cluster to which they belong—on the edge of the forest for at least the past two thousand years. These crops played no small part in clearing and occupying the forest environs, creating a subsistence economy based on yam and oil palm cultivation and animal domestication, and more importantly, institutionalizing the ritual consumption of yam and palm oil in a harvest "new year" period. The principal staple of yam was harvested between the Gregorian months of July and September, corresponding to the calendrical periods of *kitawonsa* and *ɛbɔ*. These indigenous crops were prominent during this period, and both became staple offerings to the very ancestors Kofi Dɔnkɔ habitually provided an appropriate invitation: "our ancestral spirits, come and have drink." The most fundamental ancestral food offering—and now a popular Ghanaian dish in its own right—was a meal called *ɛtɔ*, made of boiled and then mashed yams and palm oil. Eggs from the ubiquitous chicken, a staple in ritual sacrifices, were often added to this meal.

During this period of harvest and reflection on culture in the natural order of things, several kin and community healers made their transitions to asamandoɔ. Kofi Dɔnkɔ's kin and healing colleague ɔkɔmfoɔ Yaw Manu passed on 14 August 2001, just before the annual Fofie "yam" festival, where the new harvested yams were introduced and ritually consumed first by Taa Mensa Kwabena, and then by the townspeople. Senior healing colleague and close friend ɔbosomfoɔ Kofi Kyereme made his transition in August 2006. Another kin and healer, ɔkɔmfoɔ Akua Asantewaa, suffered a heart attack, went to the HFH, and passed away on 26 June 2008. Her seven-day funeral rites were held August 5–13.[80] Finally, on 3 July 2015, longtime Asubɔnten Kwabena ɔkyeame and nephew of Kofi Dɔnkɔ, Nana Kofi Ɔboɔ, was also taken to that hospital and made his transition. No theory explains the timing or meaning of these transitions. Their lives and countless others, however, represent an elongated people's history for a culture, community, and nation. As thousands of mourners representing that culture, community, and nation paid their respects as the cream-white casket was covered and the door to Kofi Dɔnkɔ's final resting room closed, what survives the mortal remains in the white casket was a quintessence of "how we go about things in our own way in this part of the world."

EPILOGUE

There's health when everything that should work together works together.
—AYI KWEI ARMAH, *The Healers*

In the preceding pages I used the optics provided by one Kofi Dɔnkɔ and his community to challenge standard accounts of Ghana's modern history and to reimagine the histories, politics, and cultures of nineteenth- and twentieth-century Africa. Chapters 1 to 7, then, narrated the story of a healer, blacksmith, farmer, drummer, and family head during shifting periods of the "colonial" and "postcolonial" world, but through the lens and interlaced evolution of kin, community, and culture. This healer was versatile, operating fluidly as custodian and interpreter of shared values, facilitator of spiritual renewal, promoter of social cohesion, settler of disputes, and assessor and planner of the community's growth. Kofi Dɔnkɔ was a marginal peasant farmer whose fortune and misfortune rode the tides of the cocoa boom, an everyday person who offered us a multiangled window into the social lives and networks of rural dwellers, and an intellectual who articulated a profound understanding of disease and therapeutics to those in West Africa and the African diaspora as well as to a group of notable scholars. Location and an integral cultural heritage stand out among several factors that shaped the life of Kofi Dɔnkɔ and his polity—a region that fell under the Asante empire and then the British empire, forming a dual colonialism. Situated in the crossroad polity of Takyiman, between the northern and southern halves of the nation, he and his polity's positionality invite scholars to think of interior Africa—rather than solely its coastal regions—as a gateway for cultural contact and the making of intra-African histories, and as a counterpoint to evangelical perspectives. Indeed, it is precisely Kofi Dɔnkɔ's deep devotion to his craft, his culture, his community that framed his life and that makes him a significant figure in African and world history, notably in relation to the twentieth-century theme of decolonization.

Although early agitations existed, the mid-twentieth-century struggle for decolonization and political independence in the British empire took formal shape in India, achieving self-rule in 1947, and in the Gold Coast, realizing the same a decade later, yet driven by the popular revolt of former servicemen, village and town dwellers, and cocoa farmers like Kofi Dɔnkɔ. The year was 1948. At that time, the existing world order began either to collapse or to reconfigure. Oscillating forces pushing toward and against empire made 1948 a watershed moment. Unlike the "big bang theory" published that year, the crucial events of 1948 did not emerge from a single explosive moment ushering in a new order. Rather, nationalist agitation, decolonization, the creation of Israel and North and South Korea, the legalization of apartheid in South Africa, the United Nations' declaration of human rights, the rebuilding of Western Europe, and the declaration of the United States as leader of the capitalist world through the Marshall Plan signaled a patchwork world where a nation was but one outcome of decolonization. Capturing all these thematic currents were the 1948 riots in the colonial capital of Accra. In February 1948 a group of unarmed former servicemen marched peacefully to petition the colonial governor for their outstanding pensions. The British colonial police fired on the former servicemen, killing three. News of the killings sparked rioting and looting throughout the capital. Soon, sympathizers-turned-rioters embraced the colony-wide riots to express grievances about unemployment, inflation, and the high price of imported European goods. The colonial authorities, naturally, suppressed the riots, appointed a commission led by Andrew Aiken Watson to investigate the unrest, and swiftly arrested nationalist leaders such as Kwame Nkrumah. Although the Commission's report paved the way for constitutional reforms, Nkrumah transformed the sentiments of unrest into a nationalist movement, leading the Gold Coast to political independence in 1957 and asserting the African's right to self-rule.

Although political independence was won, the fervor that produced it also exposed an ailment Nkrumah diagnosed as "neocolonialism," but he couldn't corral centuries of groups who pursued their own self-interests nor heal the colonized psyche of independent Ghana. The desire for British-supplied goods, notions of beauty and civilization, was not lost on the rioters, many of whom looted shops owned by foreign merchants because they *wanted* the goods and what they symbolized. Although it might be tempting to conclude that Nkrumah's control over the political levers of the nation was circumscribed through global imperialists who eventually orchestrated his overthrow, that control was fully exercised when he became president, removed the Queen of England as sovereign of Ghana, and placed the country on a path edging toward thoroughgoing independence in 1960.[1] But in this moment, and certainly during one-party rule, Nkrumah and his successors paid insufficient attention to the accumulated colonial disturbance of their people's consciousness and cultural platforms, molded through colonialism's protracted violence, traumas, and gutting of identity-affirming institutions—in short, the cascading effects of a forced intimacy occasioned by colonial rule. On this most crucial of missed opportunities for the anticolonial movement, the Watson Commission report was virtually prophetic:

> Save among the older population, there is an unconfessed desire for Europeanization, at least in many aspects. We say, unconfessed, because, while undoubtedly growing, it is not yet strong enough to cast off the shackles of tribalism. But the hands of the clock cannot be put back. The movement is gathering momentum, even if cloaked at times by anti-racial expressions. We doubt if it is sufficiently realized what problems these changes entail. Native authority in its widest sense is diminishing. *The old religions are being undermined by modern conceptions. Earlier disciplines are weakening.* Others must be devised to take their place.[2]

By "old religions" and "earlier disciplines," the Commission and the British empire targeted the real obstruction to effective foreign rule: life-sustaining ideas and practices integral to the evolution of indigenous cultures, social orders, and community life. These moral and intellectual pillars of stability and community were systematically "undermined by modern [read: European] conceptions." Although we should place undue weight on neither Nkrumah nor colonialism for the state of the colony-turned-nation during Kofi Dɔnkɔ's life, the gravity of colonialism preceded and outlived Nkrumah, making necessary a different interpretation of colonial rule and decolonization. Historian Nancy Shoemaker has produced a provisional typology of colonialism, putting in one useful document its many iterations.[3] The twelve types identified consist of settler, planter, extractive, trade, transport, imperial power, legal, rogue, missionary, romantic, postcolonial, and not-in-my-backyard colonialism. Perhaps this list is most evocative not in what it contains, but in what it suggests. Processes and impositions occasioned by colonial rule were neither inevitable nor structured uniformly, as they were for decolonization, though scholars tend to use the same word—*colonialism*.

European colonialism and the termination of colonial rule in the Gold Coast did not have to take the path it did. Whereas Iberian colonial rule in the Americas required a revamping of indigenous ideas and institutions in the image of colonists, Roman imperial rule over its colonies and Qing "foreign" rule over Han China left respective subjugated cultures and institutions largely intact, sometimes adopting them to achieve effective rule. Likewise, the product of decolonization was not always nationalism or the creation of a nation out of a colony. The nationalist ideology and practices harnessed by Nkrumah and allies was one of several intellectual and political options, and yet one that paid homage to the political and Christian architecture of European nations, including the United States, rather than the diversity and common threads of the Gold Coast/Ghana. The nationalist path of decolonization did not scrutinize how classism, racism, sexism, and religious intolerance instantiated those "model" nations, nor how nationalism creates various boundaries and exclusions based on race, religion, and other markers of politicized difference. Those who fought to decolonize, and who were celebrated for seeking the nation—a flawed archetype at that—misdiagnosed colonialism, for there was nothing new, as in *neo*colonialism, about it. In as much as nation-building arises out of intellectual work and as one kind of decolonization, colonialism is also as intellectual as it is a political project that might, given its iterations, be pluralized—or better yet, conceptualized as forced intimacy. Forced intimacy is the habitually nonconsensual sharing or laying bare of bodies, homes, ritual spaces, ecologies, and cognitive worlds under the specter of coercive power and in this case, global white supremacy. All of this was made possible by the imposition of a foreign administration—its technocrats, capitalists, missionaries and converts, schooling and medical dispensers—that provided a seductive ultimatum between their values and worldview and those of the subjugated. Survival in this cauldron, framed by this ultimatum, provided many in the Gold Coast/Ghana, including their nationalist architects, with a false choice.

As forced intimacy, European colonialism was distilled white supremacy, a tightly braided set of ideologies and enforced policies. These were less the peculiar edifices of this or that "colonial power," and even less the default staging posts from which accounting for African lives became a multiple-choice of whether they accepted, rejected, or (the fan favorite) negotiated the artificial and real terrains of forced intimacy. This forced intimacy, this colonialism, was a force and a viral disease that Kofi Dɔnkɔ diagnosed through lived experiences and patients, for whom he provided situational and institutional remedies, and for whom he forged a life in partnership, representing humanistic and transcendent values. Kofi Dɔnkɔ lived in a cultural universe Nkrumah and his "big six" co-authors of the new nation studied in books at coastal mission schools and at the colonial government–run Achimota College, and thus they were only cognitively aware of the new nation's farming, rural, non-Christian majority. Kofi Dɔnkɔ was no nationalist, no rebel against empire nor agent of colonial and religious orthodoxy. Rather, he worked against the identifiable forces wrought by forced intimacy, while Nkrumah and local critics alike failed to detect the white supremacy in the theology, in the instruments of political power hoisted above all else—"Seek ye first the political kingdom, and all else shall be added unto you," said Nkrumah, echoing almost verbatim Matthew 6:33, "But seek ye first the kingdom of God . . . and all these things shall be added unto you." Although we have seen how Kofi Dɔnkɔ led several local movements and even organizations against perceived threats to his community's values, he also strategically cooperated to preserve those values, avoiding electoral politics but remaining very much anchored in the governance and wide-angled life of an expansive community. His was a community that stretched across two empires, national borders, ecologies, polities, and racial and religious ideologies, signaling a non-national, decolonized possibility.

In the more than two decades since Kofi Dɔnkɔ's transition in 1995, his family and community have moved progressively toward the texture of life in southern Ghana, as Takyiman stands between the two halves of the nation as if it endures between two worlds. A significant number of old and middle-aged family members have transitioned as a result of poverty, state neglect, alcoholism, and the daily grind of eking out a living in rural Ghana. Others have continued along the path paved by Kofi Dɔnkɔ as best they can, in Ghana and in the African diaspora. Looking at kin and community at a crossroad, Kofi Dɔnkɔ might have uttered, "There's health when everything that should work together works together." Although axiomatically true, there is no way to know what Kofi Dɔnkɔ's rejoinder to the divergent routes taken by kin and community might have been. The layered realities of life in the crossroad town of Takyiman, and Ghana no less, cannot be bottled in a phrase, in one person, or in what I think about a place, a people, I have studied for more than a decade and a half. If I could poke at those realities, I would not lament Takyiman's independence from Asante rule or Gold Coast independence from British rule, even though both were staged for symbolic effect. Takyiman enjoys no more independence from the present configuration of Asanteman, especially in matters of chieftaincy, than Ghana exercises from England or other Group of Seven members (Group of Eight, minus Russia). I would suggest, then, an interlaced irony for further examination: First, one rooted in the theme of missed opportunities—structural occasions at broad decolonization and building a Kofi Dɔnkɔ–like community for political strangers and kinfolk. And second, an irony rooted in alternative ways of grasping these crucial moments through unlikely characters such as Kofi Dɔnkɔ, whose efficacious delivery of health with care touched over 100,000 lives regardless of religious affiliation, rank, or "ethnicity." These remain cornerstones of human flourishing in Africa and in the world.

It is deeply ironic that the forces of latent empire, colonialism, and Europeanization were unleashed on the new nation by the anticolonial figure and government of Kwame Nkrumah. Nkrumah proclaimed to build the new nation on indigenous values, but he sought to undermine local institutions underwritten by those values. Nkrumah and nationalist leaders across "independent" Africa led an anticolonial movement for political independence and made us believe that nationalism was shorthand for decolonization, but he reified rather than replaced colonial instruments of the state, at times deployed in draconian ways. Even if the artificial boundaries crisscrossing Africa might take more coordinated effort among Africans to resolve, in "independent" Ghana the tripartite colony and its colonial boundaries remain intact, with pride of place given to the colonial capital and its Christianizing environs. In 1960 the northern portions of the Northern Territories and Asante were apportioned and renamed respectively the Upper Region (divided by Rawlings into Upper East and Upper West) and the Brong-Ahafo region, while the Gold Coast Colony's three colonial provinces became regions, Greater Accra was created, and former British Togoland was renamed the Volta region. In effect, the ten administrative regions of present-day Ghana are essentially the tripartite colony, itself ironically the colonial partition of Asanteman or Greater Asante. This, then, might explain why present Asantehene Osei Tutu II rules Asanteman in ways comparable to those used by his predecessors, circumventing the Ghanaian government and securing World Bank funding and audiences with world leaders, and why nationalism and political independence were possible without decolonizing the crucial areas where forced intimacy breached. Rather than eradicate colonialism, nationalism in Ghana and in Africa writ large unleashed colonial ideas and practices reworked as signs of independence.

When Nkrumah inaugurated the new nation and a new national identity ("Ghanaian"), interlaced with a national anthem, flag, and currency, these actions gave no protection to specific cultural identities or to the ontological platforms of indigenous cultures. This, in turn, made them acutely vulnerable to predation by missionary institutions in four crucial areas of human life: spirituality/religion, education, health care, and language. Once again, mission schools rather than elders educated the young, bibles and hymnbooks were translated into indigenous languages, dictionaries and primers were created, clinics and hospitals preached the gospel to patients, and churches brought these strands together in service of the empire of "God."

We thus should read into and not gloss over Nkrumah's proclamation that Ghana's independence was impossible without the "support of God" and "God's blessing," and the ways in which anticolonialist statesmen schooled in mission settings allowed, even promoted, colonial missionary ideologies and assaults on their cultures while claiming to value things "traditional." As Nkrumah's father had placed his son on a path to Catholic priesthood, which didn't materialize, Nkrumah set Ghana on a path to political independence, and yet its decolonization awaits. There were other possibilities in the Nkrumah moment. We saw Kofi Dɔnkɔ sustain community while leading a healers' association against those assaults, protecting values and lifeways from the multitiered missions under state protection and from local officeholders who saw missions as opportunities to enhance their standing as "modern." The optics of Kofi Dɔnkɔ's actions and life work suggests that Nkrumah and his successors missed opportunities at "real" decolonization, the consequence of which were baked into the 1992 Ghana constitution. In it, for instance, individuals are guaranteed the "freedom to practice any religion and to manifest such practice," but "customary practices," which did not rise to the level of religion, that "dehumanize or are injurious to the physical and mental well-being of a person are prohibited."[4] Nothing in the constitution prohibits the dehumanization and injurious assault Christians carry out on radio, on television, and in schools against "customary practices" and their adherents. The myth of religious freedom in Ghana is of the same kind and quality as that in the United States. This should not surprise us. The 1992 Ghanaian constitution virtually counterfeited the U.S. constitution, the foundational document for a nation found recently to be the least "religiously diverse" and most religiously dogmatic.[5] If Ghanaians view the United States as "God's country," as Nkrumah saw it as a model for the Gold Coast, then perhaps it is not that forming a nation is arduous and fraught, but more crucial are the platforms or models upon which political communities are constructed.

While politicians of the independence era or the neoliberal ilk concern themselves more with the dispensation of power than with the public they claim to serve, most healers are preoccupied with the public good. A diseased society is merely a collection of traumatized bodies working against rather than with their self-healing capabilities—what scientists call immunotherapy. Such healers aptly recognize this disease or grand trauma because they see human life in the context of community and connectedness, rather than viewing people as individuals to be manipulated for the prize of power. Healers work incessantly against these forces, most often serving their communities and not their self-interest. Healers and those who seek power over people represent the fundamental tension of human life. Truth be told, both manipulate, but each works with different kinds of powers and toward radically different conclusions. The politician deploys the forces of deception and manipulation to accrue temporal power for use against other humans and with little regard for their ruin. Kofi Dɔnkɔ trained thousands of healers to understand the whole human being and what constitutes a whole human community. A healer such as Kofi Dɔnkɔ marshals the material and immaterial resources located in their ecology to restore health, repair relationships, and regenerate the self-healing capability that doggedly fights for balance within that fundamental tension. Disequilibrium is disease, and those who seek power over people thrive in diseased environments.

Most humans are politicians, with or without electoral aspirations, and so the healer fights protractedly against the politicians in us, the disease settings in which they thrive, working with forces that form the bookends of the human experience—physical forces and spiritual forces. These forces are no more than variations of the thematic interplay between energy and matter. The human being, and the world it inherits and shapes, is but a fusion of these basic root forces. Through the healer's optic, the individual and its community must work actively against the ever-present forces embodied by the politician in them. Kofi Dɔnkɔ sought to populate his world with healing and healthy people, in as much as modern societies seek to populate their roads with astute drivers to combat unsafe, intoxicated, or uninsured drivers who have a negative net effect on the disciplined, sober, and fully insured. In this metaphor, the healer promotes safe driving for all by populating the road with attentive and unimpaired drivers. The healer thus works on a logic akin to vaccination: if most people are protected against common diseases, their expansive web of immunity safeguards against those numerically few who are unprotected and thus dangerous to the community's welfare. A skilled and reputable healer such as Kofi Dɔnkɔ calibrated these forces to make a people whole, but perhaps the ills and socioeconomic forces running their course through the arteries of Takyiman and Ghana call for therapeutics beyond the capacity of one healer, however potent his cultural acumen.

I close with a big-picture, five-century view. Since the sixteenth-century global expansion of Western Europe, through which "European" colonialism was born and a white supremacist ideology became global, the Iberian leaders of this expansion built their colonial outposts and towns with a church at the center. This expansionism was also motivated by an unfinished Christian crusade. Other Europeans followed the Spanish and Portuguese overseas model for creating outposts-cum-colonies erected around ideologies of slavery, race, and variants of the Christian theology. Projecting from the church outward to the town's frontiers were the tripartite ideologies of race, religion, and slavery that structured colonial society and formed the platforms for global empires and their nation-state offspring. In the "colonial" Gold Coast, forced intimacy also inscribed those ideologies onto the tripartite colony: the Gold Coast Colony was viewed as a bastion of Christianity, mixed races, and antislavery; Asante, the "noble savages," insufficiently Christian (or Muslim) with forms of slavery; and the Northern Territories were populated by "backward tribes," relatively Islamic, and tolerant of slavery. Preceding and certainly outside of this colonial vision, the expansion of indigenous polities and empires centered on settlements ranging from modest villages to large towns, but settlements, regardless of size, erected around spiritual forces and a close-knit, temporal-spiritual understanding that formed the infrastructure of community life.

Emanating from those spiritual resources were thus transcendent values, ideologies of community bonds, and cultural codes that in their basic and idealized forms sought to balance fe/male leadership, valued community over self-interest, and offered an internalized sense of law and order. If we are to believe that British colonial success was achieved when it celebrated the undermining of "old religions" and "earlier disciplines" in 1948, then we might need to rethink the appointment of Nkrumah to head of government in 1951 and Britain granting the "model colony" independence in 1957. Here, once again, Kofi Dɔnkɔ and his community provide an alternative optic to reimagine the broader sweep of nineteenth- and twentieth-century histories, politics, and cultures under subjugation. Likewise, it is no more essentialist for scholars to keep invoking Greek democracy or the age of revolutions without Haiti or US empire and neoliberalism, and to proffer their enduring relevance than for us to do the same for African ideas and institutions in order to heal a wounded world.

NOTES

INTRODUCTION

1. Robert S. Rattray, *Ashanti* (Oxford: Clarendon Press, 1923), 114.

2. My point is this: it is not difficult to write the history of a person or a people who have left a significant documentary record to follow; if this is true—and I think it is—then the challenge for scholars is to focus more on people like Kofi Dɔnkɔ who did *not* write about themselves nor had much written about them.

3. Beyond several articles and passing references in a few books, the only substantial study of Takyiman is Dennis M. Warren, *The Techiman-Bono of Ghana: An Ethnography of an Akan Society* (Dubuque, IA: Kendall/Hunt, 1975).

4. Among these archives, I discovered that the Salvation Army only began working on the Gold Coast and in Ghana in 1922, but worked there more earnestly from 1978, when Ghana became a separate "territory," to the present. The problem for researchers is that the Ghana territory has no archives, and whatever records are kept are sent to the International Heritage Centre on an ad hoc basis.

5. The Akan/Twi language is a composite, rather than a singular, language, where four mutually intelligible variants—Bono, Asante, Akuapem, and Fante—make up the whole. Linguists have shown that a close synergy exists between the Bono and Fante variants, and those fluent in Fante have noted "the Brongs [Bono] are identical in language with Ashanti [Asante]" (TNA, CO 879/39, enclosure 1 in no. 45, Mr. Ferguson to the Acting Governor, 9 November 1893, 77). Assuming this is true, compare the following sentences in Asante, Akuapem, and Fante: Asante: *ɔbaa panin bi ne ne mmabarima baanu tenaa ase.* / Akuapem: *ɔbaa panyin bi ne ne mmabarima baanu traa ase.* / Fante: *ɔbaapanyin bi na ne mba mbarimba beenu bi tsenaa ase.* See S. K. Otoo and A. C. Denteh, *Abɔe* (Accra: Bureau of Ghana Languages, 1970), 7, 9; Ahene-Affoh, *Twi Kasakoa ne Kasatɔmmɛ s*(Tema: Ghana Publishing, 1976), v.

6. My grasp of the Akan/Twi language, especially its idiomatic phrases, has been influenced by the following texts: S. J. Kwaffo, *Fa bi Sie* (Accra: Bureau of Ghana Languages, 1997); Ahene-Affoh, *Twi Kasakoa ne Kasatɔmmɛ*; Kwabena Adi, *Mewɔ bi ka* (Accra: Bureau of Ghana Languages, 1975); Kwame Ampene, *Atetesɛm* (Accra: Waterville Publishing House, 1975); J. Yedu Bannerman, *Mfantse Akan Mbɛbusɛm* (Accra: Bureau of Ghana Languages, 1974); Ɔbɔadum Kisi, *Ɔba Nyansafoɔ* (Accra: Bureau of Ghana Languages, 1974); Ahene-Affoh, *Ɔdɔ Asaawa* (Accra: Bureau of Ghana Languages, 1973); J. Yɛboa-Dankwa, *Tete wɔ bi Kyerɛ* (Accra: Bureau of Ghana Languages, 1973); J. H. Kwabena Nketia, *Akwansosɛm bi* (Legon: Institute of African Studies, University of Ghana, 1967); J. E. Mensah, *Asantesɛm ne Mmɛbusɛm bi* (Kumasi: Author, 1966); J. Kwasi Brantuo, *Asetena mu Anwonsɛm* (Accra: Bureau of Ghana Languages, 1966); Ofei-Ayisi, *Twi Mmebusɛm wɔ Akuapem Twi mu* (Accra: Waterville Publishing House, 1966); Thomas Yao Kani, *Akanfoɔ Amammerɛ* (Accra: Bureau of Ghana Languages, 1962); Thoma Tao Kani, *Bansofo Akan Kasa mu Kasapo* (New York: Longmans, Green, 1953); Isaac D. Riverson, *Songs of the Akan Peoples* (Cape Coast, Ghana: Methodist Book Depot, 1939).

7. T. C. McCaskie, in his study of an Asante village, found "the transit from the precolonial to colonial was not a rupture with the past but a metamorphosis from it." That a prominent European/white historian did not abandon either "pre-colonial" or "colonial" trademarks—with their domineering hold on the chronology of African history—shows how entrenched both have remained, although the point about "rupture" is clear. See McCaskie, *Asante Identities: History and Modernity in an African Village, 1850–1950* (Edinburgh: Edinburgh University Press, 2000), 115.

8. On the Akan *adaduanan* calender system, see Kwasi Konadu, "The Calendrical Factor in Akan History," *International Journal of African Historical Studies* 45, no. 2 (2012): 217–46.

9. See R. Bagulo Bening, "Internal Colonial Boundary Problems of the Gold Coast, 1907–1951," *International Journal of African Historical Studies* 17, no. 1 (1984): 81–99.

CHAPTER 1. **LIBATION**

1. Richard C. Temple, "'Tout Savoir, Tout Pardonner.' An Appeal for an Imperial School of Applied Anthropology," *Man* 21, no. 10 (1921): 150–51; Robert S. Rattray, *Ashanti* (New York: Clarendon Press, 1923), 5; Ernest H. Starling, "The Report of the Royal Commission on University Education in London," *British Medical Journal* 1, no. 2735 (1913): 1168–72.

2. Temple, "Tout Savoir," 150; Rattray, *Ashanti*, 5.

3. Rattray, *Ashanti*, 5–6; Noel Machin, *"Government Anthropologist": A Life of R. S. Rattray* (Canterbury: Centre for Social Anthropology and Computing, University of Kent, 1998), 23–28, 34–36.

4. Machin, *Rattray*, 36.

5. Rattray, *Ashanti*, 8, 10; Machin, *Rattray*, 36, 89. See also Raymond Silverman, "Historical Dimensions of Tano Worship among the Asante and Bono," in *The Golden Stool: Studies of the Asante Center and Periphery*, ed. E. Schildkrout (New York: American Museum of Natural History, 1987), 272–88.

6. Machin, *Rattray*, 90, 92. The ɔkɔmfoɔ belongs to one category of healers. They can be described as spiritualist-healers. This category and others are discussed later in the chapter.

7. Rattray, *Ashanti*, 12.

8. Rattray, *Ashanti*, 12.

9. Basal Mission Archives (hereafter BMA), E-10-34-36, *Heidnische Gebete und darin enthaltene Spuren einer reineren monotheistischen Gotteserkenntnis* ("Traditional prayers and traces contained within them of a purer monotheistic recognition of God"), n.d. (probably early 1900s), 3. My translation of this record's title differs slightly from that found in Paul Jenkins, et al., *Guide to the Basel Mission's Ghana Archives*, 3rd ed. (Leipzig, Germany: Institut für Afrikanistik, Universität Leipzig, 2003), 76. On the BM in the nineteenth century see Seth Quartey, *Missionary Practices on the Gold Coast, 1832–1895: Discourse, Gaze, and Gender in the Basel Mission in Pre-Colonial West Africa* (Youngstown, NY: Cambria Press, 2007); Jon Miller, *Missionary Zeal and Institutional Control: Organizational Contradictions in the Basel Mission on the Gold Coast, 1828–1917* (Grand Rapids, MI: W. B. Eerdmans, 2003); Peter A. Schweizer, *Survivors on the Gold Coast: The Basel Missionaries in Colonial Ghana* (Accra: Smartline Limited, 2000).

10. Rattray, *Ashanti*, 54.

11. Rattray, *Ashanti*, 86.

12. Rattray, *Ashanti*, 86. Although Rattray held this view, which is accurate, he did not waiver from the "greater, because higher, ethical teachings of Christian theology" (87).

13. Rattray, *Ashanti*, 89–90.

14. Rattray, *Ashanti*, 90.

15. For a fuller account of Rattray see Theodore H. von Laue, "Anthropology and Power: R. S. Rattray among the Ashanti," *African Affairs* 75, no. 298 (1976): 33–54; T. C. McCaskie, "R. S. Rattray and the Construction of Asante History: An Appraisal," *History in Africa* 10 (1983): 187–206.

16. Interview with N. Kofi Donkor, Techiman, 20 April 1980, conducted by Raymond Silverman. I am grateful to Dr. Raymond Silverman for a typeset copy of this interview.

17. BMA, E-10-34-36, 11. See also A. A. Anti, *Obeedé* (Accra: Bureau of Ghana Languages, 1969), a novel that uses main character Kwabena Boakye, a hunter who falls into a coma and finds himself in the spirit world, to explore Akan ideas and beliefs about humans and their relation to spiritual forces and the world of ancestry.

18. For further explanations see Johann Gottlieb Christaller, *A Dictionary of the Asante and Fante Language Called Tshi (Chwee, Twi): With a Grammatical Introduction and Appendices on the Geography of the Gold Coast and Other Subjects* (Basel, Switzerland: Evangelical Missionary Society, 1881), 407–8.

19. These spirits are treated with such seriousness that the ubiquitous carved wooden stools in Akan societies are tilted to the side when not in use to prevent stray asamanbɔne or ɔtɔfo from sitting on them. Should a human sit on one before either ancestral type of spirit can escape, it is believed that person may contract pains at the waist and in the lower back (*sisi yareɛ*). Basel missionaries recorded from their informants that "Persons who committed suicide, women [who died] in childbirth, those

who died in battle [and] those who were killed through a hunting accident ... are to be buried on the high road, close to the path, so that their harmful influence is divided among all passers-by." See BMA, D-10-2-6, *Gottesnamen der Twi-Neger der Goldküste* ("Names for God of the Twi Blacks of the Gold Coast"), n.d. (probably 1920s), 11. For a counterview on humans returning to earth after death see BMA, E-10-34-36, 12, where a group of interviewed healers claimed, "When a human being dies, he or she goes to Onyame and does not return." They are partially correct in that part of the human being—the *okra* ("soul")—does not return, but other constituent parts, such as *sunsum* ("spirit"), do.

20. There seems to be several ways to reach asamandɔ. Crossing water by way of boat or raft is just one. On this see, for instance, Willem Bosman, *Nauwkeurige beschryving van de Guinese Goud- Tand- en Slave-kust*... (Utrecht: Anthony Schouten, 1704), 146 (English-spreaking readers can consult Bosman's *A New and Accurate Description of the Coast of Guinea* [London: J. Knapton, 1705], but with caution and corrections by Albert van Dantzig, "Willem Bosman's 'New and Accurate Description of the Coast of Guinea': How Accurate Is It?" *History in Africa* 1 (1974): 101–8, and subsequent issues); William Smith, *A New Voyage to Guinea* (London: J. Nourse, 1745), 214 (but Smith plagiarized Bosman, so readers should also consult H. M. Feinberg, "An Eighteenth-Century Case of Plagiarism: William Smith's 'A New Voyage to Guinea,'" *History in Africa* 6 [1979]: 45–50). In the 1920s Basel missionaries noted that the spirit of the departed had "to cross a mountain in the hereafter" (BMA, D-10-2-6, 11), or said another way, "the spirit [of a person] has to climb a steep hill on his way to the underworld" (BMA, E-10-34-36, 7). Takyiman oral histories collected in 1945 indicate when a person dies, they must "climb a hill" to get to asamandoɔ wherein a ladder is used. See the Public Records and Archives Administration Department of Ghana, Sunyani, Brong-Ahafo Regional Archives, 9/1/16 "Questions answered by the elders of Takyiman" [marked confidential], 17–20 December 1945, 2.

21. In their understanding of that life cycle, Basel missionaries wrote, "Childlessness is feared, because then no one is there to care for the obligatory ceremony at death." See BMA, D-10-2-6, 11.

22. Rattray, *Ashanti*, 96. See also T. C. McCaskie, *State and Society in Pre-colonial Asante* (New York: Cambridge University Press, 2003), 152; T. C. McCaskie, "Time and the Calendar in Nineteenth-Century Asante: An Exploratory Essay," *History in Africa* 7 (1980): 179–200.

23. Rattray, *Ashanti*, 114–18. On adae and other related ceremonies, see J. Yɛboa-Dankwa, *Tete wɔ bi kyerɛ* (Accra: Bureau of Ghana Languages, 1973), 43–46. The Pitt Rivers Museum at the University of Oxford has preserved a video of an adae ceremony Rattray recorded in the 1920s. Interested readers should consult the following link to the video: https://vimeo.com/100707923/.

24. BMA, E-10-34-36, 9.

25. BMA, E-10-34-36, 11.

26. BMA, D-10-2-6, 12.

27. See under the heading of "Education" the following consolidated colonial reports, *Colonial Reports—Annual. Nos. 360, 344, 375, 397, 426, 465, 488, 534, 573, 613, 654, 688, 725,*

770, 806. *Gold Coast. Report for 1899–1913* (London: Her Majesty's Stationery Office, 1895–1914).

28. BMA, E-10-34-36, 1.

29. Rattray, *Religion and Art in Ashanti* (London: Oxford University Press, 1927), 28, 31.

30. Rattray, *Religion and Art in Ashanti*, 27. An attempt is made to ridicule these "superstitions" through the character of Kofi Brenya in B. O. Amoako's *Ɛnɛ nso bio* (Accra: Bureau of Ghana Languages, 1976).

31. For more on mmoatia and sasabonsam in the early twentieth century see Rattray, *Religion and Art in Ashanti*, 25–30. On life in the forest see A. A. Opoku, *Mo Ahenewa* (Accra: Bureau of Ghana Languages, 1975).

32. Owusu Brempong, "They Have Used a Broom to Sweep My Womb: The Concept of Witchcraft in Ghana," *Research Review* 12, nos. 1–2 (1996): 44. The blood and saliva of humans have "soul power," but the blood of "sacrificial animals [also] has soul power, therefore smearing it on [ritual] apparatuses, therefore dripping of it onto a stone [or other ritual object]." See BMA, D-10-2-6, 8.

33. A group of healers interviewed in the early twentieth century argued, "The witches and the wizards are god's creatures. They come as such from their mother's womb. Some of them have also purchased the art from their fellowmen in order to earn something. Perhaps they are selling amulets, which one wears on one's knees, but with this one does not kill human beings. Their task is that they feed themselves on a human being. They drink his or her entire blood. If they do this to you, it does not take long and you are losing weight, become feeble and die. . . . We have to procure medicine against them. We have to drink one part of it and rub the other portion into the pricked skin. If you did that and her mouth touches you, she gets stubby teeth and does not dare anymore to come at you. Likewise if you bathe yourself with medicine and put such medicine into your house, no witch can to come to you, if she sees you she flees from you." See BMA, E-10-34-36, 12.

34. Interview with Nana Kwasi Appiah, Takyiman township, 25 December 2001.

35. The ɔbosombrafoɔ (pl. abosommerafoɔ) functions much like the human ɔbrafoɔ ("one who subdues or forbids") in the sociopolitical order: the ɔbrafoɔ is part of the state leadership's security force and an enforcer of law rather than executioner (*adumfoɔ*), hence the law enforcement functions performed by the ɔbosombrafoɔ. Abosommerafoɔ were a community's immune system, fighting internal and external forces of chaos and fracture, and thus were housed in conical buildings on the outskirts of a town, stationed on their frontiers to secure borders and confront external threat—human and immaterial. The Tanɔ abosom have a mandate to maintain peace and prosperity. Those abosom associated with the Tanɔ River made brass vessels (*nyawa*; sg. *ayawa*), after an earlier use of clay vessels, their physical abode. The Tanɔ abosom were distinguished from the abosommerafoɔ and thus kept in different quarters with their own rituals, taboos, and sacrificial preferences. The physical shrine of the abosommerafoɔ was usually an oblong wood covered with the skin of a leopard or lion and red cloth, and their akɔmfoɔ decorated themselves with charcoal or red clay (symbols of seriousness and threat), whereas the Tanɔ abosom have a distinct preference for white (symbol of purity, wellness, and victory). The Bono have an indigenous

ɔbosombrafoɔ called *Boɔtwerewa Kwaku* ("the rock born on a Wednesday will catch you"). How this anomaly came to be is not clear. On the nyawa, see Raymond Silverman, "History, Art and Assimilation: The Impact of Islam on Akan Material Culture" (PhD diss., University of Washington, 1983), 219–20.

36. Owusu Brempong, email message to author, 30 September 2010.

37. Rattray, *Ashanti*, 140.

38. Rattray, *Ashanti*, 141, 144.

39. Rattray, *Ashanti*, 148. For continued use of the caricature "sky god" by scholars see, for instance, Walter C. Rucker, *Gold Coast Diasporas: Identity, Culture, and Power* (Bloomington: Indiana University Press, 2015), 28, 58, 85–88, 209, 231–32.

40. BMA, D-10-4-1, *Sagen der Akwapim-Neger über die Erschaffung der Welt, Entstehung der Fetische* ("Tales of the Akwapim Blacks about the creation of the world, the origin of the fetishes"), n.d. (probably 1850s, though there is a penciled-in note of receiving the document in "1932"), 1–2.

41. BMA, E-10-34-36, 8.

42. BMA, D-10-4-1, 3, 10.

43. BMA, E-10-34-36, 8. See also Otto Ampofo Boateng, *Songs for Infant Schools (Twi)* (London: Oxford University Press, 1948), 31; E. M. Adu Darka, *Akanfoɔ Anwonsɛm Bi* (Tema: Ghana Publishing, 1973), 9–10.

44. In lieu of transcripts in the indigenous language, we can be certain Akan/Twi speakers supplying the information would have use the words *som* ("to serve") rather than "worship," *abosom* ("that which serves an unlimited purpose") rather than "fetish," one or more honorific for a creative force rather than "God," *asase* ("under, under" = earth) rather than "Goddess of the earth," *ɛsoro* ("sky, north, above") rather than "heaven," and gender-neutral pronouns formed by adding a prefix to the stem, indicating he/she/it rather than strictly "him/his."

45. BMA, E-10-34-36, 10.

46. BMA, E-10-34-36, 10. For a list of "praise" and proverbial by-names for this creative force which missionaries called "God," see BMA, D-10-2-6, 1–3; Christaller, *Dictionary of the Asante and Fante*, 661 (and individual entries). Compare the short lists of the BM and Christaller's dictionary with the following sample of over a hundred praise names: Onyame ("the shining one"; der. *nyam*—to shine, splendor and brightness); Odomankoma ("the benefactor of multitudes"; *dom*—to give grace; to be a benefactor; *domankoma*—multitude); Ɔdomankoma ("the only giver of grace/favor"; cf. *wo nko ara na woma yɛn adom*, "it is only you who gives favor"); Onyankopɔn ("the only great shining one"; der. *nyam* + *ko*—alone + *pɔn*—to be great); Ɔtumfoɔ ("the powerful one"); Twe(re)duampɔn ("the tree which when leaned against does not break"); Bɔrebɔre Bɔadeɛ ("the creator of all things"); Ɔdɛɛfoɔ ("the owner of all things"); Tete Botan ("the ancient rock"); Bontantim ("the immovable rock"); Tetekwaframmoa ("the one who endures for all time"); Brɛkyirihunuadeɛ ("the one who sees/knows all"); Totrobonsu ("the one who causes the rains to fall plentifully"); Abɔmmubuwafrɛ ("the one called upon in times of distress"); Amosu ("the giver of rain"); Amowia ("the giver of sunlight"); Ɔkumkɔm ("the dispeller of hunger"); Ɔkoforoboɔ ("the one who traverses great mountains during time of war"); Ɔkotwareasuo ("the one who crosses

great rivers during time of war"); Okumaniniampɔn ("the one who slays the ancient python"); and Ananse Kokroko ("the great spider"). I am grateful to Dr. Ọbádélé Kambon, who kindly shared a much longer list with me.

47. BMA, E-10-34-36, 14–15.

48. BMA, D-10-2-6, 1. I have removed the numbering from the list of sixteen items to provide for a smooth read.

49. *Colonial Report—Annual. No. 397. Gold Coast. Report for 1902* (London: Her Majesty's Stationery Office, 1903), 62.

50. BMA, E-10-34-36, 14.

51. BMA, D-10-4-1, 10.

52. Dennis M. Warren and K. Owusu Brempong, *Techiman Traditional State, Pt. II* (Legon: Institute of African Studies, University of Ghana, 1971), 87.

53. I am unsure of the origins or precise location of Mirikisi, but Boɔmuhene ("ruler inside the rock") is a recent manifestation, having revealed itself from a small lake around 1950 at Old Jama. It is an ɔbosombrafoɔ known for catching abayifoɔ and curing (unnamed) diseases, but its physical shrine is kept in an oblong leather case. Incidentally, Taa Kora is also known by the praise name "Oboɔmuhene," but this seems a generic rather than a specific honorific. See Dennis M. Warren and K. O. Brempong, *Ghanaian Oral Histories: The Religious Shrines of Techiman Traditional State* (Ames: Iowa State University Research Foundation, 1988), 3; Rattray, *Ashanti*, 183, 185–86.

54. See also T. C. McCaskie, *Asante Identities: History and Modernity in an African Village 1850–1950* (Bloomington: Indiana University Press, 2000), 83.

55. BMA, D-10-4-3a, *Der Cultus der Bewohner der Goldküste West-Afrika* ("Description of the Cults of the inhabitants of the Gold Coast, West Africa), n.d. (probably 1850), 4.

56. BMA, E-10-34-36, 14–15.

57. Rattray, *Ashanti*, 145.

58. Rattray, *Ashanti*, 145–46. I have converted the four rows on which each term was placed into one sentence and replaced the period after each with a comma. The meaning remains the same. Several odes to Tanɔ exist in the form of drum texts called *ayan*. See J. H. Kwabena Nketia, *Ayan* (Tema: Ghana Publishing, 1974), 54–55, 95–96.

59. Rattray, *Ashanti*, 146.

60. Rattray, *Ashanti*, 172. The ɔkɔmfoɔ or ɔbosomfoɔ for Taa Kora, on Rattray's 1922 visit, called Taa Kora "Odomankoma obosom," which Rattray translated as "Creator's god [=ɔbosom]." See Rattray, *Ashanti*, 178.

61. D. M. Warren and K. O. Brempong, *Techiman Traditional State, Pt. I* (Legon: Institute of African Studies, University of Ghana, 1971), 61.

62. Warren and Brempong, *Ghanaian Oral Histories*, 119.

63. The Tanɔ River measures some 249 miles from its source to the sea, whereas the Bea/Bia River measures some 186 miles. Although Bea/Bia originates in the Bono region, southwest of Takyiman, it meanders through present-day Ivory Coast before it and the Tanɔ River meet at the Aby lagoon. The Tanɔ River then enters the Atlantic

Ocean. As for Tanɔ's relation with the Bosomtwe rock and the lake of the same name, a large natural lake southeast of Kumase, see Rattray, *Ashanti*, 195–96.

64. See Rattray, *Ashanti*, 161; Warren and Brempong, *Techiman Traditional State*, Pt. II, 57, 61. On ɔbosompo see the Fante language text by J. A. Annobil, *Nana Bosompo* (Cape Coast: Methodist Book Depot, 1947).

65. Rattray, *Ashanti*, 161; A. A. Opoku, *Obi Kyerɛ* (Tema: Ghana Publishing, 1973), 74. On Rattray's trip to Tanɔboase and his visit to Taa Kora's bosomfie see Rattray, *Ashanti*, 172–202. The ɔkyeame (pl. *akyeame*) is a crucial diplomatic and communicative position within the sociopolitical structure of Akan societies. Measured by exceptional rhetorical competence, the ɔkyeame is the ruler's or leader's diplomat and orator. The ɔkyeame is also a master of Akan protocol, a walking encyclopedia of indigenous culture, and a communicative medium between the indigenous state leadership and their constituencies. See Kwesi Yankah, *Speaking for the Chief* (Bloomington: Indiana University Press, 1995); Safori Fianko, *Twifo Amammuisɛm* (London: Macmillan, 1958), 2.

66. Rattray, *Ashanti*, 200; Warren and Brempong, *Ghanaian Oral Histories*, 82; J. E. Mensah, *Asantesɛm ne Mmɛbusɛm bi* (Kumasi: Author, 1966), 32. According to Warren and Brempong, Asubɔnten Kwabena was also known by the praise name ɔ*kafena* ("when one troubles him, s/he suffers"). There are several other Asubɔnten. In addition to the ones at Kofi Dɔnkɔ's compound in Kɔmfokrom (Takyiman), Krobo, Timpanim, and Nkwaeso, others are found at Tuobodom for the Adontehene; in the Adaati stool room, taken from the Tanɔ River in Takyiman; and yet another pair of Asubɔnten, one at Mesedan/Besedan whose "father" is said to be Twumpuduo Kwadwo, and the second, whose "father" is said to be Akumsa, at the village of Akumsa Odumase in Nkoransa. In what seems like conflicting claims of "fatherhood," all rivers (at least the ones of importance) seem to fall under the "children" clause of Taa Kora. See Warren and Brempong, *Techiman Traditional State*, Pt. II, 45–47, 72, 102, 124.

67. BMA, E-10-34-36, 11. The term *master* was more than likely a translation of the Akan/Twi *owura*, which could mean "master" but also (land) "lord" and "owner." The context of the sentence suggests "landlord," in the sense that ancestors are custodians of the land and the abosom are forces of nature, hence "lords" or "owners" of lands to which humans hold not the deed but custodianship. Cf. Christaller, *Dictionary of the Asante and Fante*, 543.

68. Warren and Brempong, *Techiman Traditional State*, Pt. I, 94, 168; Warren and Brempong, *Techiman Traditional State*, Pt. II, 147.

69. The abosomma were, according to BM informants, "not created by God, but are, as their name says, children of the great fetishes [=abosompɔn]. While the former are invisible, the small fetishes [=abosomma] can appear, however not to everybody, but only to the priests, who own these fetishes and for the other priests of this second class of fetishes. The priests of this class are however no Asofo, but Akomfo, prophets. Despite the fact that the small fetishes are not created by God, but are rather children of the great fetishes, they are nevertheless sent by God to dwell among humans. They love to take up their residence in single large trees or they appear in small gleaming figures, but only to those who are already priests or priestesses or by those who they wish that

they would become their priests or priestesses by whom they then let themselves also be captured." See BMA, D-10-4-3a, 4–5.

70. BMA, D-10-4-3a, 1–2; BMA, D-10-4-1, 2.

71. BMA, D-10-4-3a, 2.

72. BMA, E-10-34-36, 7.

73. Basel missionaries claimed herbalists were "able to do magic and to soothsay. . . . They often have their amulet stuff in a gourd covered with a lid, they put this on their heads and thus let themselves receive an answer to the question." See BMA, D-10-2-6, 7.

74. BMA, E-10-34-36, 7.

75. Peter Ventevogel viewed bayi as an "evil spiritual power seen as material substance," which perverts the sunsum (spirit) of the conscious or unconscious host, transforming him or her into an ɔbayifoɔ. See Peter Ventevogel, *Whiteman's Things: Training and Detraining Healers in Ghana* (Amsterdam: Het Spinhuis, 1996), 14.

76. BMA, D-10-4-1, 15; D-10-2-6, 7. The agent-principal structure abounds in the political, social, and spiritual discourses of Akan societies, with "the use of an agent (instead of the principal) as the main focus of communication whether the principal is visible or unseen." It is from this perspective we might understand the interpretive relationship between an ɔkɔmfoɔ (agent) and an ɔbosom (principal). See Yankah, *Speaking for the Chief*, 13.

77. The ɔkɔmfoɔ can "see" and "hear" the articulations of their ɔbosom through divination. Male akɔmfoɔ did so by having a brass pan (*ayawa*) containing the masculine aspect of the ɔbosom placed on his head, on top of the *kahyire* pad made of medicines covered by *kente* cloth, whereas the feminine aspect, residing in a clay vessel (Asuo Yaa) on the floor of the bosomfie and filled with liquefied medicines, was worked by female akɔmfoɔ who stirred the contents with a ladle to "see" and "hear." Although male akɔmfoɔ can use the ayawa to divine and provide "revelations," most do not. This was reserved for the ɔbosomfoɔ.

78. When the ɔkɔmfoɔ enter spiritual communion with their ɔbosom, they first point to the sky to acknowledge Onyankopɔn, because the abosom are considered its akyeame. See Dennis M. Warren, "Disease, Medicine, and Religion among the Techiman-Bono of Ghana: A Study in Culture Change" (PhD diss., Indiana University, 1974), 56.

79. BMA, D-10-4-1, 15; D-10-4-3a, 3.

80. The abosomfoɔ do prophesize, but not by calling upon their ɔbosom and entering a trance-like state. Rather, they engage in such a state and in divination through the ayawa, but he must have the kahyire and the ayawa placed on his head—in that order—along with ritual paraphernalia affixed to the body and able shrine assistants, including the ɔkyeame that does the incantation to call the ɔbosom into the shared bodily space of the ɔbosomfoɔ. Through the ɔbosomfoɔ's muscular and nervous systems, the ɔbosom communicates with individual clients or the community.

81. BMA, D-10-4-1, 15; BMA D-10-4-3a, 3; BMA D-10-2-6, 6.

82. Kwaku Effah-Gyamfi, "Bono Manso Archaeological Research Project, 1973–1976," *West African Journal of Archeology* 9 (1979a): 173, 178; Kwaku Effah-Gyamfi, "Some Archeological Reflections on Akan Traditions of Origin," *West African Journal of Archeology* 9 (1979b): 192; Dennis M. Warren, *The Techiman-Bono of Ghana: An Ethnography of An Akan society* (Dubuque, IA: Kendall and Hunt, 1975), 2; Eva L. R. Meyerowitz,

"Bono-Mansu: The Earliest Centre of Civilisation in the Gold Coast," in *Proceedings of the Third International West African Conference, Ibadan, Nigeria, 1949* (Lagos: Nigerian Museum, 1956), 118.

83. Residents at Forikrom, an area just east of Takyiman on the Takyiman-Nkoransa road, claim the region was once thick forest. See Peter Easton, "From 'Sacrilege' to Sustainability: Reforestation and Organic Farming in Forikrom, Ghana," *IK Notes*, no. 4 (January 1999): 1.

84. Interview with Tanɔboasehene Nana Amisare Dwomo II, Tanɔboase, 12 October 1997, conducted by Kofi Sakyi Sapon.

85. On the ɛkoɔna clan see Cecilia Arthur, *Akanfoɔ Amammerɛ ho Adusua 1* (Kumasi: n.p., 2003), 5–7.

86. The hunter figure occupies a central place in the formation of settlements, not to mention their sustenance. For an excellent novel about the life and experiences of a hunter, crafted around the main character Kwasi Asiemiri and the plotline *abɔmmɔfo adwuma yɛ den* ("the work of hunters is hard/difficult"), see Edwin Efa, *Asiemiri* (London: Macmillan, 1950), 8 (quotation). J. H. Kwabena Nketia credited Efa as the first to write about the many ways of the hunter. For a rich corpus of hunters' songs, see J. H. Kwabena Nketia's *Abɔfodwom* (Tema: Ghana Publishing, 1973), v, 65–76.

87. Warren and Brempong, *Techiman Traditional State*, Pt. II, 122, 128.

88. Warren and Brempong, *Techiman Traditional State*, Pt. II, 139; T. E. Kyei, *Our Days Dwindle: Memories of My Childhood Days in Asante*, ed. and intro. Jean Allman (Portsmouth, NH: Heinemann, 2001), 37.

89. Warren and Brempong, *Ghanaian Oral Histories*, 56, 82. On the building on new settlements in Akan societies, along the lines of the discussion here, see B. S. Akuffo, *Tete Akorae* (Accra: Bureau of Ghana Languages, 1970), 7–22; A. A. Opoku, *Mpanyinsɛm* (Accra: Waterville Publishing House, 1969), 11–15; Bennett S. Akuffo, *Ahemfi Adesua (Akanfoɔ Amammerɛ)*, vol. 1 (Exeter, UK: James Townsend and Sons, 1950), 1–6.

90. Warren and Brempong, *Techiman Traditional State*, Pt. II, 34, 148.

91. Nana Akumfi Ameyaw recalled that Biakuru was located at Yɛfiri, and it was this ɔbosom that brought the people from Amowi. See Warren and Brempong, *Techiman Traditional State*, Pt. I, 94, 168.

92. Warren and Brempong, *Techiman Traditional State*, Pt. I, 28, 31, 33–34, 46, 57, 59–61, 80, 87, 98–99, 102, 132, 148, 160; Warren and Brempong, *Ghanaian Oral Histories*, 46, 102.

93. Kyei, *Our Days Dwindle*, 91, 93.

CHAPTER 2. **HOMELANDS**

1. Richard Freeman, *Travels and Life in Ashanti and Jaman* (New York: Frederick A. Stokes, 1898), 349.

2. Freeman, *Travels and Life*, 350.

3. Freeman, *Travels and Life*, 350–51, 353.

4. Public Records and Archives Administration Department of Ghana, Sunyani, Brong-Ahafo Regional Archives (hereafter BRG) 9/1/16, "Questions answered by the elders of Takyiman" [marked confidential], 17–20 December 1945, 2.

5. BRG 9/1/16, "Questions," 3. In most cases Asase Yaa is used for the earth, but in northern and some parts of southern Gold Coast/Ghana, the earth is also referred to as Asase Afua, though the same restrictions on farming apply to Asase, regardless of its natal day.

6. BRG 9/1/16, "Questions," 3.

7. BRG 1/12/122, Native Customary Law, 13 February 1961, 2, 10–11.

8. On early Bono history, language, and commerce, see Kwame Arhin, ed., *A Profile of Brong Kyempim: Essays on the Archaeology, History, Language and Politics of the Brong Peoples of Ghana* (Accra: Afram Publications and the Institute of African Studies, University of Ghana, 1979); Owusu Brempong, ed., *Oral Tradition in Ghana: The History of Bonokyempim and Techiman Politics* (Legon: Institute of African Studies, University of Ghana, 1998). More than two centuries later, Bono peoples remain acutely distrustful of those in power. Such flagrancies on the part of colonial and postcolonial officials led the Bono to refuse to pay taxes levied upon them (e.g., annual head tax and taxes on each palm tree cut, animal slaughtered, and load of cocoa, sand, or timber conveyed through Takyiman).

9. The recorded oral accounts of Baafo Pim's exploits and reward are well known. See John K. Fynn, *Asante and Its Neighbors, 1700–1807* (Evanston, IL: Northwestern University Press, 1971), 37; the National Archives of the UK, Colonial Office (CO) 879/39, enclosure 1, no. 45, Mr. Ferguson to the Acting Governor, 9 November 1893, 77; Kwame Arhin, ed., *The Papers of George Ekem Ferguson: A Fanti Official of the Government of the Gold Coast, 1890–1897* (Leiden, the Netherlands: Afrika-Studiecentrum, 1974), 35. For a little-known Twi language account see Immanuel A. Hanson, "Asantefo Atetesem Osantehene Poku Ware ne Takyimanhene Amo Yaw ntam' asem bi," *Christian Reporter for the Natives of the Gold Coast Speaking the Tshi or Asante Language* 1, no. 13 (January–March 1895): 101–16. See also H. M. J. Trutenau, "The 'Christian Messenger' and Its Successors: A Description of the First Three Series of a Missionary Periodical with Articles in Ghanaian Languages," *Mitteilungen der Basler Afrika Bibliographien* 9 (1973): 38–55.

10. Carl C. Reindorf, *The History of Gold Coast and Asante* (Basel, Switzerland: Author, 1895), 75; R. S. Rattray field notes, note block 10, "Obonus ceremony at Tekiman," Royal Anthropological Institute Library, London, MS 106, page 993. Takyiman leaders have for some time claimed that Asante literally stole, if not appropriated, many of their cultural forms, political institutions, and iconic material culture. They trace their heritage to the reign of specific Bono rulers. Bonohene Ati Kwame is credited with introducing the stool; Bonohene Boakye Tenten is credited with introducing the titles found in the Akan sociopolitical structure (e.g., Adontenhene, Nifahene, Benkumhene, Akwamuhene, Kyidomhene, Ankobeahene); and Bonohene Obunumankoma is credited with introducing the gold weights (*mmrammuo*) system, state treasury (*sanaa*), and gold dust (*sika*) as a currency that predated cowrie shells. At a time when only Takyiman and Banda engaged in cloth weaving, the Bono ancestors wore a tree-fibered cloth called *kyɛnkyɛn*, resembling an old indigenous cloth called *gagawuga*.

11. One-third of the tolls, which went to the Asante National Fund, were collected from the nine villages and paid to Asante. These villages were not only related by language, histories, and cultural forms but also by a string of related Tanɔ abosom. Using

familial language to talk about their relationships in human terms, the Bono view Taa Kora in Tanɔboase as "married" to Kranka Afua in Kranka. Their "offspring" included Twumpuduo Kwadwo at Tuobodom, Baafi Atiokosaa at Baafi, Taa Mensa Kwabena at Takyiman, and Taa Kwabena at Buoyem.

12. *Colonial Report—Annual. No. 189. Gold Coast. Report for 1895* (London: Her Majesty's Stationery Office, 1896), 7; Kwabena Adu-Boahen, "Pawn of Contesting Imperialists: Nkoransa in the Anglo-Asante Rivalry in Northwestern Ghana, 1874–1900," *Journal of Philosophy and Culture* 3, no. 2 (2006): 60, 62–63, 68–70, 73–75. Asante's economic interest in the Bono region should be understood as a prime engine of its political expansion and territorial control. Crucial to Asante interests were, for instance, the kola-producing areas of Ahafo; the Kintampo market north of Takyiman; the main route to markets in Salaga and Yendi for livestock, salt, and smelted iron; and the gold fields in western Bono territory once controlled by Manso.

13. D. J. E. Maier, "The Dente Oracle, the Bron Confederation, and Asante: Religion and the Politics of Secession," *Journal of African History* 22 (1981): 242–43. See also D. J. E. Maier, *Priests and Power: The Case of the Dente Shrine in Nineteenth-Century Ghana* (Bloomington: Indiana University Press, 1983).

14. Contemporary Gyaman is divided into two districts: one in the Ivory Coast at Bonduku and the other in the Brong-Ahafo region of Ghana at New Drobo.

15. Interview with Kofi Sakyi Sapɔn, Takyiman township, 22 December 2001.

16. CO 879/19, Further Correspondence Regarding Affairs of the Gold Coast, African (West) no. 249, June 1883, 131.

17. CO 879/19, Further Correspondence Regarding Affairs of the Gold Coast, African (West) no. 249, 12 May 1883, 140.

18. See for instance W. E. F. Ward, "Britain and Ashanti, 1874–1896," *Transactions of the Historical Society of Ghana* 15, no. 2 (1974): 131–64.

19. On apoɔ songs see Kwame Ntim-Yeboah, *Apoɔ Music* (an intensive practical work), Music Department, University of Cape Coast, Cape Coast, Ghana, May 1985, 11–13, 21; C. E. Donkoh, *Ghana Afahyɛ hodoɔ bi* (Accra: Bureau of Ghana Languages, 1969), 28–37.

20. CO 879/45, Correspondence [1896] Relative to Boundary Questions with France in the Bend of the Niger, African (West) no. 506, Gold Coast, February 1897, 277.

21. CO 879/45, Correspondence [1896] Relative to Boundary Questions with France in the Bend of the Niger, African (West) no. 506, Gold Coast, February 1897, 278.

22. CO 879/48, Further Correspondence Relative to Boundary Questions with France in the Bend of the Niger, African (West) no. 529, Gold Coast, letter dated 13 June 1897, Kumasi, 359; see also *Collection of Treaties with Native Chiefs, &c., in West Africa* (London: Colonial Office, 1914).

23. CO 879/48, letter dated 13 June 1897, Kumasi, 360.

24. CO 879/48, 361.

25. CO 879/48, 362. Signatories to the treaty included "King Kweku Yako represented by his nephew Kudjoe [Kwadwo] Konkroma of Tekiman."

26. *Colonial Report—Annual. No. 189*, 34. For context see Geoffrey Jones, *Merchants to Multinationals: British trading Companies in the Nineteenth and Twentieth Centuries* (New York: Oxford University Press, 2000); Charles Chapman, *Merchant Enterprise in*

Britain (Cambridge: Cambridge University Press, 1992); M. W. Kirby and M. B. Rose, eds., *Business Enterprise in Modern Britain from the Eighteenth to the Twentieth Centuries* (London: Routledge, 1994); William Woodruff, *The Rise of the British Rubber Industry during the Nineteenth Century* (Liverpool: Liverpool University Press, 1958).

27. CO 96/358/26, Further Correspondence Relating to Concessions and Railways: Rubber in Wenchi, Takyiman, and Nsoko, enclosure 2, no. 217, Mr. Beddington to Acting Colonial Secretary [C. Ridy Williams], 1900, 288.

28. CO 96/358/26, no. 227, Mr. Chamberlain to Governor Sir F. M. Hodgson, 18 April 1900, 297 (emphasis added).

29. Raymond E. Dumett, "The Campaign Against Malaria and the Expansion of Scientific Medical and Sanitary Services in British West Africa, 1898–1910," *African Historical Studies* 1, no. 2 (1968): 189.

30. G. B. Kay, ed., *The Political Economy of Colonialism in Ghana: A Collection of Documents and Statistics, 1900–1960* (New York: Cambridge University Press, 1972), 4–5.

31. Polly Hill, *Migrant Cocoa-Farmers of Southern Ghana: A Study in Rural Capitalism* (Cambridge: Cambridge University Press, 1963), 2–3. See also T. C. McCaskie, "Accumulation, Wealth and Belief in Asante History. I. To the Close of the Nineteenth Century," *Africa* 53, no. 1 (1983): 23–43; T. C. McCaskie, "Accumulation: Wealth and Belief in Asante History: II the Twentieth Century," *Africa* 56, no. 1 (1986): 3–23.

32. See Dumett, "Campaign Against Malaria"; Felix Ankomah Asante and Kwadwo Asenso-Okyere, "Economic Burden of Malaria in Ghana," a technical report submitted to the World Health Organization, African Regional Office, November 2003, 7–8.

33. *Colonial Report—Annual no. 189*, 27; *Colonial Report—Annual no. 220. Gold Coast. Report for 1896* (London: Her Majesty's Stationery Office, 1897), 20.

34. K. David Patterson, *Health in Colonial Ghana: Disease, Medicine, and Socio-Economic Change, 1900–1955* (Waltham, MA: Crossroads Press, 1981), 103.

35. The Gold Coast government in 1947 established the Cocoa Marketing Board, which determined the optimal conditions for producers, fixed prices locally and for distribution to the world market, and appointed agents who bought cocoa from farmers on behalf of the board. The board was or currently is the only authority to market cocoa outside of Ghana, and the Kwahuhene is the head of the board.

36. See Peter Ventevogel, *Whiteman's Things: Training and Detraining Healers in Ghana* (Amsterdam: Het Spinhuis, 1996).

37. Patterson, *Health in Colonial Ghana*, 1–4.

38. *Colonial Report—Annual. No. 573. Gold Coast. Report for 1907* (London: Her Majesty's Stationery Office, 1908), 45.

39. A. W. Cardinal, *The Gold Coast, 1931* (Accra: Government Printer, 1931), 201.

40. On the war and the person for whom it was named see A. Adu Boahen, *Yaa Asantewaa and the Asante-British War of 1900–1* (Accra: Sub-Saharan Publishers, 2003); Ivor Wilks, "Asante at the End of the Nineteenth Century: Setting the Record Straight," in *Akan Peoples in Africa and the Diaspora: A Historical Reader*, ed. Kwasi Konadu (Princeton, NJ: Markus Weiner), 168–209.

41. Yah Asantewa, letter to F. Hodgson, 19 April 1900, Ejesu [Edweso], MSS Afr. s. 1204(2), Bodleian Library of Commonwealth and African Studies at Rhodes House

(Weston Library), Oxford University, ff. 6–8. See also T. C. McCaskie, "The Life and Afterlife of Yaa Asantewaa," *Africa* 77, no. 2 (2007): 151–79.

42. David Boyle, letter to M. Perham, 10 July 1968, Ayrshire, MSS Afr. s. 1204(1), Bodleian Library of Commonwealth and African Studies at Rhodes House (Weston Library), Oxford University, ff. 1–2. This letter was found sixty-eight years after the event in an old box of papers of colonial official David Boyle. The letter was delivered to Boyle through the British resident in Kumase.

43. Jacob Simons, son of an Elmina woman and a Dutch official, was fluent in Akan/Twi and on behalf of the Dutch was dispatched on a special mission to Kumase in 1831–32. He must have heard some of these discussions in the reign of Yaw Akoto. See "Journal of Jacob Simons (1831–32)," archived at the Algemeen Rijksarchief, the Hague, Archive of the Ministry of Colonies 1813–1850, and translated by Larry Yarak as an unpublished manuscript in 1985.

44. CO 879/67, Correspondence (January 1901 to February 1902) Relating to Administration of Ashanti and the Northern Territories, enclosure 2, no. 5, Gold Coast, 4 December 1900, Kumasi, 8.

45. For more on Asante in the moment see Wilks, "Asante at the End of the Nineteenth Century," 168–209; Ivor Wilks, *Asante in the Nineteenth Century: The Structure and Evolution of a Political Order* (New York: Cambridge University Press, 1975 [1989]); Emmanuel Akyeampong, "Asante at the Turn of the Twentieth Century," *Ghana Studies* 3 (2000): 3–12; T. C. McCaskie, "The Golden Stool at the End of the Nineteenth Century: Setting the Record Straight," *Ghana Studies* 3 (2000): 61–96.

46. CO 879/67, 49–50. Other lists indicated the value of the presents only £15 (see CO 879/67, Colonial Office to Crown Agents, 13 March 1901, 55).

47. E. G. Smith, *The Laws of Ashanti, British Sphere of Togoland and Northern Territories of the Gold Coast*, vol. 1 (London: Government Printer, 1928), 1–26.

48. T. E. Kyei, *Our Days Dwindle: Memories of My Childhood Days in Asante*, ed. and intro. Jean Allman (Portsmouth, NH: Heinemann, 2001), 14. Kyei's father, whom he refers to as Papa Nkɛtia, and a group of young men his age went rubber tapping in the Bono-Takyiman area sometime during the late nineteenth century.

49. Sickle cell anemia is a hereditary condition that causes respiratory and circulation problems through acute attacks of ill health and lethargy. The condition is typically diagnosed during childhood and can be life threatening and inhibit the ability of the person to live a normal life. On this condition and the formation of Akan cultural forms in the forest see Kwasi Konadu, *The Akan Diaspora in the Americas* (New York: Oxford University Press, 2010), 37–40; Kwasi Konadu, *Akan Pioneers: African Histories, Diasporic Experiences* (New York: Diasporic Africa Press, 2018), 37–40.

50. T. E. Kyei, *Marriage and Divorce Among the Asante: A Study Undertaken in the Course of the Ashanti Social Survey (1945)* (Cambridge: African Studies Centre, 1992), 9.

51. Colonists noted, with some satisfaction, "that segregation is of the greatest efficacy in preventing the spread of malaria is now generally admitted." See *Colonial Report—Annual. No. 426. Gold Coast. Report for 1903* (London: Her Majesty's Stationery Office, 1904), 35.

52. Kwame Arhin, "Aspects of Colonial District Administration: The Case of the Northwestern District of Ashanti, 1904–1911," *Research Review* 8, no. 1 (1971): 7; *Colonial Report—Annual. No. 465. Gold Coast. Report for 1904* (London: Her Majesty's Stationery Office, 1905), 37.

53. Arhin, "Aspects of Colonial District Administration," 8, 24.

54. Francis Fuller, *A Vanished Dynasty: Ashanti* (London: J. Murray, 1921), 221–22; Basel Mission Archives (BMA), D-10-2-6, *Gottesnamen der Twi-Neger der Goldküste* ("Names for God of the Twi Blacks of the Gold Coast"), n.d. (probably 1920s), p. 4. Ongoing reappearances of Aberewa were suspected in the 1920s and beyond. See for instance BRG 28/2/7, J. W. Judd, district commissioner, Goaso, to District Commissioner, Sunyani, 12 May 1924 and 8 June 1925.

55. Jeff D. Grischow, "Tsetse and Trypanosomiasis in the Gold Coast, 1924–1954," Working Papers on Ghana: Historical and Contemporary Studies, Institute of Asian and African Studies, University of Helsinki, no. 5, 2004, 4–5.

56. *Colonial Report—Annual. No. 725. Gold Coast Report for 1911* (London: Her Majesty's Stationery Office, 1912), 14–15. Colonial officials noted, "Agriculture is the staple industry of the interior," and the cocoa "industry is almost entirely in the hands of native farmers" (18).

57. *Colonial Report—Annual. No. 725*, 28, 32. But the colonists praised themselves for "the success with which outbreaks of disease have been eradicated" (46).

58. CO 885/23/14, Correspondence (1914–15) Relating to Tropical Diseases and the Tropical Diseases Bureau, March 1914, 14.

59. CO 885/23/14, 14.

60. CO 885/23/14, 16–17.

61. For an early study on the zongos in the Gold Coast/Ghana see Enid Schildkrout, *People of the Zongo: The Transformation of Ethnic Identities in Ghana* (New York: Cambridge University Press, 1978).

62. Schildkrout, *People of the Zongo*, 21.

63. Schildkrout, *People of the Zongo*, 15.

64. BRG 28/1/8, Records of the Western Provincial Commissioner Ashanti, Native Jurisdiction Bye Laws—Cocoa Tribute, 1924–26, 15 June 1926, 1–2.

65. CO 885/23/14, 22.

66. On the clan system and aduana specifically see Cecilia Arthur, *Akanfoɔ Amammerɛ ho Adusua 1* (Kumasi: n.p., 2003), 1–7; Opoku, *Obi Kyerɛ*, 9–10, 13–15.

67. Kyei, *Our Days Dwindle*, 194; A. A. Opoku, *Obi Kyerɛ* (Tema: Ghana Publishing, 1973), 75; E. R. Addow, *Edin ne Mmrane* (Accra: Bureau of Ghana Languages, 1969), 46 ("Dɔnkɔ"), 70 ("Sakyi").

68. Basel missionaries also observed, "Such a child is called 'Blgyinaba'—'Come-and-stay-child.' Its hair is not cut and it wears all kinds of amulets in its curls. At the birth of the third, sixth or ninth child—those are lucky children—one takes some of their head hair 'spirit hair' and puts it into a special pot, the Abammo pot, which is now the place of veneration of the child's protecting deity. Of two precious pearls, one is put into the pot, the other one is affixed to the child's hair. If the child gets its hair cut, one part of it is being put into the Abammo pot. If the child dies the Abammo pot is

put into its grave with it." See BMA, E-10-34-36, *Heidnische Gebete und darin enthaltene Spuren einer reineren monotheistischen Gotteserkenntnis* ("Traditional prayers and traces contained within them of a purer monotheistic recognition of God"), n.d. (probably early 1900s), 3. See also Kyei, *Marriage and Divorce*, 139; J. E. Mensah, *Asantesɛm ne Mmɛbusɛm bi* (Kumasi: Author, 1966), 33.

69. On pregnancy and the timing and rituals between pregnancies, the BM observed, "6 month[s] after the wedding the husband has to give his wife a white wrap-around cloth and gold jewelry. For this the wife brings her husband a white chicken and eggs. He carries these to the bedroom and turns to the family spirit with the words: 'Come and receive this chicken, so that your child in the womb of its mother will be born without damage.['] Then he cuts off the chicken's head and lets some of its blood drip on the ground. After the chicken has been sacrificed he takes an Adwira [*adwera*] leaf with salt in his mouth and says: 'Kus! Kus! Kus! [*kose, kose, kose*] Tweduampong Onyame, highest God, who human beings use as support and are not brought to shame, my protecting spirit, o my soul. let this child be born in peace.' This the husband says three times, then they eat a little of the roasted chicken. The wife wears thereby her white wrap-around cloth and the gold jewelry—these things one says belong to the child in her womb. The young woman always wears a head-scarf. If a person talks to a pregnant woman about her condition, this person is held responsible if a miscarriage occurs. The wife must now don amulets to protect herself and her child against magic and bad influence. The husband is not allowed to quarrel with her during this time and she is not allowed to look at anything ugly, but must always carry an Akuaba, a black Asante doll with a slender neck and beautiful head with her, then she will also receive such a child." See BMA, E-10-34-36, 1–2.

70. BMA, E-10-34-36, 2.

71. BMA, E-10-34-36, 2.

72. Addow, *Edin ne Mmrane*, 5–8; Safori Fianko, *Twifo Amammuisɛm* (London: Macmillan, 1958), 58–63; B. S. Akuffo, *Tete Akorae* (Accra: Bureau of Ghana Languages, 1970), 71–74.

73. BMA, E-10-34-36, 3.

74. BMA, E-10-34-36, 3. Basel missionaries observed, "If it is a boy it receives the name of the paternal grandfather. . . . The infant lies thereby in the lap of the grandfather. The grandfather spits into its mouth and says: 'Father Bosontwe, my daughter N.N. has born a child and brought it to me and I am calling it now by my name N.N. Let it grow and let it stay with me and have it give me something to eat.' Then he makes him a gift. With the saliva the grandfather has put into him something of the family spirit." See also Kofi Agyekum, "The Sociolinguistic of Akan Personal Names," *Nordic Journal of African Studies* 15, no. 2 (2006): 217; Opoku, *Obi Kyerɛ*, 26, 29; Thomas Yao Kani, *Akanfoɔ Amammerɛ* (Accra: Bureau of Ghana Languages, 1962), 54–65.

75. Arthur, *Akanfoɔ Amammerɛ ho Adusua* 1, 2.

76. On the ɔkra (soul) and other constituent parts of the human being, readers can consult A. B. Ellis, *The Tshi-Speaking Peoples of the Gold Coast of West Africa* (Chicago: Benin Press, 1887 [1964]); R. S. Rattray, *Ashanti* (Oxford: Clarendon Press, 1923); R. S. Rattray, *Religion and Art in Ashanti* (Oxford: Clarendon Press, 1927); Eva L. R. Meyero-

witz, *The Akan of Ghana: Their Ancient Beliefs* (London: Faber and Faber, 1958); M. J. Field, *Search for Security: An Ethno-Psychiatric Study of Rural Ghana* (London: Faber and Faber, 1960); W. E. Abraham, *The Mind of Africa* (Chicago: University of Chicago Press, 1962); Kofi Antubam, *Ghana's Heritage of Culture* (Leipzig: Koehler and Amelang, 1963); Joseph B. Danquah, *The Akan Doctrine of God: A Fragment of Gold Coast Ethics and Religion* (London: Cass, 1968); Dennis M. Warren, *The Akan of Ghana: An Overview of the Ethnographic Literature* (Accra: Pointer Limited, 1973); Peter Sarpong, *Ghana in Retrospect: Some Aspects of Ghanaian Culture* (Tema: Ghana Publishing, 1974); Kofi A. Opoku, *West African Traditional Religion* (Accra: FEP International, 1978); Kofi Appiah-Kubi, *Man Cures, God Heals: Religion and Medical Practice among the Akan of Ghana* (New York: Friendship Press, 1981); Kwame Gyekye, *An Essay on African Philosophical Thought: The Akan Conceptual Scheme* (Philadelphia: Temple University Press, 1995).

77. A person's purpose in life was clarified through a periodic "soul-washing" ritual (*kradware*), itself accompanied by restrictions such as no palm wine before sunset, all white dress and being smeared with white clay (*hyire*), abstinence from consuming certain foods and meats, and observance of the ɔbosom associated with one's day of birth. The kradware ritual rested on a covenant between a person and a multifarious cosmic force ratified during gestation. Hence *obi kra ne Onyankopɔn na obi nnyina hɔ* ("when one takes leave of Onyankopɔn, no one stands there") and *Onyame nkrabea nni kwatibea* ("the destiny Onyame [has for someone] is unavoidable"). One *chose* the destiny or purpose (hyɛbea) they wanted in temporal life. As such, that comic force in the form of Onyankopɔn or Onyame was not liable for the "destiny" one chose, though some claim it was possible to reverse it by appealing directly to Onyame. In any case one's hyɛbea is measured by an ethical ideal and existence that is called *abrabɔ* (*ɔbra*—attitude, way of life; *bɔ*—living, existence). See Anthony Ephirim-Donkor, *African Spirituality: On Becoming Ancestors* (Trenton, NJ: Africa World Press, 1997); Opoku, *Obi Kyerɛ*, 45–47.

78. In addition to interviews and conversations over the years, I have also consulted the following on the patrilineal lines: Agyekum, "Sociolinguistic of Akan Personal Names," 218; T. C. McCaskie, *State and Society in Pre-colonial Asante* (New York: Cambridge University Press, 2003), 170–72; Gerald Pescheux, *Le Royaume Asante (Ghana): Parenté, Pouvoir, Histoire, XVIIe-XXe siècles* (Paris: Karthala Editions, 2003), 293–98; A. Abu Boahen, E. Akyeampong, N. Lawler, T. C. McCaskie, and Ivor Wilks, *"The History of Ashanti Kings and the Whole Country Itself" and Other Writing by Otumfuo Nana Agyeman Prempeh I* (New York: Oxford University Press, 2003); Opoku, *Obi Kyerɛ*, 20–23, 26–30; B. S. Akuffo, *Tete Akorae* (Accra: Bureau of Ghana Languages, 1970), 71–74; Addow, *Edin ne Mmrane*, 6; Thomas Yao Kani, *Akanfoɔ Amammerɛ* (Accra: Bureau of Ghana Languages, 1962), 54–62.

79. For further details see Dennis M. Warren, *The Techiman-Bono of Ghana: An Ethnography of an Akan Society* (Dubuque, IA: Kendall/Hunt, 1975); Dennis M. Warren, "Disease, Medicine, and Religion among the Techiman-Bono of Ghana: A Study in Culture Change" (PhD diss., Indiana University, 1974).

80. Interview with Nana Akosua Antwiwaa, Akumsa Odumase, Nkoransa, 21 March 2012.

81. Okomfoo Adwoa Akumsaa, Techiman, 15 February 1970, OT-2529, tape 36, side 1, Ghana, Brong-Ahafo region, Techiman Traditional State, Bono-Akan, 1969–71 (sound recording), collected by Dennis Michael Warren and Owusu Brempong, accession number 720249-F, Archives of Traditional Music, Indiana University. This and other recordings from the collection were recorded in Bono/Twi.

82. Interview with Nana Kwaku Sakyi, Miami, Florida, 14 June 2012.

83. Okomfoo Adwoa Akumsaa, Techiman, 15 February 1970, OT-2529. Basel missionaries described Asuo Yaa, a consecrated vessel ("a pot") used for divination, this way: "If someone wants to ask one of those prophets (*priests*) about the future he has to bring him palm wine, rum or other alcoholic beverages, which the priest pours *out onto the ground* partially in front of the fetish or in a pot, which is filled with water, herbs and all kinds of things. With a wooden or an iron spoon, *which is in the pot*, the priest then stirs together all things which are in it and finally lifts at last *with the spoon* something out of it, be it a stone, a piece of iron, wood or medicinal barks, roots, herbs or leaves which are in it. From the object, which was taken out, he *then* pretends to be to be able to give people information about their future, which he then of course communicates." See BMA, D-10–4–3a, *Der Cultus der Bewohner der Goldküste West-Afrika* ("Description of the Cults of the inhabitants of the Gold Coast, West Africa), n.d. (probably 1850.), 6.

84. See BMA, D-5–9–1, *Chronicle of the Basel Mission Out-Station in Nkoransa, 1911–1920*. I am grateful to Anne Beutter for sharing her digitized copy.

85. Warren and Brempong have him being born in Takyiman, though our dates, always approximate, do agree for his year of birth. See Dennis M. Warren and K. Owusu Brempong, *Techiman Traditional State, Pt. II* (Legon, Ghana: Institute of African Studies, University of Ghana, 1971), 45–52.

86. Interview with Nana Akosua Antwiwaa, Akumsa Odumase, Nkoransa, 21 March 2012.

87. Interview with Ama Akomaa, Takyiman township, 22 September 2012.

88. *Colonial Reports—Annual. Nos. 189, 220, 249, 271, 306, 344, 375, 397, 426, 465, 488, 534, 573, 613, 654, 688, 725, 770, 806, 859, 894. Gold Coast. Reports for 1895–1915* (London: Her Majesty's Stationery Office, 1896–1916), 8–9 (1895), 25–27 (1896), 21–22 (1897), 18–19 (1898), 14–15 (1899), 17 (1900), 26 (1901), 42 (1902), 29–30 (1903), 24–25 (1904), 27 (1905), 28–30 (1906), 31–32 (1907), 32 (1908), 32 (1909), 24–25 (1910), 19 (1913), 28–29 (1914), 20 (1915). Until the early 2000s most of Ghana's citizens had little to any English language literacy. See Kwesi Yankah, *Language, the Mass Media and Democracy in Ghana* (Accra: Ghana Academy of Arts and Sciences, 2004), 6. J. Kwasi Brantuo offered a parody of this deficiency in *Asetena mu Anwonsem* (Accra: Bureau of Ghana Languages, 1966), 24.

89. *Colonial Report—Annual. No. 344. Gold Coast. Report for 1900* (London: Her Majesty's Stationery Office, 1901), 15.

90. *Colonial Report—Annual. No. 573*, 32; *Colonial Report—Annual. No. 613*, 32 (1909).

91. *Colonial Report—Annual. No. 306*, 22. But see also the "vital statistics" section of colonial reports 189–894, ca. 1896–1916. On "colonial medicine," see Reginald Cheverton papers, MSS. Afr. s. 2276, Bodleian Library of Commonwealth and African Studies at Rhodes House (Weston Library), Oxford University.

92. *Colonial Report—Annual. No. 271*, 31.

93. *Colonial Report—Annual. No. 573*, 45; David Scott, *Epidemic Disease in Ghana, 1901–1960* (New York: Oxford University Press, 1965), 2, 4, 74, 81, 128, 187–92; K. David Patterson, "The Influenza Epidemic of 1918–19 in the Gold Coast," *Journal of African History* 24 (1983): 485–502.

94. BRG 9/1/1, Letter from Commissioner of Western Province of Ashanti to the Omanhin of Tekiman, Sunyani, 9 May 1917.

95. Dennis M. Warren and K. Owusu Brempong, *Ghanaian Oral Histories: The Religious Shrines of Techiman Traditional State*, Anthropology Program at Iowa State University, Papers in Anthropology, no. 8 (Ames: Iowa State University Research Foundation, 1988), 2, but see also pages 4, 74, 81, 128.

96. Warren and Brempong, *Techiman Traditional State, Pt. II*, 59–60.

97. Colonial penetration and its transportation networks were also at the heart of spreading another, far more deadly disease in HIV/AIDS. See Craig Timberg and Daniel Halperin, *Tinderbox: How the West Sparked the AIDS Epidemic and How the World Can Finally Overcome* (New York: Penguin Press, 2012).

CHAPTER 3. **TOOLS OF THE TRADE**

1. Thora Williamson and A. H. M. Kirk-Greene, *Gold Coast Diaries: Chronicles of Political Officers in West Africa, 1900–1919* (London: Radcliffe Press, 2000), 128.

2. Williamson and Kirk-Greene, *Gold Coast Diaries*, 192, 195.

3. On health matters see K. David Patterson, *Health in Colonial Ghana: Disease, Medicine, and Socio-Economic Change, 1900–1955* (Waltham, MA: Crossroads Press, 1981); David Scott, *Epidemic Disease in Ghana, 1901–1960* (New York: Oxford University Press, 1965).

4. Basal Mission Archives (hereafter BMA), D-5-9-1, *Chronicle of the Basel Mission Outstation in Nkoransa, 1911–1920*, 1.

5. BMA, D-5-9-1, 3. The one hundred boys requested were reduced to twenty boys and ten girls.

6. BMA, D-5-9-1, 7, 10 (quotation), 12.

7. Anne Beutter, "Church Discipline Chronicled—A New Source for Basel Mission Historiography," *History in Africa* 42 (2015): 114–15; BMA D-5-9-1, 1. The writers of the entry in the Chronicle removed pages and crossed out "fetish" content. Carl Reindorf, in his well-known *History of the Gold Coast and Asante* (1895), also cleansed his oral accounts of "fetish" content. See Heinz Hauser-Renner, "Examining Text Sediments: Commending a Pioneer Historian as an 'African Herodotus': On the Making of the New Annotated Edition of C. C. Reindorf's 'History of the Gold Coast and Asante,'" *History in Africa* 35 (2008): 241fn35.

8. BMA, D-5-9-1, 13. See also Williamson and Kirk-Greene, *Gold Coast Diaries*, 182, on "chiefs" being lectured to send children to school. The Nkoransahene's name was phonetically written "Kojoe Fah," which in the Bono region would be Kwadwo Faa. If he was in the coastal Fante area, I might suggest Kojo or a variant thereof.

9. BMA, D-5-9-1, 27.

10. BMA, D-5-9-1, 14. The Nkoransahene's oath was ɔbɔɔkyi.

11. BMA, D-5-9-1, 18.

12. BMA, D-5-9-1, 19–20.

13. BMA, D-5-9-1, 22–23.

14. BMA, D-5-9-1, 20–21.

15. BMA, D-5-9-1, 17, 33–34. The two wives' names were written phonetically as "Yah Manu" and "Ammah Tehirewah."

16. BMA, D-5-9-1, 32, 34.

17. BMA, D-5-9-1, 39, 42–43, 45, 48, 50. *Kramoni* is an Akanized term for a Muslim person. The term is ultimately of Malinke origin, deriving from the Malinke term for Muslim, *karamoko* or *nkaramo*.

18. BMA, D-5-9-1, 30, 37–38 (quotation).

19. BMA, D-5-9-1, 35.

20. BMA, D-5-9-1, 53–55. The Akan/Twi phrase *woye apō papa ntrā me sre so nsām me* should be *wɔyɛ apoɔ papa ntira, me srɛ so nsam me* ("because they do good apoɔ, I request/beg you not scatter me"). I think the catechist wrote "me sre" (my thighs) when he should have written "mesrɛ" (I request/beg), and that he wrote "so" (on) in place of "wo" (you). In his rendering, the second clause, "my thighs don't scatter me," makes little sense and bears no resemblance to any idiomatic expression known to me.

21. BMA, D-5-9-1, 59–60.

22. BMA, D-5-9-1, 64, 72.

23. BMA, D-5-9-1, 78, 89; Beutter, "Church Discipline Chronicled," 118–19; *Colonial Reports—Annual. Nos. 948, 998, 1029. Gold Coast. Reports for 1916–18* (London: Her Majesty's Stationery Office, 1917–19), 32 (1916), 36 (1917), 37 (1918). The Ewe Mission was now the Ewe Presbyterian Church and had an unnumbered amount of schools, all in the Trans-Volta district (*Colonial Report—Annual. No. 1029, 27*).

24. BMA, D-5-9-1, 93, 99.

25. *Colonial Report—Annual. No. 1066. Gold Coast. Report for 1919* (London: Her Majesty's Stationery Office, 1920), 36. Achimota College held classes in "Twi, Fanti, and Ga," with "spoken English" in all classes; its largely European staff contrasted sharply with a mostly African staff in mission schools. See *Colonial Report—Annual. No. 1386. Gold Coast. Reports for 1926–27* (London: Her Majesty's Stationery Office, 1927), 40.

26. Cati Coe, "Educating an African Leadership: Achimota and the Teaching of African Culture in the Gold Coast," *Africa Today* 49, no. 3 (2002): 24, 28, 34; Cati Coe, *Dilemmas of Culture in African Schools: Youth, Nationalism, and the Transformation of Knowledge* (Chicago: University of Chicago Press, 2005); Apollos O. Nwauwa, *Imperialism, Academe and Nationalism: Britain and University Education for Africans 1860–1960* (New York: Routledge, 2013), 55–56. On the college during its formative years see the Papers of Reverend Charles Kingsley Williams, MSS. Brit. Emp. s. 282, Bodleian Library of Commonwealth and African Studies at Rhodes House (Weston Library), University of Oxford. Williams was assistant vice-principal between 1927 and 1938.

27. James T. Campbell, *Songs of Zion: The African Methodist Episcopal Church in the United States and South Africa* (New York: Oxford University Press, 1995), 312–13 (quotation); Kobina Sekyi, *The Blinkards, a Comedy: And, the Anglo-Fanti, a Short Story* (Oxford: Heinemann, 1997); Samuel Blankson, *Fetu Afahye* (Cape Coast: University

Press, 1973), 5; Black Women Oral History Project, Interviews, 24–25 May 1978, OH-31, T-32/Abna Aggrey Lancaster. Schlesinger Library, Radcliffe Institute, Harvard University, Cambridge, MA, 2, 8.

28. G. B. Kay, ed., *The Political Economy of Colonialism in Ghana: A Collection of Documents and Statistics, 1900–1960* (New York: Cambridge University Press, 1972), 33.

29. Kay, *Political Economy*, 48–49; *Colonial Report—Annual. No. 1119. Gold Coast. Report for 1920* (London: Her Majesty's Stationery Office, 1921), 6.

30. *Colonial Report—Annual. No. 1029*, 8; *Colonial Report—Annual. No. 1066*, 7. See also A. G. Johnson, "A Contrast between Gold Coast Colony in 1850 and the Present Day," 1934, MSS. Afr. s. 845, Bodleian Library of Commonwealth and African Studies at Rhodes House (Weston Library), Oxford University, 29.

31. Kay, *Political Economy*, 143.

32. M. J. Field, *Search for Security: An Ethno-Psychiatric Study of Rural Ghana* (London: Faber and Faber, 1960), 29, 32–33. One of the principal expenses for local peoples, with or without colonial rule, was funerals. In the late 1920s the colonial authorities and indigenous officeholders created bylaws to regulate the costs of funerals in Takyiman and throughout the colony, dividing those expenses into four classes on the basis of a sociopolitical hierarchy, each with expenditure limits—"paramount chief" (ɔmanhene), "divisional chiefs" (ahene), "other persons," and "labourers." See Public Records and Archives Administration Department of Ghana, Sunyani, Brong-Ahafo Regional Archives (hereafter BRG) 28/1/32, Techiman Division (Regulation) of Funeral Custom Bye-Laws, 1929, 27 July 1929. But see also correspondence between the colonial government and local officeholders in Kumase, as the latter proposed "bye-laws to regulate expenditures on spirits in connection with funeral customs" and to curb claims of "excessive consumption of liquor at funeral ceremonies." Acting Colonial Secretary to G. C. du Boulay, acting colonial secretary, Accra, to the Chief Clerk, Kumasi, 2 November 1928, 1; John Maxwell, chief commissioner, Kumasi, to the Colonial Secretary, Accra, 15 August 1928; Chief Clerk, Kumasi, to the District Commissioner, Kumasi, 11 July 1928.

33. Colonial officials reported, "A Research Specialist from the Rockefeller Institute . . . resided in the Gold Coast during the year for the purpose of undertaking research into the causes of Yellow Fever." *Colonial Report—Annual. No. 1386*, 35; George Washington Corner, *A History of the Rockefeller Institute, 1901–1953: Origins and Growth* (New York: Rockefeller University Press, 1965), 194. See also Hideyo Noguchi papers, Rockefeller Institute for Medical Research Scientific Staff, FA121 (formerly filed under 450 N689), the Rockefeller University Archives, Sleepy Hollow, New York.

34. *Colonial Report—Annual. No. 1386*, 48.

35. Field, *Search for Security*, 50; "The Tegare Fetish," in J. A. Cowley papers, MSS. Afr. s. 1051, Rhodes House Library, Oxford University, March 1949, f. 5.

36. Around the 1920s, Basel missionaries claimed the abosommerafoɔ Aberewa (in the "colony"), Katawere of Akyem, and Otutu and Odente of Akuapem were all "destroyed by the English government." See BMA, D-10-2-6, *Gottesnamen der Twi-Neger der Goldküste* ("Names for God of the Twi Blacks of the Gold Coast"), n.d. (probably 1920s), 4; See *Colonial Report—Annual. No. 688. Gold Coast. Report for 1910* (London: Her Majesty's Stationery Office, 1911), 43. Custom ordinances also prohibited "certain

kinds of fetish worship and empowers the Chief Commissioner to make rules for suppressing or regulating certain native customs." See *Colonial Report—Annual. No. 613. Gold Coast. Report for 1908* (London: Her Majesty's Stationery Office, 1909), 30.

37. On Hwemeso's suppression see the order enacted by chief commissioner C. H. Harper on 26 February 1923, and related correspondences in BRG 28/2/19. On similarities between Hwemeso and Tigare see Emmanuel Okru, *The Rules and Byelaws of Nana Tegare* (Koforidua, Ghana: Ahao Press, n.d.), 14. On Tigare see, for instance, BRG 28/2/7, "Tigari Fetish," Chief Commissioner, Kumasi, to Commissioner of the Western Province, Sunyani, 5 September 1931; BRG 2/1/3, Native Physicians and Fetishes, vol. 2, "The Tegare Fetish," by J. A. Cowley, 1949 (cf. same essay in J. A. Cowley papers, MSS. Afr. s. 1051); Hans W. Debrunner, *Witchcraft in Ghana: A Study on the Belief in Destructive Witches and Its Effect on the Akan Tribes* (Accra: Presbyterian Book Depot, 1961), 106–8.

38. BRG 28/2/7, Father A. Mouwsen, Roman Catholic mission in Kumasi, to the District Commissioner, Kumasi, 24 April 1928, 1–2.

39. BRG 28/2/7, "Kukuro Fetish: Answers to Mr. de Graft Johnson's Questionnaire," Acting District Commissioner, Wenchi, August 1931, 2, 5 (quotation), 9; "The Use of the Fetish Kukro," [Takyimanhene] Yaw Amiyaw, Tekiman, to District Commissioner, Kumasi, 25 May 1928; Ashanti Regional Archives 1/30/1/18, "Kukuro" by W. J. Pitt, n.d.

40. John Parker, "Witchcraft, Anti-Witchcraft and Trans-Regional Ritual Innovation in Early Colonial Ghana: Sakrabundi and Aberewa, 1889–1910," *Journal of African History* 45 (2004): 393–96, 418. Parker makes two claims—"*bayi* was perceived by the Akan peoples as a destructive force" and the asuman and "witch-catching gods" could be easily bought, sold, and transported along trade routes and across frontiers—that will be addressed in this book. For more on the spread of Tigare (known by slightly modified names), see Judy Rosenthal, *Possession, Ecstasy, and Law in Ewe Voodoo* (Charlottesville: University of Virginia Press, 1998), 77, 85–86; Afeosemime Unuose Adogame, Magnus Echtler, Ulf Vierke, eds., *Unpacking the New: Critical Perspectives on Cultural Syncretization in Africa and Beyond* (Zürich: LIT Verlag Münster, 2008), 210fn6; Jean Allman and John Parker, *Tongnaab: The History of a West African God* (Bloomington: Indiana University Press, 2005), 139–40; Steven M. Friedson, *Remains of Ritual: Northern Gods in a Southern Land* (Chicago: University of Chicago Press, 2010), 197fn25.

41. In the early 1970s Nana Ogbe Dado was the ɔkɔmfoɔ for Kalasi. Born in Kayigbi, Togo, to a mother named Adwoa and a father named Dado, Ogbe became the custodian for Kalasi, who has a festival every three years. Ogbe was then married to two wives named Adwoa and Amma, though both were from Togo. See Dennis M. Warren and K. Owusu Brempong, *Ghanaian Oral Histories: The Religious Shrines of Techiman Traditional State*, Papers in Anthropology, no. 8 (Ames: Anthropology Program at Iowa State University, 1988), 132.

42. BRG 28/1/31, "Strict Compliance with the 'Rules for Residents in Residential Areas of the Gold Coast,'" Accra, 24 October 1929, Colonial Secretary, 1; "Rules for Residents in Residential Areas of the Gold Coast," n.d.; "Anthrax in the Kintampo District," J. L. Stewart, veterinary officer, to District Commissioner, Kintampo, 8–14

June 1929, 1; "Anthrax in Kintampo," J. L. Stewart, veterinary officer, to District Commissioner, Kintampo, 20 May 1928, 1 (quotation); A. G. MacPherson, medical officer, to G. H. Gibss, district commissioner, Kintampo, 15 October 1928. See also Williamson and Kirk-Greene, *Gold Coast Diaries*.

43. CO 879/120/6, Further Correspondences Relating to Medical and Sanitary Matters in Tropical Africa, December 1921, 225.

44. CO 879/120/6, 226–27.

45. Kwasi Konadu, *Indigenous Medicine and Knowledge in African Society* (New York: Routledge, 2007), 55–56; Ivor Wilks, *Asante in the Nineteenth Century: The Structure and Evolution of a Political Order* (New York: Cambridge University Press, 1989), 519–21. See also William C. Olsen, "Healing, Personhood and Power: A History of Witch-Finding in Asante" (PhD diss., Michigan State University, 1998); and Natasha A. Gray, "The Legal History of Witchcraft in Colonial Ghana: Akyem Abuakwa, 1913–1943" (PhD diss., Columbia University, 2000).

46. A statue of Guggisburg still stands outside the hospital. See Jonathan Roberts, "Remembering Korle Bu Hospital: Biomedical Heritage and Colonial Nostalgia in the 'Golden Jubilee Souvenir,'" *History in Africa* 38 (2011): 194–95. As for hospitals, there was precedence. In 1885, BM physician Rudolf Fisch came to the Gold Coast to care for missionaries through a sanatorium and a "heathen" clinic for Africans in Aburi, which grew to a small hospital in the 1900s. The BM discussed the prospect of establishing a "medical mission," precisely in the hinterland and rural areas. On Fisch see Friedrich Hermann Fischer, *Der Missionsarzt Rudolf Fisch und die Anfänge medizinischer Arbeit der Basler Mission an der Goldküste* (Herzogenrath: Murken-Altrogge, 1991).

47. Public Records and Archives Administration Department of Ghana (PRAAD), Kumase, ARG 1/3/3/40, Ohene of Agogo to District Commissioner, Juaso, December 1927; BMA, D-4-2-1, Carl B. Huppenbauer, Annual Report [for] 1931/32, 1932; BMA, D-4-6-2, Huppenbauer vor Komitee, 14 February 1934. Besides funding, conflicts between "medical" and "mission" work, and antagonism between "medical doctors" and the "mission house" remained ongoing for the BM hospital in Agogo and related facilities in the colony. See PRAAD, Accra, CSO 11/1/677, 10 April 1930; CSO 11/1/679, 20 May 1935; CSO 11/1/679, 23 August 1938; CSO 11/1/677, 13 April 1939; CSO 11/1/677, 30 May 1939.

48. For some of the general outlines of training in the early twentieth century see Rattray, *Religion and Art in Ashanti* (London: Oxford University Press), 39–47; BMA, D-10-4-1, *Sagen der Akwapim-Neger über die Erschaffung der Welt, Entstehung der Fetische* ("Tales of the Akwapim Blacks about the creation of the world, the origin of the fetishes"), n.d. (probably 1850s, although there is a penciled note of receiving the document in "1932"), 15–18; BMA, D-10-4-3a, *Der Cultus der Bewohner der Goldküste West-Afrika* ("Description of the Cults of the inhabitants of the Gold Coast, West Africa"), n.d. (probably 1850), 3–4.

49. According to an interview with Warren and Brempong, Taa Kwasi ɔbosomfoɔ Kofi Kyerere became an ɔbosomfoɔ in 1928. But the audio recording by Warren and Brempong of the Kyereme interview, held at the Archives of Traditional Music at Indiana University, indicates that he was 46 years old at the time of the 1970 interview,

which places his birth in 1924. This birth year would make it impossible to train as an ɔbosomfoɔ at four years old. Kyereme was around the same age as Kofi Dɔnkɔ, and this would speculatively place Kyereme's year of birth between 1912 and 1914.

50. Bosomfoo Kofi Kyereme, Techiman, [date inaudible] September 1970, OT-2529, tape 23, side 2, Ghana, Brong-Ahafo region, Techiman Traditional State, Bono-Akan, 1969–71 (sound recording), collected by Dennis Michael Warren and Owusu Brempong, accession number 720249-F, Archives of Traditional Music, Indiana University.

51. Kyereme, Techiman, September 1970, OT-2529.

52. Dennis M. Warren and K. Owusu Brempong, *Techiman Traditional State, Pt. II* (Legon: Institute of African Studies, University of Ghana, 1971), 67–70; interview with Nana Akosua Antwiwaa, Akumsa Odumase, Nkoransa, 21 March 2012.

53. Interview with Nana Akosua Antwiwaa, Akumsa Odumase, Nkoransa, 21 March 2012; Johann G. Christaller, *A Dictionary of the Asante and Fante Language Called Tshi (Chwee, Twi): With a Grammatical Introduction and Appendices on the Geography of the Gold Coast and Other Subjects* (Basel, Switzerland: Evangelical Missionary Society, 1881), 244.

54. On bragorɔ see A. A. Opoku, *Obi Kyerɛ* (Tema: Ghana Publishing, 1973), 30–34; Thomas Yao Kani, *Akanfoɔ Amammerɛ* (Accra: Bureau of Ghana Languages, 1962), 47–54; J. Yɛboa-Dankwa, *Tete wɔ bi Kyerɛ* (Accra: Bureau of Ghana Languages, 1973), 102–11.

55. On the Akan brass and gold weights system see G. Niangoran-Bouah, *Akan World of Gold Weights*, 3 vols. [bilingual text] (Abidjan, Ivory Coast: Les Nouvelles Editions Africaines, 1984–88); Timothy Garrard, *Akan Weights and the Gold Trade* (London: Longman, 1980); Deborah R. Fink, "Time and Space Measurement of the Bono of Ghana" (master's thesis, Iowa State University, 1974), 41; Albert Ott, "Akan Gold Weights," *Transactions of the Historical Society of Ghana* 9 (1968): 37.

56. L. M. Pole, "Decline or Survival? Iron Production in West Africa from the Seventeenth to the Twentieth Century," *Journal of African History* 23 (1982): 506–7.

57. Paul Jenkins, "The Anglican Church in Ghana, 1905–24 (I)," *Transactions of the Historical Society of Ghana* 15, no. 1 (1974): 23; Harris W. Mobley, *The Ghanaian's Image of the Missionary: An Analysis of the Published Critiques of Christian Missionaries by Ghanaians, 1897–1965* (Leiden: Brill, 1970), 28–29. See also Vincent Carretta and Ty Reese, *The Life and Letters of Philip Quaque, the First African Anglican Missionary* (Athens: University of Georgia Press, 2010).

58. John S. Pobee, *The Anglican Story in Ghana: From Mission Beginnings to Province in Ghana* (Accra: Amanza Limited, 2009), 328–29, 331 (quotation).

59. CO 96/677/12, Murder of Omanhene of Tekiman, 1928.

60. BRG 28/2/45, L. H. Wheatley, acting provincial commissioner W.P.A., Chief Commissioner's Court of Ashanti, Sunyani, 9 April 1919. The men charged were Kweku Techei (Takyi), Yao Antuma (Ankasa?), Yao Wusu, Kwami Atoa (Atua), Kojo Fojo (Kwadwo Fodwo), and Kobina Wiaa (Kra?). Though not implicated in the 1919 plot, Abina Wura was one of the persons seeking to destool Yaw Kramo in 1927 and one associated with these young men.

61. Williamson and Kirk-Greene, *Gold Coast Diaries*, 182, 195.

62. BRG 28/2/3, F. W. Applegate, acting commissioner W.P.A., to District Commissioner, Wenchi, 13 January 1928; "the Tekiman Disturbances," G. E. C. Wisdom, assistant district commissioner, to E. A. Burner, Wenchi, 27 July 1927, 1 (quotation).

63. CO 96/677/12, 28 January 1928, 2.

64. BRG 28/1/23, The re-arrangement of the districts in the western province Ashanti, 1927 ("Notes of a conference held at Sunyani on 11th March 1927 to discuss the rearrangement of the districts in the western province Ashanti").

65. CO 96/677/12. In a confidential letter from Governor to L. S. Amery, M. P., government house, Accra (28 January 1928), he discussed the matter of murder with the chief commissar of Ashanti, John Maxwell; commissioner of the western province of Ashanti, Major Ballantine; and district commissioner of Kintampo, Captain Lynch.

66. CO 96/677/12, 28 January 1928, 8.

67. CO 96/677/12, Enclosure I: Extract from Report by the Commissioner of Western Province (CWP) of Ashanti; *Colonial Report—Annual. No. 1119*, 41.

68. CO 96/677/12, Enclosure II: Road A.38—realignment of, 2.

69. CO 96/677/12, 4. Editorials in local newspapers also called the alarm about "the frequency with which chiefs are 'destooled,' leading some observers to claim that 'destoolment' seem[s] to be the order of the day." *Gold Coast Independent* 1, no. 6 (13 July 1913): 23.

70. BRG 28/2/3, F. W. Applegate, acting commissioner W.P.A., to District Commissioner, Wenchi, 13 January 1928; "the Tekiman Disturbances," G. E. C. Wisdom, assistant district commissioner, to E. A. Burner, Wenchi, 27 July 1927.

71. CO 96/677/12, Governor to L. S. Amery, 6–7.

72. CO 879/122/6, West Africa Correspondence (1921–1929) Relating to Medical Matters, African no. 1114.

73. J. A. Dadson, "The Need for the Cooperative Reorientation—The Ghana Case," in *Cooperative Revisited*, vol. 21, ed. Hans G. B. Hedlund, 173–86 (Uppsala: Nordiska Afrikainstitutet, 1988), 178. See also Amos Oppong Afriyie, Dominic Damoah, Edward Ansong, and Poakwah Gyimah, "A Conceptual Framework for Encouraging Educational Investment through 'Nnoboa' in Ghana," *International Journal of Community and Cooperative Studies* 1, no. 2 (2014): 51–58.

74. Kay, *Political Economy*, 316, 410.

75. Kay, *Political Economy*, 316.

76. BRG 28/13/1, "Return showing names of missionary societies and where they operate in the Western Province, Ashanti," n.d.; "Report on the work of the Wesleyan Mission in the Western Province of Ashanti, 1930–21," by Kenneth Horn, superintendent, n.d., 1. The mission leased land in Wankyi to be held "in trust for the [Wesleyan Methodist Missionary] Society for the period of 99 years [and renewable . . .] by rental of £1 per annum." The agreement was formulaically "read over and explained in the Twi language." See BRG 28/13/1, "Agreement between Omanhene of Wenchi and Wesleyan Mission," n.d., 1–2.

77. BRG 28/13/1, "Report on the work of the Wesleyan Mission," 1.

78. BRG 28/13/1, "Report on the work of the Wesleyan Mission," 1–2. See also C. E. Donkoh's *Aduse-Poku Kɔnkɔnko* (Accra: Bureau of Ghana Languages, 1973), 11, 37,

45–46, for his discussion of early twentieth-century missionary schools in Wankyi and attempts in Takyiman under Nana Yaw Kramo.

79. BRG 28/13/1, "Report on the work of the Wesleyan Mission," 1.

80. BRG 28/13/1, L. W. Judd, district commissioner, Goaso, to Provincial Commissioner, Sunyani, 4 April 1924, 1.

81. BRG 28/13/1, Frank A. Markin, Wesleyan mission house, Tekiman, to Provincial Commissioner, Sunyani, 24 July 1922, 1–2; Donkoh, *Aduse-Poku Kɔnkɔnko*, 41.

82. BRG 28/13/1, "Report on the visit of Evangelist Sampson Oppon to Tekieman," by Thomas Witter, superintendent of the Wenchi mission, n.d. [July 1921], 2.

83. BRG 28/13/1, Markin to Provincial Commissioner, 2; "Sampson Oppon to Tekieman," 3–4.

84. BRG 28/16/4, "1931 Census Report—Sunyani and Goaso Districts," 2; BRG 28/2/45, "Techiman Native Affairs," n.d. [1930–32], 2. Several typeset documents are marked "Techiman Native Affairs" without a date; the documents referenced here correspond to the same page.

85. Interview with N. Kofi Donkor, Techiman, 20 April 1980, conducted by Raymond Silverman.

86. Interview with N. Kofi Donkor, Techiman, 20 April 1980. The training for blacksmiths, in term of the process, had changed little since Basel missionaries observed the craft in the mid-nineteenth century. Then, they observed, "as far as the blacksmith craft is concerned, you also learn this at another. After you have completed your training the master allows you a somewhat longer stay with him, buys tools for you and with these you work and you then accept work independently, he himself gives you such work from time to time, because the blacksmith craft is not a thing, which one can immediately do for oneself alone.... The smith works under a grass roof, which is supported by bars and poles, with a small anvil and hammer and makes mostly small hatchets and bush-knives as well as other small items." See BMA, D-10-4-1, 22.

87. Interview with Kwasi Amponsa Nkron Amoah, Takyiman, 18 September 2012.

88. Interview with N. Kofi Donkor, Techiman, 20 April 1980.

89. It seems an oath, coded in the colonial understanding of indigenous oath-taking as "to take fetish," was made between healers (caricaturized as "fetish priests") and rulers of local polities sliced into "divisions." Those who did not make this oath were taxed, and this happened to one healer named Kwaku Aukra. In a letter dated 7 May 1929, from Kwame Kra of Wankyi to Takyimanhene Yaw Ameyaw, we learn that "according to customary law between Wenchi and Tekiman it is never the fraternal custom to tax any fetish priest who has been made to take fetish in the Division; this is never done in Wenchi Division, and as Wenchi and Tekiman are all one, I am aware Tekiman is the same." See BRG 9/1/1, Techiman Traditional Affairs—General (1914–49), letter from Kwame Kra [of Wankyi] to Omanhene Yao Ameyao, Tekiman, 7 May 1929.

90. Interview with Nana Akosua Antwiwaa, Akumsa Odumase, Nkoransa, 21 March 2012. Basel missionaries also noted that, "during the time of his training as prophet," the healer-to-be requires "a trained ear for the language of the fetish." See BMA, D-10-4-1, *Sagen der Akwapim-Neger über die Erschaffung der Welt, Entstehung der*

Fetische ("Tales of the Akwapim Blacks about the creation of the world, the origin of the fetishes"), n.d. (probably 1850s), 15.

91. Interview with Nana Akosua Antwiwaa, Akumsa Odumase, Nkoransa, 21 March 2012.

92. T. E. Kyei, *Our Days Dwindle: Memories of My Childhood Days in Asante*, ed. and intro. Jean Allman (Portsmouth, NH: Heinemann, 2001), 21. Kyei notes that most of these quarters (*aborɔnoo*) were named after trees planted for ritual purposes or as shade trees.

93. Dennis M. Warren, "Disease, Medicine, and Religion among the Techiman-Bono of Ghana: A Study in Cultural Change" (PhD diss., Indiana University, 1974), 176. Wells were not drilled until 1969–70. Warren successfully defended his dissertation in September 1973, but most references to it list the year 1974. Warren or his representative filed for copyright on the work in 1974. See *Catalog of Copyright Entries, Third Series: 1975: January–June* (Washington, DC: Copyright Office, Library of Congress, 1976), 2156.

94. The National Archives, War Office, 287/6, Military Report on the Gold Coast, Ashanti, the Northern Territories and Mandated Togoland (London: War Office, 1931), I: 204 (Appendix XIII, Census of Livestock).

95. On Asubɔnten's taboo of cattle see Warren and Brempong, *Techiman Traditional State, Pt. II*, 47–52. See also the following interview: Bosomfoo Kofi Donkor, Techiman, 1970, OT-2529, tape 23, side 1, Ghana, Brong-Ahafo region, Techiman Traditional State, Bono-Akan, 1969–71 (sound recording), collected by Dennis Michael Warren and Owusu Brempong, accession number 720249-F, Archives of Traditional Music, Indiana University.

96. Interview with N. Kofi Donkor, Techiman, 20 April 1980.

97. J. H. Kwabena Nketia, *Folk Songs of Ghana* (New York: Oxford University Press for the University of Ghana, Legon, 1963), 181.

98. Robert S. Rattray, *Ashanti* (London: Clarendon Press, 1923), 114 (quotation), 123 ("grey-beards").

99. Rattray, *Religion and Art in Ashanti*, 38–47.

100. BMA, D-10-4-3a, 3.

101. BMA, D-10-4-3a, 5.

102. Warren, "Disease, Medicine, and Religion," 140–41.

103. Part of the description of the kumkuma ceremony comes from Nana Kwaku Sakyi's journal, unpublished, entry dated 24 September 1998. A copy is in the author's possession.

104. Christaller defined *asubɔnten* as simply a "river" from the words for water that runs straight. See Christaller, *A Dictionary of the Asante and Fante*, 38, 461.

105. Interview with N. Kofi Donkor, Takyiman, 20 April 1980. Also associated with Asubɔnten Kwabena are the honorifics *boten* ("tall rock") and *yɛntumi* ("no one can overpower").

106. Warren and Brempong, *Techiman Traditional State, Pt. II*, 45.

107. Interview with N. Kofi Donkor, Techiman, 20 April 1980.

108. Interview with N. Kofi Donkor, Techiman, 20 April 1980; interview with Nana Kwasi Amponsah Nkron Amoah, Takyiman township, 18 September 2012. Nana Amoah

noted, "He [Kofi Donkɔ] told me their descendants came from Nkoransa before coming to Takyiman. The family first settled in or was received by the Adontenhene of Takyiman and was accepted into the Adonten royal family/house. The Adontenhene of Takyiman married one of the women from whose line Nana Donkɔ was brought forth." When in Akumsa Odumase, the shrine of Asubɔnten Kwabena was the property of the Odumasehene Bodee Dwaa; in Takyiman, possession shifted to the Takyimanhene because, as Kofi Dɔnkɔ explained, "that property is the property of the owner of the town where you take up residence."

109. Interview with N. Kofi Donkor, Techiman, 20 April 1980; Warren and Brempong, *Techiman Traditional State*, Pt. II, 45–46.

110. Warren and Brempong, *Techiman Traditional State*, Pt. II, 45–52.

111. Warren and Brempong, *Techiman Traditional State*, Pt. II, 45–52; interview with Nana Kwasi Appiah, Takyiman township, 27 September 2012.

112. Nana Kofi Dɔnkɔ Collection: Hand-written account on a five-by-eight sheet of paper dated 4 April 1977 (copy in author's possession).

113. Interview with N. Kofi Donkor, Techiman, 20 April 1980.

114. According to Kofi Ɔboɔ, the recently deceased ɔkyeame for Asubɔnten, Kofi Donkɔ's grandfather Kwadwo Owusu was Afia Fofie's uncle. He also noted Gyapon was his uncle and another Kofi Ɔboɔ was Gyapon's younger brother and Asubɔnten ɔkyeame while he briefly occupied the position of ɔbosomfoɔ. Kofi Ɔboɔ replaced his namesake (Gyapon's brother Kofi Ɔboɔ) as ɔkyeame when he, like Kofi Donkɔ, was very young. Interview with Nana Kofi Ɔboɔ (Tuffoɔ), Takyiman township, 27 March 2012.

115. Okomfoo Adwoa Akumsaa, Techiman, 15 February 1970, OT-2529, tape 36, side 1, Ghana, Brong-Ahafo region, Techiman Traditional State, Bono-Akan, 1969–71 (sound recording), collected by Dennis Michael Warren and Owusu Brempong, accession number 720249-F, Archives of Traditional Music, Indiana University.

116. Warren and Brempong, *Techiman Traditional State*, Pt. II, 45–52; BRG 1/12/112, Native Customary Letter, 13 February 1961, 10. On the *Fofie* festival, see C. E. Donkoh, *Ghana Afahyɛ hodoɔ bi* (Accra: Bureau of Ghana Languages, 1969), 17–20. At the end of its festival, Asubɔnten Kwabena was purified at the Afia Asuo River near the Takyiman market. See interview with N. Kofi Donkor, Techiman, 20 April 1980.

CHAPTER 4. **MEDICINE, MARRIAGE, AND POLITICS**

1. Okomfoo Adwoa Akumsaa, Techiman, 15 February 1970, OT-2529, tape 36, side 1, Ghana, Brong-Ahafo region, Techiman Traditional State, Bono-Akan, 1969–71 (sound recording), collected by Dennis Michael Warren and Owusu Brempong, accession number 720249-F, Archives of Traditional Music, Indiana University. On the prevalence of malaria and other diseases in the colony see *Colonial Reports—Annual. Nos. 1602, 1657, 1748, 1785, 1882. Gold Coast. Reports for 1931–38* (London: Her Majesty's Stationery Office, 1933–39), 13 (1933), 11 (1934), 16 (1936), 10 (1936), 14, 19 (1939).

2. Interview with N. Kofi Donkor, Techiman, 20 April 1980, conducted by Raymond Silverman.

3. Interview with Nana Kwaku Sakyi, Miami, Florida, 1 March 2009. Nana Sakyi was the first of several diasporic Africans residing in the Caribbean or the United States to be trained by Kofi Dɔnkɔ or, after his passing in 1995, by his relatives. In fact, Nana Sakyi was perhaps also the first diasporic African to train for a Tanɔ ɔbosom, Kwabena Bena.

4. Dennis M. Warren and K. Owusu Brempong, *Techiman Traditional State, Pt. II* (Legon: Institute of African Studies, University of Ghana, 1971), 45–52.

5. *Colonial Report—Annual. No. 1657*, 11; *Colonial Report—Annual. No. 1836. Gold Coast. Reports for 1936–37* (London: Her Majesty's Stationery Office, 1938), 22.

6. Christine Okali, "Family Labour on Cocoa Farms," *Legon Family Research Seminars*, no. 4 (Legon: Institute of African Studies, University of Ghana, 1973), 8–9.

7. Polly Hill, *The Gold Coast Cocoa Farmer: A Preliminary Survey* (London: Oxford University Press, 1956), 25–27.

8. Hill, *Gold Coast Cocoa Farmer*, 9–11, 16.

9. Ivor Wilks, *Asante in the Nineteenth Century: The Structure and Evolution of a Political Order* (New York: Cambridge University Press, [1975] 1989), 124. Meanwhile, the Northern Territories had a "gradual introduction of Indirect Rule," which involved, among others, the "task of reorganizing the tribes." *Colonial Report—Annual. No. 1559. Gold Coast. Reports for 1930–31* (London: Her Majesty's Stationery Office, 1932), 4.

10. For numerous destoolment charges and cases in Takyiman, see volumes 5–7 under Public Records and Archives Administration Department of Ghana, Sunyani, Brong-Ahafo Regional Archives (hereafter brg) 2/1/10, "Techiman Traditional Council Affairs," 8 January 1964 to 12 June 1975.

11. Takyimanhene Kwasi Twi also took the Asantehene to court over the nine villages, among other matters, in a 1935 case. See Manhyia Archives, Kumase (hereafter MAG), 1/2/2/36, Nana Kwasi Twi—Omanhene of Techiman, the Elders and the Paramount Stool of Techiman vrs. Nana Osei Agyeman Prempeh II—The Asantehene on Behalf of the Golden Stool of Asante, 1947; Documents and Letters on the Tekyiman Brong and Ashanti Dispute, files 1 and 5 (Eva L. R. Meyerowitz), MSS. Afr. s. 1447, Bodleian Library of Commonwealth and African Studies at Rhodes House (Weston Library), Oxford University, 4. As for the movement Nana Kwasi Twi spawned, Bonokyɛmpem derives from the phrase *bono kyɛ ampem dua ne kwa* ("the first created divided into a thousand and planted itself everywhere in the country"), which registers the Bono as pioneers among their Akan cohorts.

12. BRG 28/2/45, Chief Commissioner, Kumasi, to Acting Commissioner, Western Province, Sunyani, 6 May 1930.

13. "The Life and History of Nana Akumfi Ameyaw III," 25 March 1946, in MSS. Afr. s. 1447, 12, 15.

14. "The Life and History of Nana Akumfi Ameyaw III," 14.

15. CO 885/58, Miscellaneous no. 463, sub-enclosure 1 in no. 54, 58, 116.

16. Francis K. Danquah, "Sustaining A West African Cocoa Economy: Agricultural Science and the Swollen Shoot Contagion in Ghana, 1936–1965," *African Economic History* 31 (2003): 43–74.

17. G. B. Kay, ed., *The Political Economy of Colonialism in Ghana: A Collection of Documents and Statistics, 1900–1960* (New York: Cambridge University Press, 1972), 253.

18. Paulina Amponsah, Günter Leydecker, Rolf Muff, "Earthquake catalogue of Ghana for the time period 1615–2003 with special reference to the tectono-structural evolution of south-east Ghana," *Journal of African Earth Sciences* 75, no. 18 (2012): 5.

19. This section on Kofi Dɔnkɔ's marriage and early adult life relies on numerous conversations with his son, Kofi Sakyi Sapɔn, and the latter's notes and interviews about his father and larger family. Other important interviews include those with the following people: Nana Kwaku Sakyi, Miami, Florida, 14 June 2012; Nana Kwasi Amponsah Nkron Amoah, Takyiman township, 18 September 2012; Ama Akomaa, Takyiman township, 22 September 2012; Nana Kwasi Appiah, Saase, Ashanti region, 27 September 2012; Nana Kwasi Owusu, Nkukua Buoho, Kumasi, 22 March 2012; Yaa Kɔmfo, Essienimpong, Ashanti region, 24 March 2012; Nana Kofi Ɔboɔ (Tuffoɔ), Takyiman township, 27 March 2012.

20. On *asiwa awareɛ* or *awadeɛ* see Pashington Obeng, *Asante Catholicism: Religious and Cultural Reproduction among the Akan of Ghana* (Leiden: Brill, 1996), 77–78; Peter Sarpong, *Ghana in Retrospect: Some Aspects of Ghanaian Culture* (Accra: Ghana Publishing, 1974), 80; Christine Oppong, *Middle Class African Marriage: A Family Study of Ghanaian Senior Civil Servants* (New York: Cambridge University Press, 1974), 28–31.

21. Chief Commissioner W. J. A. Jones noted, "Native Law recognizes polygamy, and so therefore, does section 14 of the Marriage Ordinance." See W. J. A. Jones, Regarding Mgr. Morin's Memorandum, MSS. Afr. s. 454, Bodleian Library of Commonwealth and African Studies at Rhodes House (Weston Library), Oxford University, 8. Basel missionaries also noted, "The marriage laws of the Twi people are very strict, especially marriages among blood relatives are forbidden. A suitor has to be referred by the respective girl to the head of the family. By him the engagement is arranged." Basel Mission Archives (hereafter BMA), E-10-34-36, *Heidnische Gebete und darin enthaltene Spuren einer reineren monotheistischen Gotteserkenntnis* ("Traditional prayers and traces contained within them of a purer monotheistic recognition of God"), n.d. (probably early 1900s), 4.

22. Oppong, *Middle Class African Marriage*, 30.

23. BMA, E-10-34-36, 3–4.

24. Kofi Agyekum, "Menstruation as a Verbal Taboo among the Akan of Ghana," *Journal of Anthropological Research* 58, no. 3 (2002): 377.

25. Agyekum, "Menstruation as a Verbal Taboo," 380.

26. Nana Kofi Dɔnkɔ Collection: Nana Kofi Donkor diary/entry book, n.d. (ca. 1950s–1970s), unpaginated. The entry reads, "My wife Akosua Donkor delivered female child . . . the child is called Afua Kwafie."

27. Interview with Adowa Asamoa, Takyiman, 28 March 2012.

28. BMA, E-10-34-36, 3.

29. BRG 28/14/7, Acting Commissioner W.P.A., Sunyani, to District Commissioner, Sunyani, 13 May 1929; "Provisional Programme: Opening of the new Sunyani Hospital on 11th May, 1929."

30. Bosomfoo Kofi Kyereme, Techiman, [date inaudible] September 1970, OT-2529, tape 23, side 2, Ghana, Brong-Ahafo region, Techiman Traditional State, Bono-Akan,

1969–71 (sound recording), collected by Dennis Michael Warren and Owusu Brempong, accession number 720249-F, Archives of Traditional Music, Indiana University.

31. Bosomfoo Kofi Kyereme, Techiman, September 1970, OT-2529, tape 23, side 2.

32. 1 West African Court of Appeal [WACA] 15, Nana Sir Ofori Atta v. Nana Kwaku Amoah, Accra, 19 May 1930; Nana Kwaku Amoah II and Others v. Nana Sir Ofori Atta and Others, Accra, 24 November 1933 (1 WACA 332); and Nana Kwaku Amoah II and Others v. Nana Sir Ofori Atta and Others, Accra, 27 November 1933 (1 WACA 344); H. W. Thomas, Secretary for Native Affairs, Accra, "History of the Asamankese Dispute," 9 May 1934, MSS. Afr. s. 576, Bodleian Library of Commonwealth and African Studies at Rhodes House (Weston Library), University of Oxford; Kathryn Firmin-Sellers, *The Transformation of Property Rights in the Gold Coast: An Empirical Study Applying Rational Choice Theory* (New York: Cambridge University Press, 1996), 66–71.

33. P. A. L. Greenhalgh, *West African Diamonds, 1919–1983: An Economic History* (Manchester, UK: Manchester University Press, 1985), 102–5; Kojo Amanor, *Land, Labour and the Family in Southern Ghana: A Critique of Land Policy Under Neo-Liberalisation* (Uppsala: Nordic Africa Institute, 2001), 36–39; Emmanuel Ababio Ofosu-Mensah, "Mining and Conflict in the Akyem Abuakwa Kingdom in the Eastern Region of Ghana, 1919–1938," *Extractive Industries and Society* 2, no. 3 (2015): 480–90.

34. Richard Rathbone argues that these two forms of law became intertwined. See his *Nkrumah and the Chiefs: The Politics of Chieftaincy in Ghana, 1951–1960* (Athens: Ohio University Press, 2000), 11–16.

35. Most land in the colony and in the post-colony remains "stool land" under "chiefs," but the latter are disbarred from participating in party politics and have a status that no longer requires government recognition.

36. In 1949 Kwame Abrefa was asked to abdicate the stool so that it could be offered to Dr. Kofi Abrefa Busia. Dr. Busia declined the offer and became prime minister of Ghana between 1969 and 1972.

37. Akumfi Ameyaw III, Omanhene of Techiman (Appeal No. 66 of 1945) v. Kwasi Safo (West Africa) [1947], United Kingdom Privy Council (UKPC) 36, 22 May 1947, 5–6.

38. UKPC 36, 22 May 1947, 2–3.

39. Interview with Kwadwo Nyarko, Osei Yaw, Kwabena Adjei, Kwadwo Afram, and Kwame Yeboah, conducted by Kofi Sakyi Sapɔn, Amangoase Village, 27 October 1997.

40. Jeff Grischow and Glenn H. McKnight, "Rhyming Development: Practising Post-development in Colonial Ghana and Uganda," *Journal of Historical Sociology* 16, no. 4 (2003): 521.

41. Roger S. Gocking, *The History of Ghana* (Westport, CT: Greenwood Press, 2005), 61.

42. Firmin-Sellers, *Transformation of Property Rights in the Gold Coast*, 66; Grischow and McKnight, "Rhyming Development," 523–24.

43. The father of Ofori Atta I and J. B. Danquah was the former drummer and ɔbrafoɔ turned evangelist Yaw Boakye. On Yaw Boakye see, for instance, Richard Rathbone, *Murder and Politics in Colonial Ghana* (New Haven, CT: Yale University Press, 1993), 27–30.

44. Firmin-Sellers, *Transformation of Property Rights in the Gold Coast*, 69–71. The ordinances in question were the Peace Preservation Ordinance and the Asamankese Division Regulation Ordinance.

45. 1 WACA 332; 1 WACA 344. See also Nana Kwaku Amoah, Since Deceased (Now Represented by Yaw Ewuah), and Another v Nana Sir Ofori Atta (West Africa) [1932], UKPC 73 (21 November 1932).

46. Grischow and McKnight, "Rhyming Development," 526.

47. 1 WACA 332.

48. Grischow and McKnight, "Rhyming Development," 526.

49. M. J. Field, *Search for Security: An Ethno-Psychiatric Study of Rural Ghana* (London: Faber and Faber, 1960), 112, 117.

50. J. B. Kirk, Diary of Tours in the Gold Coast, 1942–43, MSS. Afr. s. 1368, f. 47, Bodleian Library of Commonwealth and African Studies at Rhodes House (Weston Library), Oxford University.

51. "The Life and History of Nana Akumfi Ameyaw III," in MSS. Afr. s. 1447, 9.

52. See BRG 2/2/19 Techiman State Council Affairs (1947–50).

53. For a series of relevant correspondence and petitions, see files in BRG 2/2/44 and BRG 9/1/19. The most notorious and offensive of all the insults from the Asantehene and Kumase ahene was the "feet on the head ritual," wherein the Asantehene would remove his sandals and put his left foot on the crown of the Takyimanhene's head. While the Takyimanhene squatted before the Asantehene, the Asantehene rubbed his foot three times on the crown of the Takyimanhene's head while the Kumase ahene gave the epithet, Safroadu! Safroadu! See Owusu Brempong, "Oral Tradition in Ghana: The History of Bonokyempim and Techiman Politics," *Research Review* 13 (1988): 10. For the Asantehene, this was a ritual of superiority since no Bono ɔmanhene was considered equal to him. The ritual was an insult to the Bono ɔmanhene and the Bono nation because it not only undermined the prestige and authority of the Takyimanhene, but regarded as a taboo, since nothing should touch the head of a Bono ɔmanhene once he was enstooled.

54. See, for example, BRG 2/1/10, Humble Petition of the Elders and People of Techiman Traditional Area to the Right Honourable Dr. K. A. Busia, 19 March 1970, 1–3.

55. BMA, D-18-82-10, Letter from Wilhelm Rottmann, Akropong, ca. 1902–3.

56. For letters regarding the Methodist Mission see BRG 9/1/3, Techiman Traditional Affairs—General (1933–1960).

57. "The Life and History of Nana Akumfi Ameyaw III," in MSS. Afr. S. 1447, 13.

58. BRG 9/1/13, Letter from Seventh Day Adventist Church, Forikrom, Techiman to Nana Akumfi Ameyaw III, Techimanhene and president of the Techiman State Council, Techiman, Bono State, 20 September 1950, 1; W. J. A. Jones, Regarding Mgr. Morin's Memorandum, MSS. Afr. s. 454, f. 5.

59. BRG 9/1/13, Letter from Seventh Day Adventist Church, Forikrom, Techiman to Nana Akumfi Ameyaw III, Techimanhene and president of the Techiman State Council, Techiman, Bono State, 20 September 1950, 1–3.

60. Kay, *Political Economy of Colonialism in Ghana*, 11.

61. E. D. Roberts, "The Development of Education in Pre-Independent Africa," Mss 380327, University of London, SOAS Library, Archives and Special Collections, London, 6.

62. BRG 9/2/1, Nana Akumfi Ameyaw III Papers, letter from Kofi Nsia to Nana Akumfi Ameyaw III, 5 September 1944.

63. "The Life and History of Nana Akumfi Ameyaw III," in MSS. Afr. s. 1447, 18. On radio broadcasting see Alan Wells, ed., *World Broadcasting: A Comparative View* (Norwood, NJ: Ablex Publishing, 1996), 162; Kwesi Yankah, *Language, the Mass Media and Democracy in Ghana* (Accra: Ghana Academy of Arts and Sciences, 2004), 7.

64. Letter from Tekyimanhene to Eva Meyerowitz, 7 March 1947, in MSS. Afr. s. 1447; *Spectator Daily*, 30 November 1946.

65. Letter from Techimanhene, etc., to Chief Commissioner's Office, Kumasi, 26 July 1947, in MSS. Afr. s. 1447; *Spectator Daily*, 30 November 1946, 1–2.

66. Kay, ed., *Political Economy of Colonialism in Ghana*, 81, 87, 120; Roberts, "The Development of Education in Pre-Independent Africa," 6.

67. Jean M. Allman, "The Youngmen and the Porcupine: Class, Nationalism and Asante's Struggle for Self-Determination, 1954–57," *Journal of African History* 31 (1990): 264, 267.

68. See BRG 2/2/44, Resolution of the Techiman State Council, 13 February 1956, ff. 30, 31b; BRG 1/2/8, Tekiman Native Affairs (vol. 1) and Techiman Native Affairs (vols. 2–4), for the relevant exchanges on accusations of assaults and related practices, and the numerous appeals to the Chief Commissioner of Ashanti by Takyiman, members of the Bonokyɛmpem Federation, and Asanteman. See also, in the Techiman Native Affairs files, the correspondences on the Takyiman-Tanɔso boundary dispute (in vol. 2) and the petition by Takyimanhene, Tanɔsohene, Tuobodomhene, and Offumanhene to Sir Gerald Creasy, Governor of the Gold Coast, Techiman, Ashanti, Gold Coast, July 1948; Brempong, "Oral Tradition in Ghana," 1–74.

69. Brempong, "Oral Tradition in Ghana," 6.

70. See the correspondences in BRG 2/2/44, Brong Federation Dispute Between Certain Brong Chiefs and Asanteman Council (ca. 1951–56); BRG 2/2/45, Brong Kyempem Federation: Additional Documents to the Friction between the Federation and Asanteman; BRG 1/2/106, Brong Kyempim Secession from Asanteman (10 May 1958 to 2 June 1958); BRG 1/2/105, Brong Kyempim Inquires (1955). See also "The Petition of the Tekyimanhene of Tekyiman, Tekyiman, June 1949, to His Most Excellent Majesty George the Sixth, King of Great Britain and of the British Dominions Beyond the Seas, etc.," in MSS. Afr. s. 1447. Danquah's cover letter is followed by a 115-page document, excluding two or three maps in the appendix. Meyerowitz's papers at the Bodleian Library contain two folders entitled "The Tekyiman-Brong/Ashanti Dispute in Documents and Letters written to Eva L. R. Meyerowitz."

71. See MAG 1/2/225, Techiman Native Affairs (Kwaku Gyamfi vrs. Kojo Berkor per Wusuansah), 1948–51, Letter from Kwaku Gyamfi, Tanoso, to Chief Commissioner of Ashanti, 2 September 1948, 1. In the end, on appeal, magistrate Alan Bullwinkle did not find the "charge of rebellion was proved" but that Kwaku Gyamfi was "most unwise to associate with the Tekyimanhene," although this association did not prove he was a disloyal rebel.

72. The petitions were described as "an appeal to England from the decision of the Governor of the Gold Coast, who, in December 1948 refused a Petition to him dated July 1948 which prayed for the restoration of the 9 villages and the cancellation of certain repressive steps taken by the Chief Commissioner of Ashanti to compel Techimanhene to abandon his claim." See "Memorandum concerning petitions to the King from the Techimanhene

against the allotment of 9 villages in Techiman to the Asantehene," in MSS Afr. s. 1447, 1. In in MSS Afr. s. 1447 also see Chief Commissioner [C. O. Butler], Kumasi, to Techimanhene, 1 December 1947; Techimanhene to Eva Meyerowitz, Techiman, 22 August 1948; Chief Commissioner, Kumasi, to Colonial Secretary, Accra, 17 September 1948; Eva Meyerowitz to A. Creech-Jones, Secretary of State for the Colonies, 17 September 1948.

73. BRG 9/1/29, The Memorandum to Restore Ashanti Confederacy, n.d., 11 (para. 31).

74. See, for instance, the select papers of Hebert Meyerowitz in MSS Afr. s. 793, Bodleian Library of Commonwealth and African Studies at Rhodes House (Weston Library), University of Oxford; Atta Kwami, "Kofi Antubam, 1922–1964: A Modern Ghanaian Artist, Educator, and Writer," in *A Companion to Modern African Art*, eds. Gitti Salami and Monica B. Visonà (Malden, MA: Wiley-Blackwell, 2013), 218–36; Kwame Amoah Labi, "Afro-Ghanaian Influences in Ghanaian Paintings," *Journal of Art Historiography* 9 (December 2013): 1–23.

75. See MS 598, Field Notes made by Kofi Antubam, Special Collections, University of Birmingham. In addition to Antubam's handwritten field notes made under the heading "Cultural Contributions of the Queen Mothers of Bono-Manso-Takyiman," two sets of Meyerowitz's typed notes and four photocopied letters from Antubam to her form the contents of the folder in which these materials were found.

76. BRG 9/1/19, Letter from Eva Meyerowitz, London, to Sir Gerald Creasy, Governor, Accra, 8 January 1940.

77. BRG 9/1/19, Letter from Eva Meyerowitz, London, to Nana Akumfi Ameyaw III, Techimanhene, Accra, 14 February 1949.

78. BRG 9/1/19, Letter from Nana Akumfi Ameyaw III, Accra, to Eva Meyerowitz, London, 18 February 1949.

79. BRG 9/1/19, Letter from Eva Meyerowitz, London, to Nana Akumfi Ameyaw III, Techimanhene, Accra, 22 February 1949.

80. BRG 9/1/19, Letter from Nana Akumfi Ameyaw III, Accra, to Eva Meyerowitz, London, 5 March 1949; Letter from Techiman Traditional Council (on behalf of Techiman State), Techiman, to Eva Meyerowitz, London, 24 February 1949 (quotations); Brempong, "Oral Tradition in Ghana," 38.

81. BRG 9/1/19, Letter from Eva Meyerowitz, London, to Nana Akumfi Ameyaw III, Techiman, 9 June 1949.

82. BRG 9/1/19, Letter from Nana Akumfi Ameyaw III, Techiman, to Eva Meyerowitz, London, 16 June 1949. See also CO 96/785/3–4, Petition: Paramount Chiefs of Techiman for Return of Villages, 1 January to 31 December 1949; CO 96/813/12, 1 January to 31 December 1950; CO 96/814/1, 1 January to 31 December 1951.

83. BRG 91/1/19, Letter from Nana Akumfi Ameyaw III, Techiman, to Eva Meyerowitz, London, 19 August 1949.

84. Eva L. R. Meyerowitz, *At the Court of an African King* (London: Faber and Faber, 1962), 46.

85. Eva L. R. Meyerowitz, *The Early History of the Akan States of Ghana* (London: Red Candle Press, 1974), 2.

86. Antubam, "Cultural Contributions," MS 598; Colin Flight, "The Chronology of the Kings and Queenmothers of Bono-Manso: A Reevaluation of the Evidence," *Journal*

of African History 11, no. 2 (1970): 259, 261 (quotation); Eva L. R. Meyerowitz, "Communication: The Chronology of Bono-Manso," *Journal of African History* 13, no. 2 (1972): 348 (quotation).

87. Dennis M. Warren, "A Re-appraisal of Mrs. Eva Meyerowitz's Work on the Brong," *Research Review* (Institute of African Studies, Legon) 7, no. 1 (1970): 55; David P. Henige, *The Chronology of Oral Tradition: Quest for a Chimera* (Oxford: Clarendon Press, 1974), 135.

88. Interested readers should see, for instance, Peter Pels and Oscar Salemink, eds., *Colonial Subjects: Essays on the Practical History of Anthropology* (Ann Arbor: University of Michigan Press, 1999); George W. Stocking, Jr., ed., *Colonial Situations: Essays on the Contextualization of Ethnographic Knowledge* (Madison: University of Wisconsin Press, 1991); Talal Asad, ed., *Anthropology and the Colonial Encounter* (Atlantic Highlands, NJ: Humanities Press, 1973); Diane Lewis, "Anthropology and Colonialism," *Current Anthropology* 14, no. 5 (1973): 581–602; Kathleen Gough, "Anthropology and Imperialism," *Monthly Review* 19, no. 11 (1968): 12–24.

89. On Antubam's nationalist presence see Harcourt Fuller, *Building the Ghanaian Nation-State: Kwame Nkrumah's Symbolic Nationalism* (New York: Palgrave Macmillan, 2014), 41–52.

CHAPTER 5. **INDEPENDENCES**

1. Owusu Brempong, email message to author, 30 September 2010.

2. Owusu Brempong, email message to author, 30 September 2010.

3. Owusu Brempong, email message to author, 30 September 2010.

4. Interviews with Kwaku Sakyi, Miami, Florida, 14 June 2012; Nana Kwasi Amponsah Nkron Amoah, Takyiman township, 18 September 2012; Ama Akomaa, Takyiman township, 22 September 2012; Nana Kwasi Appiah, Saase, Ashanti region, 27 September 2012; Nana Akosua Antwiwaa, Akumsa Odumase, 21 March 2012; Nana Kwasi Owusu, Takyiman township, 22 March 2012; Nana Yaa Kɔmfo, Essienimpong, Ashanti region, 24 March 2012; Nana Kofi Ɔboɔ (Tuffoɔ), Takyiman township, 27 March 2012; Adwoa Asamoaa, Takyiman township, 28 March 2012. The account of the broken leg comes from Nana Kwasi Appiah.

5. Interviews with Nana Kwasi Amponsah Nkron Amoah, Takyiman township, 18 September 2012; Ama Akomaa, Takyiman township, 22 September 2012; Nana Kwasi Owusu, Takyiman township, 22 March 2012; Nana Yaa Kɔmfo, Essienimpong, Ashanti region, 24 March 2012.

6. Interviews with Nana Kwasi Appiah, Saase, Ashanti region, 27 September 2012; Nana Akosua Antwiwaa, Akumsa Odumase, 21 March 2012.

7. Interviews with Kwaku Sakyi, Miami, Florida, 14 June 2012; Nana Kwasi Amponsah Nkron Amoah, Takyiman township, 18 September 2012; Ama Akomaa, Takyiman township, 22 September 2012; Nana Kwasi Appiah, Saase, Ashanti region, 27 September 2012; Nana Akosua Antwiwaa, Akumsa Odumase, 21 March 2012 (quotation); Nana Kwasi Owusu, Takyiman township, 22 March 2012; Nana Yaa Kɔmfo, Essienimpong, Ashanti region, 24 March 2012; Nana Kofi Ɔboɔ (Tuffoɔ), Takyiman township, 27 March 2012; Adwoa Asamoaa, Takyiman township, 28 March 2012.

8. Interviews with Nana Kwasi Appiah, Saase, Ashanti region, 27 September 2012; Nana Akosua Antwiwaa, Akumsa Odumase, 21 March 2012.

9. The Akan/Twi names for those ailments are as follows: childhood diseases, *asram*; tumor, *dobe*; chicken pox, *ntɛnkyɛm*, *borɔmpete*; convulsions, *ɛsorɔ*; guinea worm, *mfahama*; stomachache, *yafunuyareɛ*; cholera, *ayamtubrafoɔ*; gonorrhea, *babaso*; piles, *kɔkɔɔ*; menstrual pains, *anidane*.

10. Interviews with Kwaku Sakyi, Miami, Florida, 14 June 2012; Nana Kwasi Amponsah Nkron Amoah, Takyiman township, 18 September 2012; Ama Akomaa, Takyiman township, 22 September 2012; Nana Kwasi Appiah, Saase, Ashanti region, 27 September 2012; Nana Akosua Antwiwaa, Akumsa Odumase, 21 March 2012 (quotation); Nana Kwasi Owusu, Takyiman township, 22 March 2012; Nana Yaa Kɔmfo, Essienimpong, Ashanti region, 24 March 2012; Nana Kofi Ɔboɔ (Tuffoɔ), Takyiman township, 27 March 2012; Adwoa Asamoaa, Takyiman township, 28 March 2012.

11. Interviews with Nana Yaa Kɔmfo, Essienimpong, Ashanti region, 24 March 2012; Nana Kofi Ɔboɔ (Tuffoɔ), Takyiman township, 27 March 2012.

12. See the Public Records and Archives Administration Department of Ghana, Sunyani, Brong-Ahafo Regional Archives (hereafter BRG) 2/1/33, Native Physicians and Fetishes, vols. 1 and 2 (1938–49).

13. BRG 9/2/12, Visitors and Out Visitors Diary [desk diary of Akumfi Ameyaw III], entry Monday, 3 May 1948 [but possibly 1949 due to inconsistent dating in the diary].

14. Eva L. R. Meyerowitz, *At the Court of an African King* (London: Faber and Faber, 1962), 152.

15. BRG 2/1/33, "[Report] on Horo Fetish," 1 May 1949, para. 5; application letter for "Horo Fetish," by Kofi Fofie (on behalf of "Kojo Buahin"), Sunyani-Ashanti, 12 April 1949.

16. BRG 2/1/33, Letter from district commissioner, Sunyani-Ashanti, 10 May 1949.

17. BRG 9/2/11, Akumfi Ameyaw Personal Diary, entry for 9 April 1948. The seven-day Apoɔ ("apour") festival started on Friday, 2 April 1948.

18. Interviews with Nana Yaa Kɔmfo, Essienimpong, Ashanti region, 24 March 2012; Nana Kofi Ɔboɔ (Tuffoɔ), Takyiman township, 27 March 2012 (quotations). According to Warren and Brempong, Yaw Atoa or Taaho from Tunsuase in Takyiman was the nephew of Kofi Donkɔ, and he married Afua Fosuaa from Hansua, who gave birth to Adwoa Aberewa, ɔkɔmfoɔ for Kyiriakyinye at Hansua. See Dennis M. Warren and K. O. Brempong, *Ghanaian Oral Histories: The Religious Shrines of Techiman Traditional State* (Ames: Iowa State University Research Foundation, 1988), 74.

19. Because Afua/Afia Kwafie was born in an era of new mission schools in Takyiman, and if she attended one as a young girl, she would have made *awiesu* (fried cornballs) or similar snacks, sold them before and after school and on the weekends, and used the profits to pay school fees.

20. Nana Kofi Dɔnkɔ Collection: Nana Kofi Dɔnkɔ Diary, n.d. [ca. 1950–70], n.p. (hereafter, NKD Diary), entries for 5 March 1950, 23 June 1950, and 18 September 1950. The book certainly appears to be as old as the dates 1950–70 suggest.

21. NKD Diary, entries for 15 August 1954 and 21 February 1955.

22. See the *Statistical Yearbook 1970* (Accra: State Publishing Corporation, 1970).

23. BRG 2/2/44, Constitution of the Brong-Kyempem Federation, compiled 10 March 1951 and approved 25 March 1951, 1–2 (quotations); BRG 2/2/44, Committee of Enquiry into the Dispute Between the Brong Kyempem Federation, and the Asanteman Council, Formerly known as the Ashanti Confederacy Council—Memorandum by the Techimanhene, the Chiefs, and Elders and People of Techiman, 11 August 1951 [by Nana Akumfi Ameyaw III], 1–2. Takyimanhene Akumfi Ameyaw III attended a meeting of the Commission of Enquiry in Kumase on April 22–23, and of the Mate Kole Committee that was established to settle the dispute over the nine villages between Takyiman and Asante in 1951. See BRG 2/2/44, Committee of Enquiry, 3; BRG 9/2/11, Akumfi Ameyaw Personal Diary, entry for 22–23 April 1951 [misdated 1948]; *Report of the Committee on the Asanteman-Brong Dispute* (Accra: Government Printer, 1955).

24. BRG 2/2/41, Resolution by the Brong People of Tuobodom, Ofuman, Tanoso and Anyiayem (New-Techiman), 10 April 1953, 1. In a "Reply on Resolution by the Brong People of Tuobodom, Offuman, Tanoso and Ahyiayem (New Techiman)," dated 28 April 1953, an anonymous individual claimed, "Tuobodom will never on earth join hands with Techiman in politics, social, and economics again and will never think of joining the Brongkyempem Federation till the end of this present world" (1).

25. BRG 2/2/44, Resolution of the Techiman State Council, letter by Osei A. Prempeh II, president of Asanteman Council, 13 February 1956. For more on the matter of "chieftaincy" between Nkrumah and Asante, see Richard Rathbone, *Nkrumah and the Chiefs: The Politics of Chieftaincy in Ghana, 1951–1960* (Athens: University of Ohio Press, 2000).

26. Owusu Brempong, "Oral Tradition in Ghana: The History of Bonokyempim and Techiman Politics," *Research Review* 13 (1988): 10, 28; *Report of the Committee on the Asanteman-Brong Dispute*. See also the Brong-Ahafo Region Act, 1959 (No. 18 of 1959).

27. On the basis of the blank pages in his UGFCC booklet, it does not seem that Kofi Dɔnkɔ had any shares in the organization, though the booklet was used sometimes as a receipt book for transactions related to his healing work.

28. Bjorn Beckman, *Organising the Farmers: Cocoa Politics and National Development in Ghana* (Uppsala: Scandinavian Institute of African Studies, 1976), 7, 245.

29. Polly Hill, *Migrant Cocoa-Farmers of Southern Ghana: A Study in Rural Capitalism* (Cambridge: Cambridge University Press, 1963), 11.

30. Beckman, *Organising the Farmers*, 11.

31. J. A. Dadson, "The Need for the Cooperative Reorientation—The Ghana case," in *Cooperative Revisited*, vol. 21, ed. Hans G. B. Hedlund, Scandinavian Institute of African Studies (Uppsala: Nordiska Afrikainstitutet, 1988), 177–78. For a view on modern farming methods and the benefits of cooperative farming in the 1960s, see J. E. Langon's novel, *Ekuayɛ pa* (Accra: Bureau of Ghana Languages, 1963).

32. Interview with Nana Kofi Kyerere, Takyiman township, 13 December 2002.

33. BRG 1/10/3, Letter from the Holy Family Hospital Dispensary, Medical Mission Sisters, Berekum, 15 June 1952.

34. See the documents in BRG 1/10/4, Mission Hospitals—Techiman.

35. BRG 1/10/3, Letter concerning "Proposed Maternity Clinic and Dispensary—Techiman," 15 September 1953.

36. Holy Family Hospital, Techiman, Annual Report 1983, 1.

37. BRG 9/2/8, Nana Akumfi Ameyaw III, Techiman, to Seventh-Day Adventist Mission of the Gold Coast, Kumasi, 29 November 1954; Howard J. Welsh, Seventh-Day Adventist Mission, Kumasi, to Nana Akumfi Ameyaw III, Techiman, 14 December 1954.

38. BRG 9/1/44, Techiman State Council to the Clerk of Council, Techiman Local Council, 7 May 1956.

39. BMA, PSI-B05–10198, Hans Meister, *Spital Agogo. Erste Eindrücke, Gedanken und Vorschläge*, 22 April 1952.

40. Joseph B. Akamba and Isidore Kwadwo Tufuor, "The Future of Customary Law in Ghana," in *The Future of African Customary Law*, ed. Jeanmarie Fenrich, Paolo Galizzi, and Tracy E. Higgins (New York: Cambridge University Press, 2011), 211–12.

41. BRG 1/12/122, [Takyiman] Native Customary Law, 13 February 1961, 2 (quotation), 10–11.

42. For the ɔmanhene, divisional ɔhene, or *odikro* who distinguished himself in service to the polity, they would have their "white" stools ritually "blackened" upon death and kept in the respective stool house. The odikro's stool, however, required the approval of the Takyimanhene and the Takyiman Traditional Council.

43. BRG 1/12/122, [Takyiman] Native Customary Law, 10.

44. BRG 1/12/122, [Takyiman] Native Customary Law, 11, 13.

45. BRG 1/12/122, [Takyiman] Native Customary Law, 15–16.

46. BRG 1/2/122, Declaration of Customary Laws—Techiman Traditional Council, Sunyani Regional Commissioner's Office to the Principal Secretary, Ministry of Justice, Accra, 19 December 1963, 1–2.

47. See BRG 1/2/122, Modernization of Customary Laws in Brong-Ahafo Region, Brong-Ahafo House of Chiefs to Regional Administrative Office, Sunyani, 5 October 1973.

48. Herb Boyd and Ilyasah Shabazz, eds., *The Diary of Malcolm X, El-Hajj Malik El-Shabazz, 1964* (Chicago: Third World Press, 2013), 55, 165. For perspectives from prominent African American views of Nkrumah and Nkrumah's Ghana, see Kevin K. Gaines, *American Africans in Ghana: Black Expatriates and the Civil Rights Era* (Chapel Hill: University of North Carolina Press, 2006).

49. Interview with Nana Kofi Ɔboɔ (Tuffoɔ), Takyiman township, 27 March 2012.

50. Dennis M. Warren, "Disease, Medicine, and Religion among the Techiman-Bono of Ghana: A Study in Cultural Change" (PhD diss., Indiana University, 1974), 78n14. On the Akosombo project see Peter J. Bloom, Stephan F. Miescher, and Takyiwaa Manuh, eds., *Modernization as Spectacle in Africa* (Bloomington: Indiana University Press, 2014); Stephan Miescher, "'Nkrumah's Baby'": The Akosombo Dam and the Dream of Development in Ghana, 1952–1966," *Water History* 6 (2014): 341–66.

51. Kwasi Konadu, *The Akan Diaspora in the Americas* (New York: Oxford University Press, 2010), 48–50; Kwasi Konadu, *Akan Pioneers: African Histories, Diasporic Experiences* (New York: Diasporic Africa Press, 2018), 48–50.

52. BRG 9/1/1, Letter from Mallam Baba Enuwa, Hausa Zongo, Wenchi—Ashanti, to Nana Tekimanhene, Tekiman, 9 June 1949.

53. BRG 9/1/58, Techiman State—Churches and Schools, note indicating the formal opening of the Ahmadiyya Mosque in Takyiman at Otuam (Tantun), on Saturday, 1 October 1960.

54. *Colonial Report—Annual. No. 1386. Gold Coast. Reports for 19260–27* (London: Her Majesty's Stationery Office, 1927), 37.

55. For the fuller discussion of the Ahmadiyya movement in Ghana, see Maxwell Owusu, "The Muslim Factor in Akan Cultures," *Michigan Discussions in Anthropology* 4, no. 1 (1978): 75–93; E. D. Roberts, "The Development of Education in Pre-Independent Africa," MS 380327, University of London, SOAS Library, Archives and Special Collections, London, 6.

56. NKD Diary, entry for 9 October 1966.

57. "Plan of Shrub Farm the Property of Obosomfo Kofi Donkor Situates at Akenaseɛ and Agyentoa on Techiman Stool Land," field notes by Isaac Takyi Bafo, 6 March 1974, surveyed by Agyei Fetuah, licensed surveyor, Kumasi, 11 March 1974 (hereafter "Plan of Shrub Farm"). Copy of plan in author's possession.

58. BRG 1/2/122, The Techiman Fofie Yam Festival, Techiman Traditional Council to Ghana News Agency and Ghana Information Services, Sunyani, 12 September 1966. Interested researchers can find a copy of the festival's program with this file.

59. Warren, "Disease, Medicine, and Religion," 49. For recent reports on bragorɔ, see Perpetual Crentsil, "Bragoro: A Disappearing Puberty Rite of the Akan of Ghana," *Current Politics and Economics of Africa* 8, no. 2 (2015): 231–57; Paul Appiah-Sekyere and Samuel Awuah-Nyamekye, "Teenage Pregnancy in the Life and Thought of the Traditional Akan: Moral Perspectives," *Sociology Study* 2, no. 2 (2012): 129–38. More generally, see Peter Sarpong, *Girls' Nubility Rites in Ashanti* (Accra: Ghana Publishing, 1977).

60. NKD Diary, entry for 16 July 1968.

61. NKD Diary, entry for 29 December 1968.

62. In the mid-1960s and early 1970s, Warren observed that "Christian and civil-court marriages [were] rare." See Warren, "Disease, Medicine, and Religion," 88n35.

63. BRG 2/1/10, Humble Petition of the Elders and People of Techiman Traditional Area to the Right Honourable Dr. K. A. Busia, Prime Minister of Ghana, 19 March 1970, 1.

64. BRG 2/1/10, Humble Petition, 1.

65. BRG 2/1/10, Humble Petition, 2.

66. BRG 2/1/10, Humble Petition, 3.

67. BRG 2/1/10, Police Wireless Message, no. 1184, 25 December 1970 (on the matter of ɔbosomfoɔ "Kofi Mossi").

68. BRG 2/1/10, Police Wireless Message, nos. 1182–84, 25 December 1970.

69. Warren, "Disease, Medicine, and Religion," 377, 392.

70. For more details on this matter, see Warren, "Disease, Medicine, and Religion," 92–94, 94n40.

71. Dennis M. Warren, G. Steven Bova, Mary Ann Tregoning, and Mark Kliewer, "Ghanaian National Policy Towards Indigenous Healers: The Case of the Primary Health Training for Indigenous Healers (PRHETIH) Program," paper presented at the annual meeting of the Society for Applied Anthropology, Edinburgh, 12–17 April 1981, 6. A copy of this paper can be found in the Warren Collection, MsC 538, Special Collections Department, University of Iowa Libraries.

CHAPTER 6. ANTHROPOLOGIES OF MEDICINE AND AFRICA

1. Dennis M. Warren, "A Re-appraisal of Mrs. Eva Meyerowitz's work on the Brong," *Research Review* 7, no. 1 (1970): 53.

2. Dennis M. Warren, "Disease, Medicine, and Religion among the Techiman-Bono of Ghana: A Study in Cultural Change" (PhD diss., Indiana University, 1974), 2.

3. Dennis M. Warren, "The Role of Emic Analysis in Medical Anthropology: The Case of the Bono of Ghana," *Anthropological Linguistics* 17, no. 3 (1975): 118, 125.

4. Warren, "Role of Emic Analysis," 119, 123, 125.

5. Jacques Depelchin, *Silences in African History: Between the Syndromes of Discovery and Abolition* (Dar es Salaam, Tanzania: Mbuki Na Nyoto Publishers, 2005), 2.

6. Owusu Brempong, email message to author, 30 September 2010.

7. Owusu Brempong, email message to author, 30 September 2010.

8. Owusu Brempong, email message to author, 20 August 2010.

9. Interest in and a functional grasp of indigenous languages was—and remains—a serious impediment. Colonial officials working in the 1940s and 1950s, especially in the field of education/schooling, lamented, "we are severely handicapped by our ignorance of the language." See E. D. Roberts, "The Development of Education in Pre-Independent Africa," MSS. 380327, University of London, SOAS Library, Archives and Special Collections, London, 5.

10. Public Records and Archives Administration Department of Ghana, Sunyani, Brong-Ahafo Regional Archives (hereafter BRG), 2/1/10, Monthly Reports July 1974, Techiman Traditional Council, 7 August 1974, 1. It was well noted that African students, at least those from Ghana, struggled financially while studying abroad. Kwame Nkrumah was a prime example (Kwame Nkrumah, *The Autobiography of Kwame Nkrumah* [Edinburgh: Thomas Nelson and Sons, 1957], 52). For a study of the financial challenges faced by Ghanaian students abroad in 1957, see W. A. R. Walker, "A Note on Ghana Students in North America," October 1957, MSS. Afr. s. 1064, Bodleian Library of Commonwealth and African Studies at Rhodes House (Weston Library), Oxford University, 1–11.

11. Warren, "Disease, Medicine, and Religion," 253–54.

12. Warren, "Disease, Medicine, and Religion," 306n2.

13. Warren, "The Role of Emic Analyses," 118. I consulted the Archives of Traditional Music at Indiana University (Bloomington), where the tapes and notes accompanying the audio are kept, and the Warren Collection (MsC 538, Special Collections) at the University of Iowa Libraries. In fact, I was invited to catalog the Warren Collection and prepare a report on its usefulness to scholars. Because Iowa State University had an online guide to its Warren Collection (Dennis M. Warren Papers, RS 13/32/52, Special Collections Department, Iowa State University Library), I consulted that guide, which, besides some personal and family documents, had some of the same academic papers as the University of Iowa collection.

14. Warren, "The Role of Emic Analysis," 119; Peter Ventevogel, *Whiteman's Things: Training and Detraining Healers in Ghana* (Amsterdam: Het Spinhuis, 1996), 132.

15. Robert W. Wyllie, "Ghanaian Spiritual and Traditional Healers' Explanations of Illness: A Preliminary Survey," *Journal of Religion in Africa* 14, no. 1 (1983): 46–57; Helga Fink, *Religion, Disease, and Healing in Ghana: A Case Study of Traditional Dormaa Medicine* (Munich: Trickster Wissenschaft, 1990).

16. Warren, "Disease, Medicine, and Religion," 244, 246.

17. Warren, "Disease, Medicine, and Religion," 367–68.

18. Owusu Brempong, email message to author, 20 August 2010. Africans or specifically Yorùbá-speaking peoples from Nigeria were called *alatafoɔ*.

19. Warren, "Disease, Medicine, and Religion," 422–23.

20. Ivor Wilks, "Unity and Progress: Asante Politics Revisited," in *Mondes Akan: Identité et Pouvoir en Afrique Occidentale*, ed. Pierluigi Valsecchi and Fabio Viti (Paris: L'harmattan, 1999), 67. Wilks suggests that much more needs to be known about the way Akan political concepts have shifted subtly in meaning as the political landscape has changed.

21. The Takyiman market grew into the second-largest weekly market in Ghana and one of the largest in West Africa. Within the marketplace, unions were created with elected heads for traders of each commodity and heads with authority to settle small cases involving sellers within their union. These unions also served as benevolent societies with rules and regulations, attending functions together, weekly meetings (with an entrance fee), and collection at each meeting; missing meetings without an excuse carried a fine. Usually run by a woman, and following the Akan political model, the ɔhemma of each union had two assistants ("spokespersons"), treasurers and money in a bank account, and meetings of union heads. Although officers were and are predominantly female, there are a few male officers in the unions.

22. Interview with Nana Kwasi Owusu, Takyiman Township, 22 March 2012.

23. Interview with Nana Yaa Kɔmfo, Essienimpong, Ashanti region, 24 March 2012.

24. BRG 2/1/10, Monthly Reports July 1974, Techiman Traditional Council, 7 August 1974, 2–3.

25. BRG 2/1/10, Monthly Reports July 1974, 3.

26. BRG 2/1/10, Monthly Reports July 1974, 4.

27. Dennis M. Warren, G. Steven Bova, Sr. Mary Ann Tregoning, and Mark Kliewer, "Ghanaian National Policy Towards Indigenous Healers: The Case of the Primary Health Training for Indigenous Healers (PRHETIH) Program," paper presented at the annual meeting of the Society for Applied Anthropology, Edinburgh, April 12–17, 1981, 24–25. This paper was published as "Ghanaian National Policy toward Indigenous Healers: The Case of the Primary Health Training for Indigenous Healers (PRHETIH) Program," *Social Science and Medicine* 16, no. 21 (1982): 1873–81. See also D. M. Warren and Mary Ann Tregoning, "Indigenous Healers and Primary Health Care in Ghana," *Medical Anthropology Newsletter* 11, no. 1 (1979): 11–13.

28. Interview with Nana Kofi Owusu, Pomakrom (Takyiman Township), 18 December 2002.

29. HFH, Techiman, Annual Report 1990, 1, 9.

30. BRG 1/10/5, Holy Family Hospital, Techiman, Annual Report 1976, 12.

31. HFH, Techiman, Annual Report 1990, 5.

32. HFH, Techiman, Annual Report 1990, 2.
33. Warren et al., "Ghanaian National Policy Towards Indigenous Healers," 8.
34. Warren et al., "Ghanaian National Policy Towards Indigenous Healers," 2.
35. BRG 1/10/5, Holy Family Hospital, Techiman, Annual Report 1977, 4.
36. BRG 1/10/5, Holy Family Hospital, Techiman, Annual Report 1977, 5.
37. BRG 1/10/5, Holy Family Hospital, Techiman, Annual Report 1977, 2.
38. BRG 1/10/5, Holy Family Hospital, Techiman, Annual Report 1977, 3.
39. BRG 1/10/5, Holy Family Hospital, Techiman, Annual Report 1977, 4.
40. BRG 1/10/5, Holy Family Hospital, Techiman, Annual Report 1977, 4. Between Kofi Donkɔ's passing in 1995 and 2001, malaria OPD cases rose from 1.5 million to 3 million in Ghana. See Felix Ankomah Asante and Kwadwo Asenso-Okyere, "Economic Burden of Malaria in Ghana," a technical report submitted to the World Health Organization, African Regional Office, November 2003, 11.
41. BRG 1/10/5, Holy Family Hospital, Techiman, Annual Report 1978, 1.
42. BRG 1/10/5, Holy Family Hospital, Techiman, Annual Report 1978, 2.
43. BRG 1/10/5, Holy Family Hospital, Techiman, Annual Report 1978, 7.
44. Interested readers can watch a short video of this transition: "J.J. Rawlings–Handover to Hilla Limann, 1979," YouTube, https://www.youtube.com/watch?v=PbuGZVosum4/.
45. Nana Kofi Dɔnkɔ Collection: Letter from Aribert Keil, Castrop—Rauxel, East Germany, to Nana Kofi Donkor, Techiman, n.d. (copy in author's possession).
46. Nana Kofi Effa traveled to the United States with Michael Warren and Sr. Elaine Khol of the Medical Mission Sisters and the HFH to present a conference paper on the PRHETIH (ca. 1981). He stayed at the Medical Mission Sisters's North American headquarters in Philadelphia. S. Elaine Khols, email message to author, 20–21 August 2013.
47. Warren et al., "Ghanaian National Policy Towards Indigenous Healers," 18.
48. Nana Kofi Dɔnkɔ Collection: S. Oduro-Sarpong, field Coordinator PRHETIH, "Fact Sheet: Primary Health Training for Indigenous Healers (PRHETIH) Project. Holy Family Hospital," April 1991, 1–2 (copy in author's possession).
49. S. Elaine Khols, email message to author, 21 August 2013. Sr. Elaine Khols joined the Medical Mission Sisters in 1955 at age eighteen. Her first overseas assignment was to Ghana and the HFH hospitals in Berekum and Takyiman; she spent two years in the former and thirteen years in the latter location (i.e., 1970–83). She left Ghana for Ethiopia in 1984.
50. Interview with Nana Kwasi Appiah, Saase, Ashanti region, 27 September 2012.
51. Warren et al., "Ghanaian National Policy Towards Indigenous Healers," 12.
52. Warren et al., "Ghanaian National Policy Towards Indigenous Healers," 14.
53. Warren et al., "Ghanaian National Policy Towards Indigenous Healers," 21, 24.
54. Warren et al., "Ghanaian National Policy Towards Indigenous Healers," 4.
55. HFH, Techiman, Annual Report 1981.
56. HFH, Techiman, Annual Report 1981, 2.
57. HFH, Techiman, Annual Report 1981, 1.
58. HFH, Techiman, Annual Report 1981, 3.
59. *Study Guide for the film Bono Medicines* (Lone Rock, IA: Scott Dodds Productions, 1982), 1 [part 1] (emphasis added).

60. *Bono Medicines*, 3 (part 1).
61. *Bono Medicines*, 2 (part 2).
62. *Bono Medicines*, 2 (part 2).
63. *Bono Medicines*, 6 (part 2).
64. *Bono Medicines*, 9 (part 2).
65. *Bono Medicines*, 2 (part 2).
66. Conversation with Sister Elaine Kohls, electronic communication, 21 August 2013. She believes that the "young healer" in her story was Nana Kofi Effa, Nana Kofi Dɔnkɔ's son, but this is speculation for now: "Yes, I think the healer who went with us to the States may have been Kofi Dɔnkɔ's son. He certainly was younger."
67. Interview with Yaa Kɔmfo, Essienimpong, Ashanti region, 24 March 2012.
68. Samuel Gyanfosu, "A Traditional Religion Reformed: Vincent Kwabena Damuah and the Afrikania Movement, 1982–2000," in *Christianity and the African Imagination: Essays in Honour of Adrian Hastings*, ed. David Maxwell and Ingrid Lawrie (Boston: Brill, 2002), 271–72. See also Marleen de Witte, "Afrikania's Dilemma: Reframing African Authenticity in a Christian Public Sphere," *Etnofoor* 17, nos. 1–2 (2004): 133–55; Marleen de Witte, "Neo-traditional Religions," in *The Wiley-Blackwell Companion to African Religions*, ed. Elias Kifon Bongmba (Oxford: John Wiley, 2012), 173–83.
69. Kwabena Damuah, *Miracle at the Shrine* (Accra: Afrikania Mission, 1990), 11, 54, 64.
70. Damuah, *Miracle at the Shrine*, 14.
71. Nana Kofi Dɔnkɔ Collection: Bye-Laws for the welfare of the members of Afrikania Mission—Techiman district branch, n.d., 2.
72. Bye-Laws for the welfare of the members of Afrikania Mission, 1.
73. Bye-Laws for the welfare of the members of Afrikania Mission, 1.
74. Gerrie Ter Haar, "A Wondrous God: Miracles in Contemporary Africa," *African Affairs* 102 (2003): 423; Damuah, *Miracle at the Shrine*, 99. Damuah completed his doctoral dissertation on religion in Wassa in the Department of African Studies at Howard University in 1971. Gyanfosu claims that Damuah obtained his PhD in theology. Damuah is also a founding member of the PNDC under Jerry Rawlings, and was a PNDC member before he resigned to take charge of his religious movement.
75. Damuah, *Miracle at the Shrine*, 99.
76. Haar, "A Wondrous God," 424.
77. Haar, "A Wondrous God," 425.
78. Gyanfosu, "A Traditional Religion Reformed," 284.
79. "Osofo Komfo Kove Is New Head of Afrikania Religion," GhanaWeb, 25 April 2004, access 22 September 2015, http://www.ghanaweb.com/GhanaHomePage/economy/artikel.php?ID=56619/.
80. The Afrikania movement/mission claims 4 million followers, according to the U.S. Department of State "International Religious Freedom Report 2003: Ghana," accessed 22 September 2015, http://www.state.gov/g/drl/rls/irf/2003/23710.htm/. No mention is made of Afrikania in the 2013 and subsequent versions of this report.

CHAPTER 7. **UNCERTAIN MOMENTS AND MEMORY**

1. Cited in Kwame Akonor, *Africa and IMF Conditionality: The Unevenness of Compliance, 1983–2000* (New York: Routledge, 2013), 72. See also Ransford E. V. Gyampo, "Student Activism and Democratic Quality in Ghana's Fourth Republic," *Journal of Student Affairs in Africa* 1, nos. 1–2 (2013): 49–66; John L. Adedeji, "The Legacy of J. J. Rawlings in Ghanaian Politics," *African Studies Quarterly* 5, no. 2 (2001): 1–27.

2. See "Ghana: Roots of Student Protest," *West Africa*, 6 June 1983, 1343–45.

3. Peter Blackburn, "Coup-prone Ghana: Once-rising African Star Fades," *Christian Science Monitor*, 21 June 1983, accessed 22 September 2015, http://www.csmonitor.com/1983/0621/062150.html.

4. *Travel Account for the Film Bono Medicines* (Lone Rock, IA: Scott Dodds Productions, 1982), 3.

5. Peter Easton, "From 'Sacrilege' to Sustainability: Reforestation and Organic Farming in Forikrom, Ghana," *IK Notes*, no. 4 (January 1999): 1.

6. This episode about Nana Dɔnkɔ's land and farming in 1983 is based on a set of conversations—rather than formal interviews—with Kofi Sakyi Sapɔn and his family in July 2009 and again in January 2011.

7. Holy Family Hospital, Techiman, Annual Report 1983, 1.

8. Holy Family Hospital, Techiman, Annual Report 1983, 4.

9. Holy Family Hospital, Techiman, Annual Report 1983, 6.

10. Holy Family Hospital, Techiman, Annual Report 1983, 5.

11. Mirjam C. Manni, "Local Ideas and Practices in Relation with Anaemia and the Nutrition-Pattern in the Techiman-District (Ghana)" (master's thesis, University of Leiden, 1996), 173.

12. For more on these committees, see, for instance, Kevin Shillington, *Ghana and the Rawlings Factor* (New York: St. Martin's Press, 1992); Naomi Chazan, "Ghana: Problems of Governance and the Emergence of Civil Society," in *Democracy in Developing Countries: Africa*, vol. 2, ed. Larry Diamond, Iuan I. Linz, and Seymour M. Lipset (Boulder, CO: Lynne Rienner Publishers, 1988); Colin Legum, ed., *Africa Contemporary Record: Annual Survey and Documents 1984–1985* (London: Africana Publishing, 1986).

13. Holy Family Hospital, Techiman, Annual Report 1985, 4.

14. Nana Kofi Dɔnkɔ Collection: Letter from Nana Kofi Donkor, Techiman, to the Controller of Posts, P&T Corporation, Kumase, 28 May 1985 (copy in author's possession).

15. Holy Family Hospital, Techiman, Annual Report 1985, 1.

16. Interview with Kofi Sakyi Sapɔn, Yaw Badu, and Afia Takyiwaa, Takyiman township, 13–14 June 2015.

17. Holy Family Hospital, Techiman, Annual Report 1985, 1.

18. According to HFH records, the general outpatient department attendance for 1985 was 65,346, or 250 outpatients per day. Both yearly and daily totals were down 17 percent compared to those in the previous year. See Holy Family Hospital, Techiman, Annual Report 1985, 7, 21.

19. Holy Family Hospital, Techiman, Annual Report 1985, 11.
20. Holy Family Hospital, Techiman, Annual Report 1986, 4.
21. Holy Family Hospital, Techiman, Annual Report 1985, 15.
22. Holy Family Hospital, Techiman, Annual Report 1985, 16.
23. Holy Family Hospital, Techiman, Annual Report 1985, 19.
24. Nana Kofi Dɔnkɔ Collection: S. Oduro-Sarpong, "Primary Health Training for Indigenous Healers (PRHETIH) Project. Holy Family Hospital," April 1991, unpublished document, 1 (copy in author's possession).
25. Holy Family Hospital, Techiman, Annual Report 1985, 4.
26. Holy Family Hospital, Techiman, Annual Report 1985, 2.
27. Holy Family Hospital, Techiman, Annual Report 1985, 6
28. Conversation with Sister Therese Tindirugamu, electronic communication, 11 January 2012.
29. Conversation with Sister Therese Tindirugamu, electronic communication, 15 January 2012.
30. Holy Family Hospital, Techiman, Annual Report 1985, 9.
31. Holy Family Hospital, Techiman, Annual Report 1986, 6.
32. Holy Family Hospital, Techiman, Annual Report 1986, 4.
33. Holy Family Hospital, Techiman, Annual Report 1986, 5, 8. Many children who get measles also get malaria.
34. Holy Family Hospital, Techiman, Annual Report 1986, 7.
35. *Travel Account for the Film Bono Medicines*, 5. The sacrificial use of goat is inaccurate. Asubɔnten Kwabena taboo goat, and so the visitor misidentified the animal used.
36. *Travel Account for the Film Bono Medicines*, 5–6.
37. *Travel Account for the Film Bono Medicines*, 6.
38. *Travel Account for the Film Bono Medicines*, 13–14.
39. *Travel Account for the Film Bono Medicines*, 7.
40. Interview with N. Kofi Donkor, Techiman, 20 April 1980, conducted by Raymond Silverman.
41. Interview with Nana Kwaku Sakyi, Miami, Florida, 14 June 2012.
42. Nana Kofi Dɔnkɔ Collection: "Kofi Donkor Herbalist Clinic Nyafoma—Techiman B.A.," unpublished record books. I have transcribed both books and created a Microsoft Excel file compiling data from each. The statistical analysis that appears in this section of the book derives from these files. These data sets are in my possession.
43. Nana Kofi Dɔnkɔ Collection: Ghana Psychic and Traditional Healers Association's Certificate of Competence and Authority (registered no. 3377) to "Oduyefo—Okomfo Kofi Donkor," 1988 (copy in author's possession).
44. Copies of the certificate and card are in the author's possession.
45. Funeral announcement for Akosua Antwiwaa, 15 December 1984 (copy in author's possession). Kofi Dɔnkɔ or a scribe dated the events in his life on the back of these announcement cards, which are not the same as the date of the actual funeral. I have used the date for the actual funeral, and this dating system applies to all such cards.
46. Funeral announcement for Kwadwo Krah, 15 November 1980 (copy in author's possession).

47. Invitation and program for Mr. J. K. Tuffour, 2 September 1990 (copy in author's possession).
48. Holy Family Hospital, Techiman, Annual Report 1990, 13.
49. Holy Family Hospital, Techiman, Annual Report 1990, 8.
50. Holy Family Hospital, Techiman, Annual Report 1990, 2, 15.
51. Holy Family Hospital, Techiman, Annual Report 1990, 15–16, 18.
52. Margaret Yeakel-Twum, "Medicinal Plants and Traditional Healers in Ghana, West Africa," unpublished paper, University of Minnesota, 1991, 9.
53. Yeakel-Twum, "Medicinal Plants," 12.
54. Yeakel-Twum, "Medicinal Plants," 13.
55. Yeakel-Twum, "Medicinal Plants," 13.
56. Yeakel-Twum, "Medicinal Plants," 14.
57. Nana Kofi Dɔnkɔ Collection: Letter from Nana Kofi Donkor to [unnamed], Techiman, 22 December 1991.
58. Interview with Nana Kwasi Appiah, Takyiman, 25 December 2001; interview with Nana Kwasi Owusu, Takyiman, 25 December 2001.
59. Oduro-Sarpong, "Primary Health Training for Indigenous Healers (PRHETIH) Project," 1.
60. The certificate received by healers who completed the PRHETIH program was standardized and only the name of each recipient changed. The back of each had the following:

> This traditional medical practitioner has taken part in a 15 week training programme including the following topics:
> The traditional medical practitioner in primary health care.
> The hygienic preparation and storage of medicinal herbs.
> The work of the health inspector [and]/worms, mosquitos, flies and the spread of disease. The importance of proper and well-maintained latrines, proper disposal of garbage and clean houses and surroundings.
> The work of the medical field unit (M.O.H.). How to give a traditional immunization hygienically.
> The causes, symptoms and prevention of typhoid and cholera/diarrhea, dehydration and rehydration
> Measles. How to protect children against measles and serious complications such as convulsions, pneumonia and malnutrition.
> Basic nutrition, including the three main food groups—body-building foods, foods that help to prevent disease, and energy-giving foods. Prevention of Kwashiorkor, marasmus and night-blindness.
> Preservation of medicinal herbs in liquid form.
> Sexually transmitted diseases. The causes, types, symptoms and prevention
> Basic family planning
> First solid food for babies who are 4 or more months old, and who need to start taking food besides mother's milk.
> Basic first aid for bleeding, snakes' bites, dog bites and convulsions.

Leprosy. The cause, mode of transmission, and early diagnosis/recognition.
Safe dosages for medicinal herbs.
Primary health care and community development.

This is *not* a license. It is a certificate showing that this traditional medical practitioner has taken part in a continuous cooperative training programme in the Techiman district, Brong-Ahafo region, Ghana. All questions should be addressed to the coordinator, PRHETIH Project, c/o Holy Family Hospital, P. O. Box 36, Takyiman. See the Nana Kofi Dɔnkɔ Collection: Nana Kwaku Buadu's PRHETIH program handbook and certificate, n.d.

61. Oduro-Sarpong, "Primary Health Training for Indigenous Healers (PRHETIH) Project," 2.

62. For a mid-twentieth-century report on the Dagomba as a "warring tribe," see Arthur W. Davies, "The History and Organization of the 'Kambonse' in Dagomba," June 1948, MSS. Afr. s. 189, Bodleian Library of Commonwealth and African Studies at Rhodes House (Weston Library), Oxford University.

63. On the 1994 conflict see Benjamin Talton, *Politics of Social Change in Ghana: The Konkomba Struggle for Political Equality* (New York: Palgrave Macmillan, 2010); Artur Bogner, "The 1994 Civil War in Northern Ghana: The Genesis and Escalation of a 'Tribal' Conflict," in *Ethnicity in Ghana: The Limits of Invention*, ed. Carola Lentz and Paul Nugent (New York: Palgrave Macmillian, 2000), 183–203.

64. Holy Family Hospital, Techiman, Annual Report 1994, 13.

65. Holy Family Hospital, Techiman, Annual Report 1994, 3.

66. Holy Family Hospital, Techiman, Annual Report 1994, 3, 20.

67. Holy Family Hospital, Techiman, Annual Report 1990, 5; Holy Family Hospital, Techiman, Annual Report 1994, 5.

68. Holy Family Hospital, Techiman, Annual Report 1994, 7, 12, 18.

69. Holy Family Hospital, Techiman, Annual Report 1994, 6, 12, 15–16 (quotation). For a critique of the PRHETIH program and of healers as partners in health delivery systems, see PeterVentevogel, *Whiteman's Things: Training and Detraining Healers in Ghana* (Amsterdam: Het Spinhuis, 1996), 54, 95, 118, 123, 137.

70. Holy Family Hospital, Techiman, Annual Report 1994, 19.

71. Holy Family Hospital, Techiman, Annual Report 1994, 9.

72. Interview with Kofi Sakyi Sapɔn and family, July 2009, January 2011.

73. Interview with Nana Yaw Mensa, Takyiman township, 22 December 2001.

74. Interview with Nana Kofi Ɔboɔ, Takyiman township, 10 December 2002.

75. Kofi Sakyi Sapɔn Collection: "Asubonten annual Kwabena festival," 16 September 1998 (unpublished notebook).

76. IRB—Immigration and Refugee Board of Canada: Krotia Royal Family at Tuobodom . . . [GHA34834.E], 13 July 2000, accessed 17 October 2015, http://www.ecoi.net/local_link/177052/279273_en.html/.

77. U.S. Department of State, "Ghana Country Report on Human Rights Practices for 1996," Bureau of Democracy, Human Rights and Labor, 30 January 1997 (accessed 17 October 2015, https://1997-2001.state.gov/global/human_rights/1996_hrp_report

/ghana.html); Napoleon Abdulai, ed., *Ghana, the Kume Preko Demonstrations: Poverty, Corruption and the Rawlings Dictatorship* (London: Africa Research and Information Bureau, 1995); "Ghana: Kume Preko—Kill Me Now," *Africa Confidential Magazine*, 26 May 1995.

78. Holy Family Hospital, Techiman, Annual Report 1996, 4.

79. Holy Family Hospital, Techiman, Annual Report 1996, 4, 8, 31.

80. Nana Kofi Dɔnkɔ Collection: Celebration of Life of the Late Nana Okomfo Akua Asantewa Funerary Program, n.d. (copy in author's possession).

EPILOGUE

1. For more on Nkrumah and his use of Ghana to fulfill his vision of African unity, see Lansiné Kaba, *Kwame Nkrumah and the Dream of African Unity* (New York: Diasporic Africa Press, 2017).

2. Kwasi Konadu and Clifford Campbell, eds., *The Ghana Reader: History, Culture, Politics* (Durham, NC: Duke University Press, 2016), 262 (emphasis added).

3. Nancy Shoemaker, "A Typology of Colonialism," *Perspectives on History* 53, no. 7 (2015): 29–30.

4. See https://www.judicial.gov.gh/index.php/fundamental-human-rights-and-freedom (accessed 25 December 2015).

5. See David Sehat, *The Myth of American Religious Freedom* (New York: Oxford University Press, 2011); Pew Research Center, "Global Religious Diversity: Half of the Most Religiously Diverse Countries are in Asia-Pacific Region," 4 April 2014, accessed 25 December 2015, http://www.pewforum.org/2014/04/04/global-religious-diversity/.

BIBLIOGRAPHY

ARCHIVAL SOURCES

ENGLAND

Royal Anthropological Institute Library, London
Robert Sutherland Rattray Papers, MS 106
　University of Birmingham, Special Collections, Birmingham
Field Notes made by Kofi Antubam, MS 598
　Oxford University, Bodleian Library of Commonwealth and African Studies (Weston Library), Oxford
　MSS. Afr. s. 189
　MSS. Afr. s. 454
　MSS. Afr. s. 506
　MSS. Afr. s. 576
　MSS. Afr. s. 793
　MSS. Afr. s. 845
　MSS. Afr. s. 1051
　MSS. Afr. s. 1064.
　MSS. Afr. s. 1204(2)
　MSS. Afr. s. 1368
　MSS. Afr. s. 1447
　MSS. Afr. s. 1856
　MSS. Afr. s. 2276
　MSS. Brit. Emp. s. 282
　MSS. Perham/MSS. Afr. s. 1204(1)

University of London, SOAS Library, Archives and Special Collections, London
Notes of E. D. Roberts, MS 380326
Frederick William Migeod Papers, PP MS 59
The National Archives, Kew, Colonial Office (CO), War Office (WO)
  CO 96/358/26
  CO 96/358/26
  CO 96/677/12
  CO 96/785/3–4
  CO 96/813/12
  CO 96/814/1
  CO 879/120/6
  CO 879/19
  CO 879/39
  CO 879/45
  CO 879/48
  CO 879/67
  CO 885/23/14
  CO 885/58
  CO 1069/42/89
  WO 287/6

SWITZERLAND

The Basel Mission Archives, Basel, Switzerland
  D-10-2-6, *Gottesnamen der Twi-Neger der Goldküste*, n.d.
  D-10-4-1, *Sagen der Akwapim-Neger über die Erschaffung der Welt, Entstehung der Fetische*, n.d.
  D-10-4-3a, *Der Cultus der Bewohner der Goldküste West-Afrika*
  D-5-9-1, *Chronicle of the Basel Mission Out-Station in Nkoransa, 1911–1920*
  D-4-2-1, Carl B. Huppenbauer, *Annual Report [for] 1931/32*, 1932
  D-4-6-2, *Huppenbauer vor Komitee*, 14 February 1934
  D-18-82-10, Letter from Wilhelm Rottmann, Akropong, ca. 1902–3
  E-10-34-36, *Heidnische Gebete und darin enthaltene Spuren einer reineren monotheistischen Gotteserkenntnis*, n.d.
  PS1-B05-03-10198, Hans Meister, *Spital Agogo. Erste Eindrücke, Gedanken und Vorschläge*, 22 April 1952

GHANA

Public Records and Archives Administration Department of Ghana (PRAAD), Brong-Ahafo Regional Archives (BRG), Sunyani
  BRG 1/10/3
  BRG 1/10/4
  BRG 1/10/5
  BRG 1/12/112

BRG 1/12/122
BRG 1/2/8
BRG 1/2/105
BRG 1/2/106
BRG 1/2/122
BRG 2/1/3
BRG 2/1/10
BRG 2/1/33
BRG 2/2/19
BRG 2/2/41
BRG 2/2/44
BRG 2/2/45
BRG 28/1/23
BRG 28/1/31
BRG 28/1/32
BRG 28/2/3
BRG 28/2/7
BRG 28/2/45
BRG 28/13/1
BRG 28/14/7
BRG 28/16/4
BRG 9/1/1
BRG 9/1/3
BRG 9/1/13
BRG 9/1/16
BRG 9/1/19
BRG 9/1/29
BRG 9/1/44
BRG 9/1/58
BRG 9/2/1
BRG 9/2/8
BRG 9/2/11
BRG 9/2/12
BRG 28/2/19
PRAAD, Colonial Secretary's Office (CSO), Accra
CSO 11/1/677, 10 April 1930
CSO 11/1/677, 13 April 1939
CSO 11/1/677, 30 May 1939
CSO 11/1/679, 20 May 1935
CSO 11/1/679, 23 August 1938
PRAAD, Ashanti Regional Archives (ARG), Kumase
ARG 1/3/3/40, December 1927
ARG 1/30/1/18, n.d.
Manhyia Archives (MAG), Kumase

MAG 1/2/2/36, Nana Kwasi Twi—Omanhene of Techiman, the Elders and the Paramount Stool of Techiman vrs. Nana Osei Agyeman Prempeh II—The Asantehene on Behalf of the Golden Stool of Asante, 1947

MAG 1/2/225, Techiman Native Affairs (Kwaku Gyamfi vrs. Kojo Berkor per Wusuansah), 1948–1951

Holy Family Hospital Records Office, Takyiman
Holy Family Hospital, Takyiman, Annual Report 1976
Holy Family Hospital, Takyiman, Annual Report 1977
Holy Family Hospital, Takyiman, Annual Report 1978
Holy Family Hospital, Takyiman, Annual Report 1981
Holy Family Hospital, Takyiman, Annual Report 1983
Holy Family Hospital, Takyiman, Annual Report 1985
Holy Family Hospital, Takyiman, Annual Report 1986
Holy Family Hospital, Takyiman, Annual Report 1990
Holy Family Hospital, Takyiman, Annual Report 1994
Holy Family Hospital, Takyiman, Annual Report 1995

UNITED STATES

Archives of Traditional Music, Indiana University, Bloomington
Bosomfoo Kofi Donkor, Techiman, 1970, OT-2529, tape 23, side 1, Ghana, Brong-Ahafo region, Techiman Traditional State, Bono-Akan, 1969–1971 (sound recording), collected by Dennis Michael Warren and Owusu Brempong, accession number 720249-F
Bosomfoo Kofi Kyereme, Techiman, [date inaudible] September 1970, OT-2529, tape 23, side 2, Ghana, Brong-Ahafo region, Techiman Traditional State, Bono-Akan, 1969–1971 (sound recording), collected by Dennis Michael Warren and Owusu Brempong, accession number 720249-F
Okomfoo Adwoa Akumsaa, Techiman, 15 February 1970, OT-2529, tape 36, side 1, Ghana, Brong-Ahafo region, Techiman Traditional State, Bono-Akan, 1969–1971 (sound recording), collected by Dennis Michael Warren and Owusu Brempong, accession number 720249-F
Schlesinger Library, Radcliffe Institute, Harvard University, Cambridge, MA
Black Women Oral History Project, Interviews, 24–25 May 1978. OH-31, T-32/Abna Aggrey Lancaster
Special Collections Department, Iowa State University Library, Ames
Dennis M. Warren Papers, RS 13/32/52
Rockefeller University Archives, New York
Hideyo Noguchi Papers, Rockefeller Institute for Medical Research Scientific Staff, FA121 (formerly 450 N689)
Special Collections Department, University of Iowa Libraries, Iowa City
Warren Collection, MsC 538

UNPUBLISHED COLLECTIONS

Kofi Sakyi Sapɔn Collection, Takyiman, Ghana, in private hands
Nana Kofi Dɔnkɔ Collection, Takyiman, Ghana, in private hands
Nana Kwaku Sakyi Collection, Miami, Florida, in private hands

INTERVIEWS

All interviews were conducted by author unless otherwise noted.
Akomaa, Ama, Takyiman township, 22 September 2012
Amoah, Kwasi Amponsah Nkron, Takyiman township, 18 September 2012
Appiah, Kwasi, Saase, Ashanti region, 27 September 2012
Appiah, Kwasi, Takyiman township, 25 December 2001
Asamoaa, Adwoa, Takyiman township, 28 March 2012
Asantewaa, Akua, Takyiman township, 21 December 2001
Atta, Kofi, Takyiman township, 10 December 2002
Donkor, Kofi, interview by Raymond Silverman, Techiman, 20 April 1980
Dwomo II, Tanɔboasehene Amisare, interview by Kofi Sakyi Sapɔn, Tanɔboase, 12 October 1997
Kɔmfo, Yaa, Essienimpong, Ashanti region, 24 March 2012
Kyerere, Kofi, Takyiman township, 13 December 2002
Mensa, Yaw, Takyiman township, 22 December 2001
Nyarko, Kwadwo, Osei Yaw, Kwabena Adjei, Kwadwo Afram, and Kwame Yeboah, interview by Kofi Sakyi Sapɔn, Amangoase village, Takyiman, 27 October 1997
Ɔboɔ, Kofi, Takyiman township, 10 December 2002
Ɔboɔ, Kofi, Takyiman township, 27 March 2012
Owusu, Kofi, Pomakrom (Takyiman township), 18 December 2002
Owusu, Kwasi, Nkukua Buoho, Kumase, 22 March 2012
Owusu, Kwasi, Takyiman township, 25 December 2001
Sakyi, Kwaku, Miami, Florida, 1 March 2009 and 14 June 2012
Sapɔn, Kofi Sakyi, Takyiman township, 22 December 2001
Sapɔn, Kofi Sakyi, and family, July 2009 and January 2011
Sapɔn, Kofi Sakyi, Yaw Badu, and Afia Takyiwaa, Takyiman township, 13–14 June 2015

PUBLISHED SOURCES

AKAN/TWI LANGUAGE SOURCES

Addow, E. R. *Edin ne Mmrane*. Accra: Bureau of Ghana Languages, 1969.
Adi, Kwabena. *Mewɔ bi ka*. Accra: Bureau of Ghana Languages, 1975.
Ahene-Affoh. *Ɔdɔ Asaawa*. Accra: Bureau of Ghana Languages, 1973.
Ahene-Affoh. *Twi Kasakoa ne Kasatɔmme*. Tema: Ghana Publishing Corp., 1976.
Akuffo, B. S. *Tete Akorae*. Accra: Bureau of Ghana Languages, 1970.
Akuffo, B. S. *Ahemfi Adesua (Akanfoɔ Amammerɛ)*, vol. 1. Exeter, UK: James Townsend and Sons, 1950.
Amoako, B. O. *Ɛnnɛ nso bio*. Accra: Bureau of Ghana Languages, 1976.

Ampene, Kwame. *Ateteswm*. Accra: Waterville Publishing House, 1975.
Annobil, J. A. *Nana Bosompo*. Cape Coast: Methodist Book Depot, 1947.
Anti, A. A. *Obeedé*. Accra: Bureau of Ghana Languages, 1969.
Arthur, Cecilia. *Akanfoɔ Amammerɛ ho Adusua 1*. Kumasi: n.p., 2003.
Bannerman, J. Yedu. *Mfantse Akan Mbɛbusɛm*. Accra: Bureau of Ghana Languages, 1974.
Blankson, Samuel. *Fetu Afahye*. Cape Coast: University Press, 1973.
Brantuo, J. Kwasi. *Asetena mu Anwonsɛm*. Accra: Bureau of Ghana Languages, 1966.
Darka, E. M. Adu. *Akanfoɔ Anwonsɛm Bi*. Tema: Ghana Publishing, 1973.
Donkoh, C. E. *Aduse-Poku Kɔnkɔnko*. Accra: Bureau of Ghana Languages, 1973.
Donkoh, C. E., *Ghana Afahyɛ hodoɔ bi*. Accra: Bureau of Ghana Languages, 1969.
Efa, Edwin. *Asiemiri*. London: Macmillan, 1950.
Fianko, Safori. *Twifo Amammuisɛm*. London: Macmillan, 1958.
Hanson, Immanuel A. "Asantefo Atetesem Osantehene Poku Ware ne Takyimanhene Amo Yaw ntam' asem bi," *Christian Reporter for the Natives of the Gold Coast Speaking the Tshi or Asante Language* 1, no. 13 (January–March 1895): 101–16.
Kani, Thomas Yao. *Akanfoɔ Amammerɛ*. Accra: Bureau of Ghana Languages, 1962.
Kani, Thomas Yao. *Bansofo Akan Kasa mu Kasapo*. New York: Longmans, Green, 1953.
Kisi, Ɔbɔadum. *Ɔba Nyansafoɔ*. Accra: Bureau of Ghana Languages, 1974.
Kwaffo, S. J. *Fa bi Sie*. Accra: Bureau of Ghana Languages, 1997.
Langon, J. E. *Ekuayɛ pa*. Accra: Bureau of Ghana Languages, 1963.
Mensah, J. E. *Asantesɛm ne Mmɛbusɛm bi*. Kumasi: Author, 1966.
Nketia, J. H. Kwabena. *Abɔfodwom*. Tema: Ghana Publishing, 1973.
Nketia, J. H. Kwabena. *Akwansosɛm bi*. Legon: Institute of African Studies, University of Ghana, 1967.
Nketia, J. H. Kwabena. *Ayan*. Tema: Ghana Publishing, 1974.
Ofei-Ayisi. *Twi Mmebusem wɔ Akuapem Twi mu*. Accra: Waterville Publishing House, 1966.
Opoku, A. A. *Mo Ahenewa*. Accra: Bureau of Ghana Languages, 1975.
Opoku, A. A. *Mpanyinsɛm*. Accra: Waterville Publishing House, 1969.
Opoku, A. A. *Obi Kyerɛ*. Tema: Ghana Publishing, 1973.
Otoo, S. K., and A. C. Denteh. *Abɔe*. Accra: Bureau of Ghana Languages, 1970.
Yɛboa-Dankwa, J. *Tete wɔ bi Kyerɛ*. Accra: Bureau of Ghana Languages, 1973.

COLONIAL REPORTS

Colonial Report—Annual. No. 189. Gold Coast. Report for 1895. London: Her Majesty's Stationery Office, 1896.
Colonial Report—Annual. No. 220. Gold Coast. Report for 1896. London: Her Majesty's Stationery Office, 1897.
Colonial Report—Annual. No. 249. Gold Coast. Report for 1897. London: Her Majesty's Stationery Office, 1898.
Colonial Report—Annual. No. 271. Gold Coast. Report for 1898. London: Her Majesty's Stationery Office, 1899.
Colonial Report—Annual. No. 306. Gold Coast. Report for 1899. London: Her Majesty's Stationery Office, 1900.

Colonial Report—Annual. No. 344. Gold Coast. Report for 1900. London: Her Majesty's Stationery Office, 1901.
Colonial Report—Annual. No. 375. Gold Coast. Report for 1901. London: Her Majesty's Stationery Office, 1902.
Colonial Report—Annual. No. 397. Gold Coast. Report for 1902. London: Her Majesty's Stationery Office, 1903.
Colonial Report—Annual. No. 426. Gold Coast. Report for 1903. London: Her Majesty's Stationery Office, 1904.
Colonial Report—Annual. No. 465. Gold Coast. Report for 1904. London: Her Majesty's Stationery Office, 1905.
Colonial Report—Annual. No. 488. Gold Coast. Report for 1905. London: Her Majesty's Stationery Office, 1906.
Colonial Report—Annual. No. 534. Gold Coast. Report for 1906. London: Her Majesty's Stationery Office, 1907.
Colonial Report—Annual. No. 573. Gold Coast. Report for 1907. London: Her Majesty's Stationery Office, 1908.
Colonial Report—Annual. No. 613. Gold Coast. Report for 1908. London: Her Majesty's Stationery Office, 1909.
Colonial Report—Annual. No. 654. Gold Coast. Report for 1909. London: Her Majesty's Stationery Office, 1910.
Colonial Report—Annual. No. 688. Gold Coast. Report for 1910. London: Her Majesty's Stationery Office, 1911.
Colonial Report—Annual. No. 725. Gold Coast. Report for 1911. London: Her Majesty's Stationery Office, 1912.
Colonial Report—Annual. No. 770. Gold Coast. Report for 1912. London: Her Majesty's Stationery Office, 1913.
Colonial Report—Annual. No. 806. Gold Coast. Report for 1913. London: Her Majesty's Stationery Office, 1914.
Colonial Report—Annual. No. 859. Gold Coast. Report for 1914. London: Her Majesty's Stationery Office, 1915.
Colonial Report—Annual. No. 894. Gold Coast. Report for 1915. London: Her Majesty's Stationery Office, 1916.
Colonial Report—Annual. No. 948. Gold Coast. Report for 1916. London: Her Majesty's Stationery Office, 1917.
Colonial Report—Annual. No. 998. Gold Coast. Report for 1917. London: Her Majesty's Stationery Office, 1918.
Colonial Report—Annual. No. 1029. Gold Coast. Report for 1918. London: Her Majesty's Stationery Office, 1919.
Colonial Report—Annual. No. 1066. Gold Coast. Report for 1919. London: Her Majesty's Stationery Office, 1920.
Colonial Report—Annual. No. 1119. Gold Coast. Report for 1920. London: Her Majesty's Stationery Office, 1921.
Colonial Report—Annual. No. 1154. Gold Coast. Report for 1921. London: Her Majesty's Stationery Office, 1922.

Colonial Report—Annual. No. 1207. Gold Coast. Report for 1922–3. London: Her Majesty's Stationery Office, 1924.
Colonial Report—Annual. No. 1255. Gold Coast. Report for 1923–4. London: Her Majesty's Stationery Office, 1925.
Colonial Report—Annual. No. 1333. Gold Coast. Report for 1925–6. London: Her Majesty's Stationery Office, 1926.
Colonial Report—Annual. No. 1386. Gold Coast. Report for 1926–7. London: Her Majesty's Stationery Office, 1927.
Colonial Report—Annual. No. 1418. Gold Coast. Report for 1927–8. London: Her Majesty's Stationery Office, 1929.
Colonial Report—Annual. No. 1464. Gold Coast. Report for 1928–9. London: Her Majesty's Stationery Office, 1929.
Colonial Report—Annual. No. 1504. Gold Coast. Report for 1929–30. London: Her Majesty's Stationery Office, 1930.
Colonial Report—Annual. No. 1559. Gold Coast. Report for 1930–31. London: Her Majesty's Stationery Office, 1932.
Colonial Report—Annual. No. 1602. Gold Coast. Report for 1931–2. London: Her Majesty's Stationery Office, 1933.
Colonial Report—Annual. No. 1657. Gold Coast. Report for 1932–3. London: Her Majesty's Stationery Office, 1934.
Colonial Report—Annual. No. 1748. Gold Coast. Report for 1934–5. London: Her Majesty's Stationery Office, 1936.
Colonial Report—Annual. No. 1785. Gold Coast. Report for 1935–6. London: Her Majesty's Stationery Office, 1936.
Colonial Report—Annual. No. 1836. Gold Coast. Report for 1936–7. London: Her Majesty's Stationery Office, 1938.
Colonial Report—Annual. No. 1882. Gold Coast. Report for 1937–8. London: Her Majesty's Stationery Office, 1939.
Colonial Report—Annual. No. 1919. Gold Coast. Report for 1938–9. London: Her Majesty's Stationery Office, 1939.

COURT CASES

Akumfi Ameyaw III, Omanhene of Techiman v. Kwasi Safo, United Kingdom Privy Council (UKPC) 36, 22 May 1947, Appeal No. 66 of 1945. London: His Majesty's Stationery Office Press, 1947.
Nana Kwaku Amoah, since deceased (now represented by Yaw Ewuah) and another v. Nana Sir Ofori Atta, UKPC 73, 21 November 1932.
Nana Kwaku Amoah II and Others v. Nana Sir Ofori Atta and Others, Accra, 1 West African Court of Appeal (WACA) 332, 24 November 1933.
Nana Kwaku Amoah II and Others v. Nana Sir Ofori Atta and Others, Accra, 1 WACA 344, 27 November 1933.
Nana Sir Ofori Atta v. Nana Kwaku Amoah, Accra, 1 West African Court of Appeal (WACA) 15, 19 May 1930.

Techimanhene v. Wenchihene, UKPC 42, 9 July 1956, Appeal No. 42 of 1954. London: His Majesty's Stationery Office Press, 1956.

NEWSPAPERS

Gold Coast Independent
Spectator Daily

SECONDARY SOURCES

Abdulai, Napoleon, ed. *Ghana, the Kume Preko Demonstrations: Poverty, Corruption and the Rawlings Dictatorship*. London: Africa Research and Information Bureau, 1995.

Abraham, W. E. *The Mind of Africa*. Chicago: University of Chicago Press, 1962.

Adedeji, John L. "The Legacy of J. J. Rawlings in Ghanaian Politics." *African Studies Quarterly* 5, no. 2 (2001): 1–27.

Adogame, Afeosemime Unuose, Magnus Echtler, and Ulf Vierke, eds. *Unpacking the New: Critical Perspectives on Cultural Syncretization in Africa and Beyond*. Zürich: LIT Verlag Münster, 2008.

Adu-Boahen, Kwabena. "Pawn of Contesting Imperialists: Nkoransa in the Anglo-Asante Rivalry in Northwestern Ghana, 1874–1900." *Journal of Philosophy and Culture* 3, no. 2 (2006): 55–85.

Afriyie, Amos Oppong, Dominic Damoah, Edward Ansong, and Poakwah Gyimah. "A Conceptual Framework for Encouraging Educational Investment through 'Nnoboa' in Ghana." *International Journal of Community and Cooperative Studies* 1, no. 2 (2014): 51–58.

Agyekum, Kofi. "Menstruation as a Verbal Taboo among the Akan of Ghana." *Journal of Anthropological Research* 58, no. 3 (2002): 367–87.

Agyekum, Kofi. "The Sociolinguistic of Akan Personal Names." *Nordic Journal of African Studies* 15, no. 2 (2006): 206–35.

Akamba, Joseph B., and Isidore Kwadwo Tufuor. "The Future of Customary Law in Ghana." In *The Future of African Customary Law*, edited by Jeanmarie Fenrich, Paolo Galizzi, and Tracy E. Higgins, 202–24. New York: Cambridge University Press, 2011.

Akonor, Kwame. *Africa and IMF Conditionality: The Unevenness of Compliance, 1983–2000*. New York: Routledge, 2013.

Akyeampong, Emmanuel. "Asante at the Turn of the Twentieth Century." *Ghana Studies* 3 (2000): 3–12.

Allman, Jean, and John Parker. *Tongnaab: The History of a West African God*. Bloomington: Indiana University Press, 2005.

Allman, Jean M. "The Youngmen and the Porcupine: Class, Nationalism and Asante's Struggle for Self-Determination, 1954–57," *Journal of African History* 31 (1990): 263–79.

Amanor, Kojo. *Land, Labour and the Family in Southern Ghana: A Critique of Land Policy Under Neo-Liberalisation*. Uppsala: Nordic Africa Institute, 2001.

Amponsah, Paulina, Günter Leydecker, and Rolf Muff. "Earthquake Catalogue of Ghana for the Time Period 1615–2003 with Special Reference to the Tectonostructural Evolution of South-east Ghana." *Journal of African Earth Sciences* 75, no. 18 (2012): 1–13.

Antubam, Kofi. *Ghana's Heritage of Culture*. Leipzig: Koehler and Amelang, 1963.

Appiah-Kubi, Kofi. *Man Cures, God Heals: Religion and Medical Practice among the Akan of Ghana*. New York: Friendship Press, 1981.

Appiah-Sekyere, Paul, and Samuel Awuah-Nyamekye. "Teenage Pregnancy in the Life and Thought of the Traditional Akan: Moral Perspectives." *Sociology Study* 2, no. 2 (2012): 129–38.

Arhin, Kwame. "Aspects of Colonial District Administration: The Case of the Northwestern District of Ashanti, 1904–1911." *Research Review* 8, no. 1 (1971): 1–30.

Arhin, Kwame, ed. *The Papers of George Ekem Ferguson: A Fanti Official of the Government of the Gold Coast, 1890–1897*. Leiden, Netherlands: Afrika-Studiecentrum, 1974.

Arhin, Kwame, ed. *A Profile of Brong Kyempim: Essays on the Archaeology, History, Language and Politics of the Brong Peoples of Ghana*. Accra: Afram Publications and the Institute of African Studies, University of Ghana, 1979.

Armah, Ayi Kwei. *The Healers*. London: Heinemann, 1979.

Asad, Talal, ed. *Anthropology and the Colonial Encounter*. Atlantic Highlands, NJ: Humanities Press, 1973.

Asante, Felix Ankomah, and Kwadwo Asenso-Okyere. "Economic Burden of Malaria in Ghana." A technical report submitted to the World Health Organization, African Regional Office, November 2003.

Beckman, Bjorn. *Organising the Farmers: Cocoa Politics and National Development in Ghana*. Uppsala: Scandinavian Institute of African Studies, 1976.

Bening, R. Bagulo. "Internal Colonial Boundary Problems of the Gold Coast, 1907–1951." *International Journal of African Historical Studies* 17, no. 1 (1984): 81–99.

Beutter, Anne. "Church Discipline Chronicled—A New Source for Basel Mission Historiography." *History in Africa* 42 (2015): 109–38.

Blackburn, Peter. "Coup-prone Ghana: Once-rising African Star Fades." *Christian Science Monitor*, 21 June 1983. Accessed 22 September 2015. http://www.csmonitor.com/1983/0621/062150.html/.

Bloom, Peter J., Stephan F. Miescher, and Takyiwaa Manuh, eds. *Modernization as Spectacle in Africa*. Bloomington: Indiana University Press, 2014.

Boahen, A. Adu. *Yaa Asantewaa and the Asante-British War of 1900–1*. Accra: Sub-Saharan Publishers, 2003.

Boahen, A. Adu, E. Akyeampong, N. Lawler, T. C. McCaskie, and Ivor Wilks. *"The History of Ashanti Kings and the Whole Country Itself" and Other Writing by Otumfuo Nana Agyeman Prempeh I*. New York: Oxford University Press, 2003.

Boateng, Otto Ampofo. *Songs for Infant Schools (Twi)*. London: Oxford University Press, 1948.

Bogner, Artur. "The 1994 Civil War in Northern Ghana: The Genesis and Escalation of a 'Tribal' Conflict." In *Ethnicity in Ghana: The Limits of Invention*, edited by Carola Lentz and Paul Nugent, 183–203. New York: Palgrave Macmillian, 2000.

Bosman, Willem. *Nauwkeurige beschryving van de Guinese Goud- Tand- en Slave-kust....* Utrecht, Netherlands: Anthony Schouten, 1704.

Bosman, Willem. *A New and Accurate Description of the Coast of Guinea.* London: J. Knapton, 1705.

Boyd, Herb, and Ilyasah Shabazz, eds. *The Diary of Malcolm X, El-Hajj Malik El-Shabazz, 1964.* Chicago: Third World Press, 2013.

Brempong, Owusu, ed. "Oral Tradition in Ghana: The History of Bonokyempim and Techiman Politics." *Research Review* 13 (1988): 1–73.

Brempong, Owusu, ed. *Oral Tradition in Ghana: The History of Bonokyempim and Techiman Politics.* Legon: Institute of African Studies, University of Ghana, 1998.

Brempong, Owusu. "They Have Used a Broom to Sweep My Womb: The Concept of Witchcraft in Ghana." *Research Review* 12, nos. 1–2 (1996): 42–50.

Campbell, James T. *Songs of Zion: The African Methodist Episcopal Church in the United States and South Africa.* New York: Oxford University Press, 1995.

Cardinal, A. W. *The Gold Coast, 1931.* Accra: Government Printer, 1931.

Carretta, Vincent, and Ty Reese. *The Life and Letters of Philip Quaque, the First African Anglican Missionary.* Athens: University of Georgia Press, 2010.

Catalog of Copyright Entries, Third Series: 1975: January–June. Washington, DC: Copyright Office, Library of Congress, 1976.

Chapman, Charles. *Merchant Enterprise in Britain.* Cambridge: Cambridge University Press, 1992.

Chazan, Naomi. "Ghana: Problems of Governance and the Emergence of Civil Society." In *Democracy in Developing Countries: Africa*, vol. 2, edited by Larry Diamond, Iuan I. Linz, and Seymour M. Lipset, 93–139. Boulder, CO: Lynne Rienner Publishers, 1988.

Christaller, Johann Gottlieb. *A Dictionary of the Asante and Fante Language Called Tshi (Chwee, Twi): With a Grammatical Introduction and Appendices on the Geography of the Gold Coast and Other Subjects.* Basel, Switzerland: Evangelical Missionary Society, 1881.

Coe, Cati. *Dilemmas of Culture in African Schools: Youth, Nationalism, and the Transformation of Knowledge.* Chicago: University of Chicago Press, 2005.

Coe, Cati. "Educating an African Leadership: Achimota and the Teaching of African Culture in the Gold Coast." *Africa Today* 49, no. 3 (2002): 23–46.

Collection of Treaties with Native Chiefs, &c., in West Africa. London: Colonial Office, 1914.

Corner, George Washington. *A History of the Rockefeller Institute, 1901–1953: Origins and Growth.* New York: Rockefeller University Press, 1965.

Crentsil, Perpetual. "Bragoro: A Disappearing Puberty Rite of the Akan of Ghana." *Current Politics and Economics of Africa* 8, no. 2 (2015): 231–57.

Dadson, J. A. "The Need for the Cooperative Reorientation—The Ghana Case." In *Cooperative Revisited*, edited by Hans G. B. Hedlund, 173–86. Uppsala: Nordiska Afrikainstitutet, 1988.

Damuah, Kwabena. *Miracle at the Shrine.* Accra: Afrikania Mission, 1990.

Danquah, Francis K. "Sustaining A West African Cocoa Economy: Agricultural Science and the Swollen Shoot Contagion in Ghana, 1936–1965." *African Economic History* 31 (2003): 43–74.

Danquah, Joseph B. *The Akan Doctrine of God: A Fragment of Gold Coast Ethics and Religion*. London: Cass, 1968.

Debrunner, Hans W. *Witchcraft in Ghana: A Study on the Belief in Destructive Witches and Its Effect on the Akan Tribes*. Accra: Presbyterian Book Depot, 1961.

Depelchin, Jacques. *Silences in African History: Between the Syndromes of Discovery and Abolition*. Dar es Salaam, Tanzania: Mbuki Na Nyoto Publishers, 2005.

Dumett, Raymond E. "The Campaign against Malaria and the Expansion of Scientific Medical and Sanitary Services in British West Africa, 1898–1910." *African Historical Studies* 1, no. 2 (1968): 153–97.

Easton, Peter. "From 'Sacrilege' to Sustainability: Reforestation and Organic Farming in Forikrom, Ghana." *IK Notes*, no. 4 (January 1999): 1–4.

Effah-Gyamfi, Kwaku. "Bono Manso Archeological Research Project, 1973–1976." *West African Journal of Archeology* 9 (1979): 176–86.

Effah-Gyamfi, Kwaku. "Some Archeological Reflections on Akan Traditions of Origin." *West African Journal of Archeology* 9 (1979): 189–94.

Ellis, A. B. *The Tshi-Speaking Peoples of the Gold Coast of West Africa*. Chicago: Benin Press, [1887] 1964.

Ephirim-Donkor, Anthony. *African Spirituality: On Becoming Ancestors*. Trenton, NJ: Africa World Press, 1997.

Feinberg, H. M. "An Eighteenth-Century Case of Plagiarism: William Smith's 'A New Voyage to Guinea.'" *History in Africa* 6 (1979): 45–50.

Field, M. J. *Search for Security: An Ethno-Psychiatric Study of Rural Ghana*. London: Faber and Faber, 1960.

Fink, Deborah R. "Time and Space Measurement of the Bono of Ghana." Master's thesis, Iowa State University, 1974.

Fink, Helga. *Religion, Disease, and Healing in Ghana: A Case Study of Traditional Dormaa Medicine*. Munich: Trickster Wissenschaft, 1990.

Firmin-Sellers, Kathryn. *The Transformation of Property Rights in the Gold Coast: An Empirical Study Applying Rational Choice Theory*. New York: Cambridge University Press, 1996.

Fischer, Friedrich Hermann. *Der Missionsarzt Rudolf Fisch und die Anfänge medizinischer Arbeit der Basler Mission an der Goldküste*. Herzogenrath, Germany: Murken-Altrogge, 1991.

Flight, Colin. "The Chronology of the Kings and Queenmothers of Bono-Manso: A Reevaluation of the Evidence." *Journal of African History* 11, no. 2 (1970): 259–68.

Freeman, Richard. *Travels and Life in Ashanti and Jaman*. New York: Frederick A. Stokes, 1898.

Friedson, Steven M. *Remains of Ritual: Northern Gods in a Southern Land*. Chicago: University of Chicago Press, 2010.

Fuller, Francis. *A Vanished Dynasty: Ashanti*. London: J. Murray, 1921.

Fuller, Harcourt. *Building the Ghanaian Nation-State: Kwame Nkrumah's Symbolic Nationalism*. New York: Palgrave Macmillan, 2014.

Fynn, John K. *Asante and Its Neighbors, 1700–1807*. Evanston, IL: Northwestern University Press, 1971.

Gaines, Kevin K. *American Africans in Ghana: Black Expatriates and the Civil Rights Era.* Chapel Hill: University of North Carolina Press, 2006.
Garrard, Timothy. *Akan Weights and the Gold Trade.* London: Longman, 1980.
"Ghana: Kume Preko—Kill Me Now." *Africa Confidential Magazine,* 26 May 1995.
"Ghana: Roots of Student Protest." *West Africa,* 6 June 1983, 1343–45.
Gocking, Roger S. *The History of Ghana.* Westport, CT: Greenwood Press, 2005.
Gough, Kathleen. "Anthropology and Imperialism." *Monthly Review* 19, no. 11 (1968): 12–24.
Gray, Natasha A. "The Legal History of Witchcraft in Colonial Ghana: Akyem Abuakwa, 1913–1943." PhD dissertation, Columbia University, 2000.
Greenhalgh, P. A. L. *West African Diamonds, 1919–1983: An Economic History.* Manchester, UK: Manchester University Press, 1985.
Grischow, Jeff, and Glenn H. McKnight. "Rhyming Development: Practising Post-development in Colonial Ghana and Uganda." *Journal of Historical Sociology* 16, no. 4 (2003): 517–49.
Grischow, Jeff D. "Tsetse and Trypanosomiasis in the Gold Coast, 1924–1954." Working Papers on Ghana: Historical and Contemporary Studies, no. 5. Helsinki: Institute of Asian and African Studies, University of Helsinki, 2004.
Gyampo, Ransford E. V. "Student Activism and Democratic Quality in Ghana's Fourth Republic." *Journal of Student Affairs in Africa* 1, nos. 1–2 (2013): 49–66.
Gyanfosu, Samuel. "A Traditional Religion Reformed: Vincent Kwabena Damuah and the Afrikania Movement, 1982–2000." In *Christianity and the African Imagination: Essays in Honour of Adrian Hastings,* edited by David Maxwell and Ingrid Lawrie, 271–94. Boston: Brill, 2002.
Gyekye, Kwame. *An Essay on African Philosophical Thought: The Akan Conceptual Scheme.* Philadelphia: Temple University Press, 1995.
Haar, Gerrie Ter. "A Wondrous God: Miracles in Contemporary Africa." *African Affairs* 102 (2003): 409–28.
Hauser-Renner, Heinz. "Examining Text Sediments: Commending a Pioneer Historian as an 'African Herodotus': On the Making of the New Annotated Edition of C. C. Reindorf's 'History of the Gold Coast and Asante.'" *History in Africa* 35 (2008): 231–99.
Henige, David P. *The Chronology of Oral Tradition: Quest for a Chimera.* Oxford: Clarendon Press, 1974.
Hill, Polly. *The Gold Coast Cocoa Farmer: A Preliminary Survey.* London: Oxford University Press, 1956.
Hill, Polly. *Migrant Cocoa-Farmers of Southern Ghana: A Study in Rural Capitalism.* Cambridge: Cambridge University Press, 1963.
Jenkins, Paul. "The Anglican Church in Ghana, 1905–24 (I)." *Transactions of the Historical Society of Ghana* 15, no. 1 (1974): 23–39.
Jenkins, Paul, et al. *Guide to the Basel Mission's Ghana Archives,* 3rd ed. Leipzig, Germany: Institut für Afrikanistik, Universität Leipzig, 2003.
Jones, Geoffrey. *Merchants to Multinationals: British Trading Companies in the Nineteenth and Twentieth Centuries.* New York: Oxford University Press, 2000.

Kaba, Lansiné. *Kwame Nkrumah and the Dream of African Unity*. New York: Diasporic Africa Press, 2017.

Kay, G. B., ed. *The Political Economy of Colonialism in Ghana: A Collection of Documents and Statistics, 1900–1960*. New York: Cambridge University Press, 1972.

Kirby, M. W., and M. B. Rose, eds. *Business Enterprise in Modern Britain from the Eighteenth to the Twentieth Centuries*. London: Routledge, 1994.

Konadu, Kwasi. *The Akan Diaspora in the Americas*. New York: Oxford University Press, 2010.

Konadu, Kwasi. *Akan Pioneers: African Histories, Diasporic Experiences*. New York: Diasporic Africa Press, 2018.

Konadu, Kwasi. "The Calendrical Factor in Akan History." *International Journal of African Historical Studies* 45, no. 2 (2012): 217–46.

Konadu, Kwasi. *Indigenous Medicine and Knowledge in African Society*. New York: Routledge, 2007.

Konadu, Kwasi, and Clifford Campbell, eds. *The Ghana Reader: History, Culture, Politics*. Durham, NC: Duke University Press, 2016.

Kwami, Atta. "Kofi Antubam, 1922–1964: A Modern Ghanaian Artist, Educator, and Writer." In *A Companion to Modern African Art*, edited by Gitti Salami and Monica B. Visonà, 218–36. Malden, MA: Wiley-Blackwell, 2013.

Kyei, T. E. *Marriage and Divorce among the Asante: A Study Undertaken in the Course of the Ashanti Social Survey (1945)*. Cambridge: African Studies Centre, 1992.

Kyei, T. E. *Our Days Dwindle: Memories of My Childhood Days in Asante*, edited and introduction by Jean Allman. Portsmouth, NH: Heinemann, 2001.

Labi, Kwame Amoah. "Afro-Ghanaian Influences in Ghanaian Paintings." *Journal of Art Historiography* 9 (2013): 1–23.

Legum, Colin, ed. *Africa Contemporary Record: Annual Survey and Documents 1984–1985*. London: Africana Publishing, 1986.

Lewis, Diane. "Anthropology and Colonialism." *Current Anthropology* 14, no. 5 (1973): 581–602.

Machin, Noel. *"Government Anthropologist": A Life of R. S. Rattray*. Canterbury: Centre for Social Anthropology and Computing, University of Kent, 1998.

Maier, D. J. E. "The Dente Oracle, the Bron Confederation, and Asante: Religion and the Politics of Secession." *Journal of African History* 22 (1981): 242–43.

Maier, D. J. E. *Priests and Power: The Case of the Dente Shrine in Nineteenth-Century Ghana*. Bloomington: Indiana University Press, 1983.

Manni, Mirjam C. "Local Ideas and Practices in Relation with Anaemia and the Nutrition-Pattern in the Techiman-District (Ghana)." Master's thesis, University of Leiden, 1996.

McCaskie, T. C. "Accumulation, Wealth and Belief in Asante History: I. To the Close of the Nineteenth Century." *Africa* 53, no. 1 (1983): 23–43.

McCaskie, T. C. "Accumulation: Wealth and Belief in Asante History: II. The Twentieth Century." *Africa* 56, no. 1 (1986): 3–23.

McCaskie, T. C. *Asante Identities: History and Modernity in an African Village, 1850–1950*. Edinburgh: Edinburgh University Press, 2000.

McCaskie, T. C. "The Golden Stool at the End of the Nineteenth Century: Setting the Record Straight." *Ghana Studies* 3 (2000): 61–96.

McCaskie, T. C. "The Life and Afterlife of Yaa Asantewaa." *Africa* 77, no. 2 (2007): 151–79.

McCaskie, T. C. "R. S. Rattray and the Construction of Asante History: An Appraisal." *History in Africa* 10 (1983): 187–206.

McCaskie, T. C. *State and Society in Pre-colonial Asante*. New York: Cambridge University Press, 2003.

McCaskie, T. C. "Time and the Calendar in Nineteenth-Century Asante: An Exploratory Essay." *History in Africa* 7 (1980): 179–200.

Miescher, Stephan. "'Nkrumah's Baby': The Akosombo Dam and the Dream of Development in Ghana, 1952–1966." *Water History* 6 (2014): 341–66.

Meyerowitz, Eva L. R. *The Akan of Ghana: Their Ancient Beliefs*. London: Faber and Faber, 1958.

Meyerowitz, Eva L. R. *Akan Traditions of Origin*. London: Faber and Faber, 1952.

Meyerowitz, Eva L. R. *At the Court of an African King*. London: Faber and Faber, 1962.

Meyerowitz, Eva L. R. "Bono-Mansu: The Earliest Centre of Civilisation in the Gold Coast." In *Proceedings of the Third International West African Conference, Ibadan, Nigeria, 1949*. Lagos: Nigerian Museum, 1956.

Meyerowitz, Eva L. R. "Communication: The Chronology of Bono-Manso." *Journal of African History* 13, no. 2 (1972): 348–50.

Meyerowitz, Eva L. R. *The Early History of the Akan States of Ghana*. London: Red Candle Press, 1974.

Meyerowitz, Eva L. R. *The Sacred State of the Akan*. London: Faber and Faber, 1951.

Miller, Jon. *Missionary Zeal and Institutional Control: Organizational Contradictions in the Basel Mission on the Gold Coast, 1828–1917*. Grand Rapids, MI: W. B. Eerdmans, 2003.

Mobley, Harris W. *The Ghanaian's Image of the Missionary: An Analysis of the Published Critiques of Christian Missionaries by Ghanaians, 1897–1965*. Leiden: Brill, 1970.

Niangoran-Bouah, G. *Akan World of Gold Weights*, 3 vols. Abidjan: Les Nouvelles Editions Africaines, 1984–88.

Nketia, J. H. Kwabena. *Folk Songs of Ghana*. New York: Oxford University Press for the University of Ghana, Legon, 1963.

Nkrumah, Kwame. *The Autobiography of Kwame Nkrumah*. Edinburgh: Thomas Nelson and Sons, 1957.

Ntim-Yeboah, Kwame. *Apoɔ Music (An Intensive Practical Work)*. Cape Coast: Music Department, University of Cape Coast, 1985.

Nwauwa, Apollos O. *Imperialism, Academe and Nationalism: Britain and University Education for Africans 1860–1960*. New York: Routledge, 2013.

Obeng, Pashington. *Asante Catholicism: Religious and Cultural Reproduction among the Akan of Ghana*. Leiden: Brill, 1996.

Ofosu-Mensah, Emmanuel Ababio. "Mining and Conflict in the Akyem Abuakwa Kingdom in the Eastern Region of Ghana, 1919–1938." *Extractive Industries and Society* 2, no. 3 (2015): 480–90.

Okali, Christine. "Family Labour on Cocoa Farms." *Legon Family Research Seminars*, no. 4. Legon: Institute of African Studies, University of Ghana, 1973.

Okru, Emmanuel. *The Rules and Byelaws of Nana Tegare*. Koforidua, Ghana: Ahao Press, n.d.

Olsen, William C. "Healing, Personhood and Power: A History of Witch-Finding in Asante." PhD dissertation, Michigan State University, 1998.

Opoku, Kofi A. *West African Traditional Religion*. Accra: FEP International, 1978.

Oppong, Christine. *Middle Class African Marriage: A Family Study of Ghanaian Senior Civil Servants*. New York: Cambridge University Press, 1974.

Ott, Albert. "Akan Gold Weights." *Transactions of the Historical Society of Ghana* 9 (1968): 17–42.

Owusu, Maxwell. "The Muslim Factor in Akan Cultures." *Michigan Discussions in Anthropology* 4, no. 1 (1978): 75–93.

Parker, John. "Witchcraft, Anti-Witchcraft and Trans-Regional Ritual Innovation in Early Colonial Ghana: Sakrabundi and Aberewa, 1889–1910." *Journal of African History* 45 (2004): 393–420.

Patterson, K. David. *Health in Colonial Ghana: Disease, Medicine, and Socio-Economic Change, 1900–1955*. Waltham, MA: Crossroads Press, 1981.

Patterson, K. David. "The Influenza Epidemic of 1918–19 in the Gold Coast." *Journal of African History* 24 (1983): 485–502.

Pels, Peter, and Oscar Salemink, eds. *Colonial Subjects: Essays on the Practical History of Anthropology*. Ann Arbor: University of Michigan Press, 1999.

Pescheux, Gerald. *Le Royaume Asante (Ghana): Parenté, Pouvoir, Histoire, XVIIe-XXe siècles*. Paris: Karthala Editions, 2003.

Pobee, John S. *The Anglican Story in Ghana: From Mission Beginnings to Province in Ghana*. Accra: Amanza Limited, 2009.

Pole, L. M. "Decline or Survival? Iron Production in West Africa from the Seventeenth to the Twentieth Century." *Journal of African History* 23 (1982): 503–13.

Quartey, Seth. *Missionary Practices on the Gold Coast, 1832–1895: Discourse, Gaze, and Gender in the Basel Mission in Pre-Colonial West Africa*. Youngstown, NY: Cambria Press, 2007.

Rathbone, Richard. *Murder and Politics in Colonial Ghana*. New Haven, CT: Yale University Press, 1993.

Rathbone, Richard. *Nkrumah and the Chiefs: The Politics of Chieftaincy in Ghana, 1951–1960*. Athens: Ohio University Press, 2000.

Rattray, Robert S. *Ashanti*. New York: Clarendon Press, 1923.

Rattray, Robert S. *Ashanti Law and Constitution*. London: Clarendon Press, 1929.

Rattray, Robert S. *Religion and Art in Ashanti*. London: Oxford University Press, 1927.

Reindorf, Carl C. *The History of the Gold Coast and Asante*. Basel, Switzerland: Author, 1895.

Report of the Committee on the Asanteman-Brong Dispute. Accra: Government Printer, 1955.

Riverson, Isaac D. *Songs of the Akan Peoples*. Cape Coast, Ghana: Methodist Book Depot, 1939.

Roberts, Jonathan. "Remembering Korle Bu Hospital: Biomedical Heritage and Colonial Nostalgia in the 'Golden Jubilee Souvenir.'" *History in Africa* 38 (2011): 193–226.

Rosenthal, Judy. *Possession, Ecstasy, and Law in Ewe Voodoo*. Charlottesville: University of Virginia Press, 1998.

Rucker, Walter C. *Gold Coast Diasporas: Identity, Culture, and Power*. Bloomington: Indiana University Press, 2015.

Sarpong, Peter. *Ghana in Retrospect: Some Aspects of Ghanaian Culture*. Tema: Ghana Publishing Corp., 1974.

Sarpong, Peter. *Girls' Nubility Rites in Ashanti*. Accra: Ghana Publishing Corp., 1977.

Schildkrout, Enid. *People of the Zongo: The Transformation of Ethnic Identities in Ghana*. New York: Cambridge University Press, 1978.

Schweizer, Peter A. *Survivors on the Gold Coast: The Basel Missionaries in Colonial Ghana*. Accra: Smartline, 2000.

Scott, David. *Epidemic Disease in Ghana, 1901–1960*. New York: Oxford University Press, 1965.

Sehat, David. *The Myth of American Religious Freedom*. New York: Oxford University Press, 2011.

Sekyi, Kobina. *The Blinkards, a Comedy: And, the Anglo-Fanti, a Short Story*. Oxford: Heinemann, 1997.

Shillington, Kevin. *Ghana and the Rawlings Factor*. New York: St. Martin's Press, 1992.

Shoemaker, Nancy. "A Typology of Colonialism." *Perspectives on History* 53, no. 7 (2015): 29–30.

Silverman, Raymond. "Historical Dimensions of Tano Worship among the Asante and Bono." In *The Golden Stool: Studies of the Asante Center and Periphery*, edited by E. Schildkrout, 272–88. New York: American Museum of Natural History, 1987.

Silverman, Raymond. "History, Art and Assimilation: The Impact of Islam on Akan Material Culture." PhD dissertation, University of Washington, 1983.

Smith, E. G. *The Laws of Ashanti, British Sphere of Togoland and Northern Territories of the Gold Coast*. London: Government Printer, 1928.

Smith, William. *A New Voyage to Guinea*. London: J. Nourse, 1745.

Starling, Ernest H. "The Report of the Royal Commission on University Education in London." *British Medical Journal* 1, no. 2735 (1913): 1168–72.

Statistical Yearbook 1970. Accra: State Publishing Corp., 1970.

Stocking, George W., Jr., ed. *Colonial Situations: Essays on the Contextualization of Ethnographic Knowledge*. Madison: University of Wisconsin Press, 1991.

Study Guide for the film Bono Medicines. Lone Rock, IA: Scott Dodds Productions, 1982.

Talton, Benjamin. *Politics of Social Change in Ghana: The Konkomba Struggle for Political Equality*. New York: Palgrave Macmillan, 2010.

Temple, Richard C. "'Tout Savoir, Tout Pardonner.' An Appeal for an Imperial School of Applied Anthropology." *Man* 21, no. 10 (1921): 150–55.

Timberg, Craig, and Daniel Halperin. *Tinderbox: How the West Sparked the AIDS Epidemic and How the World Can Finally Overcome*. New York: Penguin Press, 2012.

Travel Account for the Film Bono Medicines. Lone Rock, IA: Scott Dodds Productions, 1982.

Trutenau, H. M. J. "The 'Christian Messenger' and Its Successors: A Description of the First Three Series of a Missionary Periodical with Articles in Ghanaian Languages." *Mitteilungen der Basler Afrika Bibliographien* 9 (1973): 38–55.

van Dantzig, Albert. "Willem Bosman's 'New and Accurate Description of the Coast of Guinea': How Accurate Is It?" *History in Africa* 1 (1974): 101–8 et seq.

Ventevogel, Peter. *Whiteman's Things: Training and Detraining Healers in Ghana.* Amsterdam: Het Spinhuis, 1996.

von Laue, Theodore H. "Anthropology and Power: R. S. Rattray among the Ashanti." *African Affairs* 75, no. 298 (1976): 33–54.

Ward, W. E. F. "Britain and Ashanti, 1874–1896." *Transactions of the Historical Society of Ghana* 15, no. 2 (1974): 131–64.

Warren, Dennis M. *The Akan of Ghana: An Overview of the Ethnographic Literature.* Accra: Pointer, 1973.

Warren, Dennis M. "Disease, Medicine, and Religion among the Techiman-Bono of Ghana: A Study in Culture Change." PhD dissertation, Indiana University, 1974.

Warren, Dennis M. "A Re-appraisal of Mrs. Eva Meyerowitz's Work on the Brong." *Research Review* 7, no. 1 (1970): 53–76.

Warren, Dennis M. "The Role of Emic Analysis in Medical Anthropology: The Case of the Bono of Ghana." *Anthropological Linguistics* 17, no. 3 (1975): 117–26.

Warren, Dennis M. *The Techiman-Bono of Ghana: An Ethnography of an Akan Society.* Dubuque, IA: Kendall/Hunt, 1975.

Warren, Dennis M., G. Steven Bova, Mary Ann Tregoning, and Mark Kliewer. "Ghanaian National Policy toward Indigenous Healers: The Case of the Primary Health Training for Indigenous Healers (PRHETIH) Program." Paper presented at the annual meeting of the Society for Applied Anthropology, Edinburgh, April 12–17, 1981.

Warren, Dennis M., G. Steven Bova, Mary Ann Tregoning, and Mark Kliewer. "Ghanaian National Policy toward Indigenous Healers: The Case of the Primary Health Training for Indigenous Healers (PRHETIH) Program." *Social Science and Medicine* 16, no. 21 (1982): 1873–81.

Warren, Dennis M., and K. O. Brempong. *Ghanaian Oral Histories: The Religious Shrines of Techiman Traditional State.* Ames: Iowa State University Research Foundation, 1988.

Warren, Dennis M., and K. Owusu Brempong, *Techiman Traditional State, Pt. I.* Legon: Institute of African Studies, University of Ghana, 1971.

Warren, Dennis M., and K. Owusu Brempong, *Techiman Traditional State, Pt. II.* Legon: Institute of African Studies, University of Ghana, 1971.

Warren, Dennis M., and Mary Ann Tregoning. "Indigenous Healers and Primary Health Care in Ghana." *Medical Anthropology Newsletter* 11, no. 1 (1979): 11–13.

Wells, Alan, ed. *World Broadcasting: A Comparative View.* Norwood, NJ: Ablex Publishing, 1996.

Wilks, Ivor. "Asante at the End of the Nineteenth Century: Setting the Record Straight." In *Akan Peoples in Africa and the Diaspora: A Historical Reader*, edited by Kwasi Konadu, 168–209. Princeton, NJ: Markus Weiner, 2013.

Wilks, Ivor. *Asante in the Nineteenth Century: The Structure and Evolution of a Political Order.* New York: Cambridge University Press, [1975] 1989.

Wilks, Ivor. "Unity and Progress: Asante Politics Revisited." In *Mondes Akan: Identité et Pouvoir en Afrique Occidentale*, edited by Pierluigi Valsecchi and Fabio Viti, 151–79. Paris: L'harmattan, 1999.

Williamson, Thora, and A. H. M. Kirk-Greene. *Gold Coast Diaries: Chronicles of Political Officers in West Africa, 1900–1919*. London: Radcliffe Press, 2000.

Witte, Marleen de. "Afrikania's Dilemma: Reframing African Authenticity in a Christian Public Sphere." *Etnofoor* 17, nos. 1–2 (2004): 133–55.

Witte, Marleen de. "Neo-traditional Religions." In *The Wiley-Blackwell Companion to African Religions*, edited by Elias Kifon Bongmba, 173–83. Oxford: John Wiley and Sons, 2012.

Woodruff, William. *The Rise of the British Rubber Industry during the Nineteenth Century*. Liverpool: Liverpool University Press, 1958.

Wyllie, Robert W. "Ghanaian Spiritual and Traditional Healers' Explanations of Illness: A Preliminary Survey." *Journal of Religion in Africa* 14, no. 1 (1983): 46–57.

Yankah, Kwesi. *Language, the Mass Media and Democracy in Ghana*. Accra: Ghana Academy of Arts and Sciences, 2004.

Yankah, Kwesi. *Speaking for the Chief*. Bloomington: Indiana University Press, 1995.

INDEX

Page numbers followed by *f* indicate figures; page numbers followed by *t* indicate tables.

Abrafi, Akua, 200, 203
Abrefa, Kwame, 123
Accra, 62, 130, 141, 182, 214; 1948 riots, 229; colonial administration, 52–53; government hospital, 58, 83; Greater Accra, 233; plague outbreak, 59; religious fervor, 174; social unrest, 129, 131, 195–96, 225
Acheampong, Ignatius, 165, 180
Achimota College, 79–80, 133
Adomaa, Abena, 117
aduto vs. *aduro* (medicine), 206, 210
Afia Ankomaa (ancestral figure), 39–41, 42
Afrikania Mission, 191–94
Aggrey, James Kwegyir, 80
Agogo hospital, 83, 152, 179, 183
Ahmad, Hazrat Mirza Ghulam, 157–58
Ahmadiyyans, 116t, 140, 157–58, 174, 175, 187
Akɔm, Yaw (first child of Kofi Dɔnkɔ), 119, 120
Akoto, Baffour Osei, 131
Akuapem area, 27, 38, 54, 74, 193, 217
Akuffo, William, 180
Akumsa, Adwoa (sister of Kofi Dɔnkɔ), 105, 107, 113; Ameyaw III prophecy, 143–45; family migration to Takyiman, 103, 104; as mother of Yaw Mensa, 222–23; retirement party, attending, 213; as sister of Kofi Dɔnkɔ, 26, 67, 69, 139
Akumsa Odumase village, 6, 13, 67–69, 78, 85–87, 93, 102–3, 105
Akwatia village, 124
Alliance for Change, *Kume Preko* campaign, 225
Amangoase village dispute, 123–24
Amankwa, Kofi, 124
Ameve, Kofi, 194
Ameyaw, Yaw, 68, 84, 105
Ameyaw, Akumfi, III, 149, 161, 162; abdication, 127, 136; Adwoa Akumsa, prophesizing safe return of, 143–44; Amangoase, claiming stool of, 123–24; Kofi Dɔnkɔ and, 137, 174–75; Kwakye Ameyaw II as successor, 157; Meyerowitz and, 132, 133, 135; Okoyo stool, creating, 130; Seventh Day Adventist Mission, reaching out to, 152; Takyiman Traditional Council, chairing, 154
A.M.E. Zion mission, 80, 114–16t
Amoah, Kwaku, 125
Amoah, Kwasi Amponsa Nkron (cousin of Kofi Dɔnkɔ), 93
Ampofo, Oku, 179

Amponsa, Kwame (uncle of Kofi Dɔnkɔ), 86, 92–93, 113, 116, 118–19
Ampromfi, Amea, 32–33, 102
Anane, Akua (Asantewaa), 105, 226
Anglican presence, 86, 111, 114–16t
Aning, Kwadwo, 124
Ankomah, J. K., 133, 136
Ankrah, Joseph, 155
Antubam, Kofi, 133, 136
Antwiwaa, Akosua, 85, 93
Apoɔ state festival, 47, 50–51, 74, 77, 105, 142–43, 153, 164, 225
Appiah, Kwasi, 184, 217
Asamankese-Akwatia case, 124–26
Asamoaa, Adwoa, 119
Asamoah, J. A., 111
Asante, 74, 90, 236; Agyeman Perempe, as leader of, 49–50; Akumfi Ameyaw III, seceding from, 143; Anglican missionary efforts on Gold Coast, 86; anti-Asante sentiments, 89, 132–33; Asante language, Takyiman replacing with Brong, 146; Asante overlordship and British colonial control, 57; Ashanti theological beliefs, 32–33, 35; Bono revolts against, 47–48; chieftaincy as problematic, 147; colonial anthropology in, 18–19; meningitis epidemic, 82; missionary activity, 56; NLM and, 131–32; Opoku Ware II as Asantehene, 174; patients from Asante region, 208, 209–10, 211, 217; Takyiman tensions, 47–48, 83, 101, 104, 110–11, 142, 223–24; witchcraft eradication efforts, 59
Asubɔnten, Afia (sister of Kofi Dɔnkɔ), 67, 68, 69, 113, 116
Atta, S. Ammiah, 78
Atta, Ofori, I, 123, 124, 125
Aye, Hanson, 74

Baafi village, 101, 179, 180, 198
Badu, Joseph, 77
Badu, Kwaku, 84, 90, 93, 96, 99, 109
Badu, Kwasi, 71, 198
Badu, Yaa, 162
Badu, Yaw (father of Kofi Dɔnkɔ), 4, 5, 17, 62–66, 69, 85, 113
Bagyei, Akosua, 76–77
Bagyei, Arku (grandmother of Kofi Dɔnkɔ), 39, 101, 102–4, 105

Bannerman, Robert, 179, 182
Basel mission (BM), 19, 29; Agogo mission hospital, constructing, 83; Akuapem area, settling into, 193; Anglican missionary efforts, restrained by, 86; ethnographic observations, 23, 27–28, 35, 63–64, 99, 113; herbalists, on the work of, 37–38; inspection findings, 114–16t; outstations, 56, 68, 74–78, 112
Beddington, Claude, 52
bin Adam, Maulvi Abdul Wahab, 157
blacksmithing, craft of, 85–86, 94–96
Boahen, Albert Adu, 218
Boahen, Kwadwo, 141
Boakye, Kwame, 57
Boere, Magda, 189, 205
Boere, Willem, 189, 205
Bonne, Nii Kwabena, III, 130
Bonokyɛmpem movement (Bono Federation), 14, 111, 132, 139, 146–47
Bono Medicines (film), 182, 187–88
Bova, G. Steven, 182, 185
Boyle, David, 88
Bremen mission, 23, 114–16t
Brempong, Owusu (kin of Kofi Dɔnkɔ), 137, 138, 161; as assistant to Dennis Warren, 136, 166, 169–73, 182
British Togoland, 13, 148, 233. See also Ghana
Brong-Ahafo, 147, 179, 187, 191–92, 201, 208–9, 220, 233
Brong-Ahafo Regional House of Chiefs, 153, 154, 157, 163
Brong-Ahafo Rural Integrated Development Project, 182
Buruwaa, Akosua (fourth wife of Kofi Dɔnkɔ), 119
Busia, Kofi, 131, 162, 163, 164–65, 174

Cannon, Harold L., 188
Carriage of Goods Road Ordinance, 112
Catholic presence, 192, 209, 234; attempted conversion of Kofi Dɔnkɔ, 221; Basel mission, forbidding marriage with Catholics, 77; Cathedral of St. Paul, completion of, 152; Catholic mission hospital of Brong-Ahafo, 220; Damuah, suspended for political affiliation, 193; Gold Coast school inspection data, 114–16t; HFH transfer of ownership to Diocese of Sunyani, 179; Medical Mission

Sisters, 120, 151, 179, 183, 203; Nkrumah, affinity to Catholic missions, 153; schools, establishing, 111, 127; Society of Catholic Medical Missionaries (SCMM), 151
Christian Health Association of Ghana, 197
Church of England. *See* Anglican presence
Clerk, Alexander Worthy, 74
Clerk, Nicholas Timothy, 74
cocoa, 57, 61, 163; *abusa* system, cocoa farms managed under, 109; Accra as a cocoa-producing area, 52; cocoa boom, 6, 7, 60, 121, 125, 174, 228; cocoa farmers, investment choices of, 81; Cocoa Marketing Board (CMB), 130–31, 148; colonial control over cocoa industry, 45, 53–54, 55; deforestation in Takyiman region, 180; forest fires, crops affected by, 197; great cocoa rush, 80; *nkokouano* laborers, 109; *nnoboa* labor exchange system, 90; one-third system applied to, 46; plant sanitation campaign, 86; prosperity of the Takyiman region due to, 71, 89, 122, 184; sale of cocoa plantations to private buyers, 214; swollen shoot disease, crops affected by, 112, 123, 129; Takyiman, cocoa produced in, 14, 122, 146
colonialism: Accra riots, colonial government suppressing, 229; anticolonialism of Nkrumah, 148–49, 233; Bono Federation, anticolonial sentiments of, 146; cocoa industry, asserting control over, 54, 55; colonial anthropology, 17–18; colonialism as witchcraft, 126; colonial policies on traditional healers, 141; dual colonialism of the tripartite region, 228; forced intimacy of colonial rule, 15, 230, 231–32, 234, 236; Ghana as a model colony, 237; Gold Coast colony, establishment of, 48–49, 50–53; malnutrition of colonial children, 57–58; mission schools, providing grants to, 37; neocolonial laws of Rawlings administration, 218; Sleeping Sickness Bureau, establishment of, 59; transition of Takyiman from colonial rule, 147. *See also* Basel mission
Convention People's Party (CPP), 131–32, 147–49
Cudjoe, P. R., 89

Damuah, Vincent Kwabena, 191–95
Dangel, Anna, 151
Danquah, J. B., 124–25, 130, 149
Dapa, Afua, 74, 78
Democratic Alliance of Ghana, 214
Dokyi, Henry, 78
Dɔnkɔ, Akosua (third wife of Kofi Dɔnkɔ), 118–19, 120, 145
Dɔnkɔ, Kofi, 148, 181, 209; Afrikania Mission, as a member of, 191–92; Asubɔnten Kwabena as ɔbosom, 18–19, 32, 62, 92, 93, 97, 101–5, 107, 108, 204; birth and early years, 4–5, 17, 62–68; as a blacksmith, 85, 90, 92, 94, 96, 109; certificate of competence, 211–12; cocoa farming, 80, 90, 109, 112, 122, 197, 229; death of, 1–3, 196, 221–22, 223, 232; diary entries, 145; Donkor Herbalist Clinic, 198–99, 208, 215–17; dual colonialism, living under, 62, 228–29; as a healer, 86, 107–9, 139, 177, 205–7, 233, 235, 236; Holy Family Hospital stays, 218, 221; initiation and training, 83–85, 87, 96–97, 99–101; Kwadwo Owusu, inheriting position from, 137–38; land disputes and, 200–202; marriages and children, 118–21; Muslims, popularity among, 158–59; "old man" as nickname, 2, 213; PRHETIH program participation, 185–88; ritual practices of *mpaeɛ*, 20–23, 26–28, 33–36; *tumi* (power) of, 100, 140; Warren, dissertation work on, 167–73. *See also* Monofie, Afia
Dɔnkɔ, Kwadwo, 84
Donkor, James, 165, 187, 203
Dwamena, Elizabeth, 203, 217

Effa, Kofi, 119, 121–22, 126, 182–83
Enuwa, Mallam Bana, 156–57

Feintim, Ama, 155
Field, Margaret, 126, 167
Fink, Helga, 172
Fofie, Kwabena, 48, 104
Fofie yam festival, 105, 153, 161, 226
Foot, Michael, 132
Forikrom Health Center, 176
Foulkes, Roland A., 189
Freeman, Richard A., 44

Ghana: administrative regions, 214, 233; Christianization of, 91, 218; cocoa, as a global producer of, 184; economic

Ghana (continued)
decline, 213–14; electricity in, 177, 185; ɛtɔ as ancestral food offering, 226; Ghanaian constitution, 234–35; health concerns, 175, 182, 183, 198; Malcolm X, visit to, 155; northern conflicts, 219–20, 224, 225; political independence, 139, 148, 149–50, 193, 230, 233; population growth, 199, 209; repatriation of Ghanaians from Nigeria, 190. *See also* Asante; colonialism; Takyiman

Ghana Psychic and Traditional Healers Association (GPTHA), 165, 179, 203, 211–12
gold prospecting, 45–46, 53, 57
Guggisburg, Gordon, 83
Gya, Amma, 76
Gyako, Kwaku, II, 50, 51
Gyako, Kwaku, III, 111, 126–27
Gyamfi, Kofi Adu, 192
Gyantrubi, Kwasi, 47–48
Gyare, Owusu, 201

Healers of Ghana (film), 182, 188
Hodgson, Frederic M., 52, 56
Holy Family Hospital (HFH), 120, 165, 185, 214; Abosomankotere credit union, developing, 220; Committee for the Defense of the Revolution, forming, 200; as district hospital for Takyiman, 151–52, 175–76, 219; electricity connection, 177; Elizabeth Dwamena as matron, 203, 217; Kofi Dɔnkɔ and, 139, 186–87, 202, 205, 215, 218, 221, 222; management shift, 179; PRHETIH project, 182, 216–17, 221; sanitation concerns, 176, 180, 202, 204; supply shortages, 197–98; traditional healers, relationship with, 183, 189, 196, 225–26
Hwemeso movement, 81

International Monetary Fund (IMF), 190, 195, 199, 214, 225

Kalasi movement, 82
Kinghorn, Dr., 60–61
Kleiwer, Mark, 185, 187
Kohls, Elaine, 180, 189
Kɔmfo, Amma (daughter of Kofi Dɔnkɔ), 119, 120

Kɔmfo, Yaa, 190
Kompan Adɛ Pa association, 149
Konkroma, Kwadwo, 51
Korsah, K. A., 124
Kove, Atsu, 194
Kramo, Yaw, 84, 87–89, 90, 92, 116, 117, 127
Kukuro, 81–82
Kuma, Kwasi, 125
Kumase, 111, 131, 136, 157, 176; Ameyaw III trial held in, 143; Anglican presence, 86; as Asante capital, 19, 225; British occupation, 74; Christian missions, 75, 81–82, 152; colonial administration, 50, 52, 57; Gyako II, detention of, 51; illnesses passing through trade route, 82; Kofi Dɔnkɔ, traveling to, 139; Kumase roads, 42, 44, 60, 73, 155; Perempe I as Kumasehene, 83; tax collection duties, 47
Kwakye, Ameyaw, 47
Kyei, Thomas, 43
Kyereme, Kofi, 100f, 223, 226; Afrikania Mission, membership in, 192; as healing colleague of Kofi Dɔnkɔ, 83–85, 93; pride in indigenous therapeutics, 120–21; Takyiman market, helping to create, 174
Kyereme, Kofi (elder), 89, 116–17
Kyereme, Kwaku, 111, 126, 133

Lancaster, Abena Aggrey, 80
Limann, Hilla, 181, 184, 218
Lonsdale, Rupert LaTrobe, 48

Malik, Abdul, 196
Manu, Yaw, 145, 226
Mate Kole Commission, 147
Medical Mission Sisters, 120, 151, 179, 183, 203
Mensa, Kwabena, 163, 188, 192, 223
Mensa, Kwasi, 123
Mensa, Yaw, 222–23
menstruation ritual, 113, 116
Methodist presence, 50, 76, 78; Methodist middle school, opening of, 127; Methodist visitors to Kofi Dɔnkɔ, 209; Takyiman Wesleyan mission, 91–92, 111; Wesleyan mission schools, 23, 73, 74, 114t, 116t
Meyerowitz, Eva, 6, 132, 133–36, 140, 169, 170
Meyerowitz, Herbert V., 133
Mframa, Akosua, 177
Mframa, Kwabena, 201

mmoatia (forest spirits), 24, 25
Monofie, Afia (first wife of Kofi Dɔnkɔ), 108, 213, 221; asiwa marriage arrangement, 113, 116; children, 119–20, 145; cocoa farm and, 109, 122; as a healer, 121; trading experience, 117–18
Mosi, Kofi, 141, 142f, 161, 162, 163, 164
Movement for Freedom and Justice, 214
Muslims: Ahmadiyyans, 140, 157–58, 174, 175, 187; Gold Coast school inspection data, 114–16t; Kofi Dɔnkɔ, seeking treatments from, 158–59; marriage with Christians as discouraged, 76; Northern Territories, presence in, 71; "wicked Muslims," invoking protection against, 22, 23, 24; in zongo communities, 156

Na, Ya, 219
National Democratic Congress (NDC), 218
National Liberation Council (NLC), 155–56
National Liberation Movement (NLM), 131, 147
National Union of Ghana Students, 195
New Taakofiano, 177
Nigeria, 82, 168, 173–74, 190, 196
Nkoransa, 83, 88, 141; Anglican presence in, 86, 111; Asubɔnten Kwabena and, 101–2; Baafo Pim as leader of, 47; Basel mission school, located in, 112; failure of rebellion against Asante, 48; insult songs, targeted by, 50; mission (outstation), 68, 75–78; as natal town of Kofi Dɔnkɔ, 6, 13, 17, 45, 62, 86; Queen mother of, 56, 77; roads east, protected by Taa Atoa, 42; Takyiman, rivalry with, 74; treaty signed in, 51
Nkrumah, Kwame, 184, 193, 231; arrest of, 229; Bonokyempem Federation, partnering with, 14, 139, 146; Catholic missions, affinity for, 153; Convention People's Party and, 131–32, 147–49; as head of state, 230, 233–34, 237; missionary schooling, as a product of, 150, 232; as a nationalist, 136; as overthrown by coup, 155, 164; UGCC, as general secretary of, 130–31; United States, using as a model for the Gold Coast, 235
Nyantakyi, Godfrid, 68, 74, 75–76

Ɔboɔ, Kofi, 144, 145, 223, 226
Oduro-Sarpong, Samuel, 214, 217

Oforikrom village culture clash, 127–29
Opare, William, 76, 77
Opoku, Kwame, 163
Opokuaa, Adwoa (second wife of Kofi Dɔnkɔ), 118, 119
Opon, Sampson, 91–92
Ormsky-Gore, William G. A., 80–81
Owusu, D. K., 136, 169–70
Owusu, Kofi, 177, 188
Owusu, Kwadwo (grandfather of Kofi Dɔnkɔ), 69, 169; as a blacksmith, 94; as invoked by Kofi Dɔnkɔ, 21–23; as succeeded by Kofi Dɔnkɔ, 93, 113, 137–38
Owusu, Kwaku, 105, 123
Owusu, Kwasi, 174–75, 217

Pentecostal presence, 161, 174, 194, 208, 218
Perempe, Agyeman, 49–50, 82–83, 110
Pim, Baafo, 47, 74
Pomaa, Akosua, 141
Prempe, Osei, II, 147
Presbyterians, 78, 116f, 127, 209
Preventive Detention Act, 149
Primary Health Training for Indigenous Healers (PRHETIH), 179, 186, 216; asymmetrical interaction with healers, 182–83, 185, 191; HFH participation, 187, 189, 203, 221; revival of program, 214, 217; training sessions held at compound of Kofi Dɔnkɔ, 188
Provisional National Defense Council (PNDC): compulsory land registration, instituting, 202; constitutional immunity, receiving, 218; Damuah as a member of, 193, 281n74; Economic Recovery Program, implementing, 190–91; HFH salaries subsidized by, 200; Rawlings, established by, 184; student uprising against, 195–96

Quashie, Sydney Andrew, 86, 111

Rattray, Robert S., 96, 111; on Asante spiritual beliefs, 23, 24, 27–29, 32–33; as a colonial anthropologist, 6, 17–21, 101
Rawlings, Jerry: Armed Forces Revolutionary Council, establishing, 180–81; coup attempt, 180, 184, 185, 192; farmers, reducing government assistance to, 201;

Rawlings, Jerry (continued)
  IMF, obtaining loans from, 199; National Commission for Democracy, work of, 214; PNDC and, 184, 190, 191, 195, 202; as president of Ghana, 15, 218; re-installment of government, 219; Upper Region, dividing, 233; VAT tax introduction, 225
Roman Catholics. *See* Catholic presence

Safo, Kwame, 124
Sakyi, Kwaku, 3, 108
Salawuh, Mary, 166
Sapɔn, Kofi Sakyi, 4–5, 119, 120, 156, 197
sasabonsam (forest spirits), 24, 25
Scott Dodds Productions, 187–88
Sekyi, Kobina, 80, 124–25
Sekyi, W. E., 124–25
Seventh-Day Adventists, 127, 129, 152, 209
Shoemaker, Nancy, 230–31
Slater, Alexander Ransford, 123
Stein, Jeff M., 187
Stewart, D., 51, 57
Sunyani General Hospital (SGH), 120

Taa Kofi (ɔbosom), 32, 33, 42–43, 84, 102
Taa Kora (ɔbosom), 41, 45, 47, 98, 164; in Asante spiritual beliefs, 32–33, 35; caves, association with, 36, 39–40; as embodiment of Tanɔ River, 46; as invoked by Kofi Dɔnkɔ, 30, 31; Tanɔboase and, 42, 102
Taa Kwasi (ɔbosom), 32, 42, 83–84, 223
Taa Mensa Kwabena (ɔbosom), 47, 50, 102, 163, 223; adherents of, 100f, 142f; Adonten royal family as custodians, 41–42; authority of, 38–39, 90–91, 92, 164; Fofie yam festival and, 105, 153, 161, 226; Kofi Dɔnkɔ and, 92, 99, 101; ritual petition of, 97; as state ɔbosom, 104, 172; Taa Kwasi as first offspring, 84; as third-born of Taa Kora, 32, 33
Takyi, Kwabena, 116–17
Takyi Firi (ancestral figure), 39–41, 42, 161
Takyiman, 32, 74, 94; agricultural conditions, 58–59; Asante rivalry, 47–48, 83, 101, 104, 110–11, 127, 142, 223–24; British control over regional cocoa trade, 57; as a crossroads, 44, 69, 155, 196, 220, 229, 232, 233; district restructuring, 214; electricity arrival to area, 177; as gateway between northern/southern Ghana, 6, 7, 200; as a gold-mining area, 45–46; healers, favorable stance toward, 141, 145; health care in district, 178, 182, 187, 205, 225; HFH as district hospital, 151–52, 175–76, 196, 219; influenza epidemic in Northern Territories, 71–72; as a market town, 174–75, 196–97, 202, 204, 220; nationalistic sentiments, 139, 146; origin story, 39–41; road construction, 73, 88; sanitation challenges, 126, 176, 180, 202, 204; Taa Mensa Kwabena as national ɔbosom, 33, 38–39, 41–42, 50; Takyiman Local Council (TLC), 151; Tigare movement originating in, 82; Wesleyan missionary activity, 91–92; *zongo* settlements, 60–61, 73
Temple, Richard C., 17–18
Tigare, 81–82
Tindirugamu, Therese, 203
Toa, Akosua (mother of Kofi Dɔnkɔ), 4, 5, 17, 62–63, 67–69
Togo, 82, 190, 196, 219
Treaty of Fomena, 48–49
Tregoning, Mary Ann, 185, 189
Tunsuase, 42, 93–95, 116, 118, 121, 144–45
Tutu II, Osei, 234
Twi, Kwasi, 111

United Ghana Farmers Council (UGFC), 148–49
United Gold Coast Convention (UGCC), 130–31

Ware, Opoku, 47
Ware, Opoku, II, 174, 224
Warren, Dennis Michael (Mike): Brempong as research assistant, 137–38, 169–70; dissertation work, 166–68, 171; Healing Association fraud, exposing, 165; indigenous medicine, investigating, 182, 185; Kofi Dɔnkɔ, as witness to healing work of, 14, 172–73; Meyerowitz, reviewing anthropological work of, 136; PRHETIH project, helping to initiate, 203
Waterworth, W. G., 91
Watson, Andrew Aiken, 229
Watson Commission report, 229–30

Welsh, Howard J., 152
Wesleyans. *See* Methodists
white supremacy, 231–32, 236
World Bank, 6, 190, 195, 214, 225, 234
World Health Organization (WHO), 179
Wyllie, Robert W., 172

X, Malcolm, 155

Yaa Asantewaa war, 55–56
Yeakel-Twum, Margaret, 215

zongo settlements, 60–61, 73, 80, 156, 158–59

www.ingramcontent.com/pod-product-compliance
Lightning Source LLC
Chambersburg PA
CBHW070751230426

43665CB00017B/2328